Ethical and Psychosocial Aspects of Genomics in the Neonatal Period

Ethical and Psychosocial Aspects of Genomics in the Neonatal Period

Guest Editors

Lynn Wein Bush
Olaf Bodamer

MDPI

Basel • Beijing • Wuhan • Barcelona • Belgrade • Novi Sad • Cluj • Manchester

Guest Editors
Lynn Wein Bush
Pediatrics and Center for Bioethics
Harvard Medical School
Boston
USA

Olaf Bodamer
Department of Pediatrics
Boston Children's Hospital
Boston
USA

Editorial Office
MDPI AG
Grosspeteranlage 5
4052 Basel, Switzerland

This is a reprint of the Special Issue, published open access by the journal *International Journal of Neonatal Screening* (ISSN 2409-515X), freely accessible at: https://www.mdpi.com/journal/IJNS/special_issues/ethical_psychosocial_genomics.

For citation purposes, cite each article independently as indicated on the article page online and as indicated below:

Lastname, A.A.; Lastname, B.B. Article Title. *Journal Name* **Year**, *Volume Number*, Page Range.

ISBN 978-3-7258-7693-8 (Hbk)
ISBN 978-3-7258-7694-5 (PDF)
https://doi.org/10.3390/books978-3-7258-7694-5

Contents

About the Editors

Lynn Wein Bush

Lynn Wein Bush is a bioethicist, developmental scientist, and educator on the faculty of the Department of Pediatrics and the Division of Genetics and Genomics at Boston Children's Hospital. She serves as an affiliate faculty member of the Translational Neuroscience Center, a member of the BCH Fetal Therapy Board, and a collaborator with the Yu Lab, where she focuses on the bioethical aspects of individualized genomic interventions for ultra-rare "n-of-1" conditions. At Harvard Medical School, Dr. Bush is an Instructor in Pediatrics, a member of the HMS Center for Bioethics, a faculty member of the HMS Genetics Training Program, and a member of the Academy. Dr. Bush earned her PhD in Clinical Psychology (pediatric and neuropsychology subspecialty) from Columbia University, alongside graduate degrees in bioethics and in developmental science. She then completed clinical and research Fellowships, followed by further training in neuroscience, fetology, genomics, and public health. She has expertise in qualitative, longitudinal, mixed-methodologies, the Delphi process, narrative case-based pedagogy, and neurodevelopmental assessment. For the past four decades, Dr. Bush has used the term *diagnostic odyssey continuum* as she focused on the complexities and uncertainties during the prenatal–neonatal–pediatric *developmental continuum*, particularly bioethical, psychosocial, and policy aspects of rare neurogenetic conditions, developmental disorders, and translational technologies in the context of screening, diagnosis, prognosis, and treatment. Dr. Bush co-authored (with Prof. Karen Rothenberg) *The Drama of DNA: Narrative Genomics*, Oxford University Press, which includes a chapter on Newborn Screening. She was honored with the Declan Hurley Endowed Bioethics Visiting Professorship at Children's Hospital Los Angeles, the Strouck Memorial Endowed Visiting Professorship at Children's National Hospital, DC, and the 2023 BCH Academy Ambassador Award for Distinguished Contribution to Educational Excellence.

Olaf Bodamer

Olaf Bodamer obtained his M.D. degree from the University of Heidelberg. Following pediatric residencies in Germany and at Great Ormond Street Hospital in London, he moved to the United States for a fellowship in Clinical and Biochemical Genetics at Baylor College of Medicine, Houston, Texas. After serving as the Director of the Austrian Newborn Screening Program, he returned to the United States in 2010 to join the University of Miami as the founding Chief of the Division of Clinical and Translational Genetics and Director of the Medical Genetics Laboratories. Dr. Bodamer was recruited to Boston Children's Hospital as Associate Chief for Genetics and Genomics (2015–2023), where he established a research laboratory, a multidisciplinary Kabuki syndrome program, and the NORD Center of Excellence for Rare Disorders. He is a member of the Rare Disease Council of Massachusetts and a member of the Massachusetts Newborn Screening Advisory Council. Dr. Bodamer maintains a busy clinical practice at Boston Children's Hospital where he specializes in treating individuals with complex genetic disorders.

Preface

As the application of genomics in the neonatal period accelerates, it is critical for the global community to examine the ethical and psychosocial implications—both potential benefits and potential harms—shaped by the scientific and resource allocation landscapes of the early 2020s. Genome-based technologies, ranging from large targeted panel screens to comprehensive whole genome sequencing and innovative therapies, pose contextually nuanced opportunities and challenges, while the calculus shifts when utilized in a neonatal intensive care unit versus a mandated public health (PH) screening program. Navigating the complexities of decision-making and counseling is essential for both ill and healthy neonates, especially when faced with high levels of clinical variability and uncertainty, or limited access to care.

We are delighted to present this diverse collection of scholarly submissions relating to these and other ethical and psychosocial aspects of neonatal genomics. The scope of inquiry for this Special Issue is broad, including substantive peer-reviewed empirical research (quantitative, qualitative, or mixed methodologies), reports of developing novel approaches to better evaluate or minimize psychological distress, updated literature reviews, and brief commentaries with an ethical analysis.

In this Special Issue, themes of interest involving genomics in the PH NBS and/or NICU settings include the following:

- International, regional, cultural, and comparative perspectives.
- Newborn population-based research on neurological, auditory, or other conditions not currently screened for, with some not manifesting until later in childhood.
- Implications of secondary and incidental findings.
- Impact of variable phenotypes and uncertain prognosis, including age of onset.
- Uncertain or unknown genotype–phenotype correlation.
- Disclosure of adult-onset conditions.
- Balancing the best interests of the child with the interests and perspectives of the family and society.
- Identifying and disclosing carrier status, including distinctions between true carriers and individuals with variant risk alleles (1 or 2).
- Financial/reimbursement issues with universal health care systems versus non-government run programs.
- Informed consent issues for public health initiative.
- Identification of risk when the diversity of the population is not yet adequately reflected in the variant databases, including ascertainment bias.
- Criteria decision-point to expand conditions using newborn genome panels.
- Blurring the distinction between health, illness, disability, normalcy, and rarity.
- Diagnostic odyssey and "the diagnostic odyssey continuum" (the latter term used by Bush since the 1980s to reflect the potential for uncertainty beyond diagnosis, extending to prognosis and treatment).

- Genomic information to eventually shift diagnosis or therapy to the prenatal period.
- Sequencing to inform management, including new genetic therapies.

Lynn Wein Bush and Olaf Bodamer

Guest Editors

International Journal of
Neonatal Screening

MDPI

Commentary

Ethical and Psychosocial Implications of Genomic Newborn Screening

Harvey L. Levy [1,2]

[1] Division of Genetics and Genomics, Boston Children's Hospital, Boston, MA 02115, USA; Harvey.Levy@childrens.harvard.edu
[2] Department of Pediatrics, Harvard Medical School, Boston, MA 02115, USA

Abstract: The potential for genomic screening of the newborn, specifically adding genomic screening to current newborn screening (NBS), raises very significant ethical issues. Regardless of whether NBS of this type would include entire genomes or only the coding region of the genome (exome screening) or even sequencing specific genes, the ethical issues raised would be enormous. These issues include the limitations of bioinformatic interpretation of identified variants in terms of pathogenicity and accurate prognosis, the potential for substantial uncertainty about appropriate diagnosis, therapy, and follow-up, the possibility of much anxiety among providers and parents, the potential for unnecessary treatment and "medicalizing" normal children, the possibility of adding large medical costs for otherwise unnecessary follow-up and testing, the potential for negatively impacting medical and life insurance, and the almost impossible task of obtaining truly-informed consent. Moreover, the potentially-negative consequences of adding genomic sequencing to NBS might jeopardize all of NBS which has been and continues to be so beneficial for thousands of children and their families throughout the world.

Keywords: genomic sequencing; ethics; interpretation; newborn screening

1. Evolution of Newborn Screening

Dr. Robert Guthrie, the founder of newborn screening (NBS), and I were sharing a taxi in New York in the late 1980's or early 1990's heading for the airport when again he brought up the subject of NBS for histidinemia. He had modified his famous bacterial inhibition assay, the one he had developed for phenylalanine to identify phenylketonuria (PKU), so that maple syrup urine disease (MSUD) and homocystinuria (HCU) could be added to NBS. This latest modification semi-quantitatively measured histidine so that now histidinemia could be added to NBS. But I knew histidinemia very well. In the Massachusetts NBS Program we had identified many cases through urine screening [1] and in my follow-up of these children I knew that histidinemia was benign [2], a disorder that Archibald Garrod would have defined as a "metabolic sport" [3]. So I argued that histidinemia should not be added to NBS, that screening for it would be of no benefit and that indeed, it would result in much anxiety to the parents and clinicians, would "medicalize" the children by falsely labeling then as having a disease, might result in their being unnecessarily put on a difficult and expensive diet and therefore, it would be unethical to screen for histidinemia. Guthrie was a brilliant medical researcher but he was not a clinician and had never seen a child with histidinemia. Nevertheless, he was so dedicated to preventing intellectual disability that he believed every case report of disability, however misleading, and rejected every study to the contrary. NBS at that time was only possible for disorders that led to disabilities, such as PKU, MSUD, HCU, congenital hypothyroidism, congenital adrenal hyperplasia, and sickle cell disease so ethics and psychosocial issues had not yet become major considerations.

A few years later, however, tandem mass spectrometry (MS-MS), which greatly expanded NBS, came into being. With this technology a single assay could screen for many metabolic disorders rather than each disorder requiring its own assay. It soon became clear that although this technology added many important disorders to NBS and prevented substantial disability as well as sudden death, expanded NBS (ENBS) also resulted in identifying benign disorders and benign mild variants of otherwise disabling disorders. In fact, it is likely that the majority of infants identified by MS-MS have a benign finding [4–6]. This raised issues such as what to report to attending physicians, which findings should be called to the attention of parents, which findings required confirmatory assessment and perhaps treatment, and how parents received and perceived this information. Thus, ethical and psychosocial concerns became major considerations in NBS [7,8].

Robert Guthrie was a genius. Like so many geniuses he came to an idea and then devoted his life to making this idea a reality that changed the world. His development of newborn screening required two components—a test which was the bacterial inhibition assay that semi-quantitatively measured phenylalanine and a blood specimen that could easily and safely be obtained from the newborn infant and readily transported to a central laboratory [9]. Of these two components, Guthrie maintained that the one he would be best remembered for was the filter paper blood specimen, for he correctly recognized that the bacterial assay would be replaced but the dried blood specimen would remain and allow for many additional tests that would benefit babies and their families [10]. Indeed, that has been true. From its beginning as a single screening for PKU, additional tests were added in stages. First, in the mid- and late-1960's bacterial assays that would identify galactosemia, MSUD, and HCU, then, in the mid 1970's, a test for congenital hypothyroidism was added, followed by tests for sickle cell disease and congenital adrenal hyperplasia in the late 1970's, biotinidase deficiency in the 1980's and early 1990's, cystic fibrosis and then tandem mass spectrometry in the late 1990's and early 2000's, and, most recently, NBS for severe combined immunodeficiency, Pompe disease, adrenoleukodystrophy, mucopolysaccharidosis type 1, and spinal muscular atrophy. However, even Guthrie could but imagine how valuable the blood "spot" would turn out to be and that it would be used for many things beyond NBS, including genomic sequencing.

In 1987 McCabe and colleagues set the stage for sequencing by recognizing that since the blood impregnated within the filter paper was whole blood it contained DNA. They then developed a method for extracting the DNA [11]. Subsequently, dried blood in filter paper became used for molecular diagnosis in patients with clinical symptoms [12] and, most recently, a number of studies have examined next-generation sequencing in the dried blood specimens for the possibility that it could be used in NBS [13–16].

2. Potential Applications of Genomics Screening

There are several potential applications of next-generation sequencing in NBS [17,18].

2.1. Targeted Genotyping

This application would be to either analyze a panel of known pathogenic gene variants in a single gene or to sequence the entire coding sequence of a selected set of genes. The former is used today in some NBS programs for second-tier screening, i.e., to follow an abnormal initial NBS result for cystic fibrosis, galactosemia, or medium chain acyl-CoA dehydrogenase deficiency in order to better define the initial abnormality. Sequencing an entire coding sequence of selected genes would, of course, potentially identify more infants with genetic disorders than NBS currently identifies but might also result in identifying many more infants with benign disorders as well as infants with variants of undefined significance (VUS), the vast majority of which are simply normal nucleotide variations but for which required costly and lengthy follow-up and continued uncertainty could overwhelm the system.

2.2. Genome-Wide Sequencing

This could be either whole-exome sequencing (WES), i.e., sequencing only the coding sequences (exons) in the genome or whole-genome sequencing (WGS), i.e., sequencing the entire genome, all three billion nucleotides. Both of these possibilities offer the advantage of detecting virtually any genetic disorder but the very significant disadvantage of resulting in even many more VUSs than sequencing only selected genes (see above) and requiring confirmatory evaluations and likely still-inconclusive results with perhaps long periods of follow-up and additional testing in very large numbers of clinically-normal infants. If targeted sequencing could overwhelm the follow-up system, the far more extensive demands for follow-up of genome-wide sequencing could not imaginably be accommodated by the current follow-up system.

3. Ethical and Psychosocial Implications

The potential for genomic NBS has raised ethical and psychosocial concerns to a new level. The original NBS included only a very few disorders. ENBS included many more disorders but all of a metabolic nature. Genomic NBS, however, could expand NBS beyond anything originally imagined. Certainly, many more metabolic disorders could be identified but beyond metabolics, genomic NBS could include a huge number of non-metabolic clinical genetic disorders such as developmental defects, cerebral malformations, genetic causes of epilepsy, immunologic disorders, and hematologic disorders. One can imagine the ethical and psychosocial concerns raised by this degree of NBS expansion. Among the questions would be the purpose of identifying so many of these disorders in phenotypically-normal newborn infants, whether the negative effects would outweigh any good from genomic sequencing, whether bioinformatics would allow the precision of interpretation required to identify important findings and exclude insignificant changes, whether interpretation of the genotypic results could predict outcomes with any degree of accuracy, how the information derived from genomic sequencing could be best acted upon, and how the information would be received and perceived by physicians and, especially, by parents.

Thus it is fitting for the *International Journal of Neonatal Screening* (*IJNS*) to devote this issue to ethical and psychosocial issues of NBS. These issues include the diagnostic and prognostic dilemmas of variant interpretation, how to handle the identification of carriers, identifying benign variants with the inevitable uncertainty and anxiety that this produces, unnecessary treatment, the potential for very large additional medical costs of confirmatory testing and unnecessary treatment, the identification of late-onset disorders with the need for continuous follow-up and uncertainty of early therapy, the need for informed consent and the difficulty of providing the correct information for appropriate consenting, the potential for adverse long-term consequences of insurance for the family as well as the infant, the need for additional geneticists and other specialists to handle, educate, and treat these newly-detected newborns, and the dreaded possibility that standard NBS for PKU, congenital hypothyroidism, and other well-established screening might be threatened [17–19]. All of these and many more issues must be carefully examined [20,21], as they will be in this special issue of the *IJNS*.

Funding: This research received no external funding.

Conflicts of Interest: The authors declare no conflict of interest.

References

1. Levy, H.L.; Coulombe, J.T.; Shih, V.E. Newborn urine screening. In *Neonatal Screening for Inborn Errors of Metabolism*; Bickel, H., Guthrie, R., Hammersen, G., Eds.; Springer: Berlin/Heidelberg, Germany, 1980; pp. 89–103.
2. Levy, H.L.; Shih VEMadigan, P.M. Routine urine screening for histidinemia—Clinical and biochemical results. *N. Engl. J. Med.* **1974**, *291*, 1214–1219. [CrossRef] [PubMed]
3. Garrod, A.E. The incidence of alkaptonuria: A study in chemical individuality. *Lancet* **1902**, 2, 1616–1620. [CrossRef]

4. Hoffmann, L.; Haussmann, U.; Mueller, M.; Spiekerkoetter, U. VLCAD enzyme activity determinations in newborns identified by screening: A valuable tool for risk assessment. *J. Inherit. Metab. Dis.* **2012**, *35*, 269–277. [CrossRef] [PubMed]
5. Ensenauer, R.; Vockley, J.; Willard, J.M.; Huey, J.C.; Sass, J.O.; Edland, S.D. A common mutation is associated with a mild, potentially asymptomatic phenotype in patients with isovaleric acidemia diagnosed by newborn screening. *Am. J. Hum. Genet.* **2004**, *75*, 1136–1142. [CrossRef] [PubMed]
6. Chien, Y.-H.; Abdenur, E.; Biom, H.J. Mudd's disease (MAT I/III deficiency: A survey of data for MATIA homozygotes and compound heterozygotes. *Orphanet J. Rare Dis.* **2015**, *10*, 99. [CrossRef] [PubMed]
7. Buchbinder, M.; Timmermans, S. Newborn screening for metabolic disorders: Parental perceptions of the initial communication of results. *Clin. Pediatr.* **2012**, *51*, 739–744. [CrossRef] [PubMed]
8. Hewlett, J.; Waisbren, S. A review of the psychosocial effects of false-positive results on parents and current communications practices in newborn screening. *J. Inherit. Metab. Dis.* **2006**, *29*, 677–682. [CrossRef] [PubMed]
9. Guthrie, R.; Susi, A. A simple phenylalanine method for detecting phenylketonuria in large populations of newborn infants. *Pediatrics* **1963**, *32*, 338–342. [PubMed]
10. Guthrie, R. The origin of newborn screening. *Screening* **1992**, *1*, 5–15. [CrossRef]
11. McCabe, E.R.; Huang, S.Z.; Seltzer, W.K.; Law, M.L. DNA microextraction from dried blood spots on filter paper blotters: Potential applications to newborn screening. *Hum. Genet.* **1987**, *75*, 213–216. [CrossRef] [PubMed]
12. Uttayamakul, S.; Likanonsakul, S.; Sunthornkachit, R.; Kuntiranont, K.; Louisirochanakul, S.; Chaovavanich, A.; Thiamchai, V.; Tanprasertsuk, S.; Sutthent, R. Usage of dried blood spots for molecular diagnosis and monitoring HIV-1 infection. *J. Virol. Methods* **2005**, *128*, 128–134. [CrossRef] [PubMed]
13. Cantarel, B.L.; Lei, Y.; Weaver, D.; Zhu, H.; Farrell, A.; Benstead-Hume, G.; Reese, J.; Fennell, R.H. Analysis of archived residual newborn screening blood spots after whole genome amplification. *BMC Genom.* **2015**, *16*, 602. [CrossRef] [PubMed]
14. Hollegaard, M.V.; Gauholm, J.; Nielsen, J.; Mandrup, S.; Hougaard, M. Archived neonatal dried blood spot samples can be used for accurate whole genome and exome-targeted next-generation sequencing. *Mol. Genet. Metab.* **2013**, *110*, 65–72. [CrossRef]
15. Poulsen, J.B.; Lescai, F.; Grove, J.; Baekvad-Hansen, M.; Christiansen, M.; Hagen, C.M.; Maller, J.; Stevens, C.; Li, S.; Li, Q.; et al. High-quality exome sequencing of whole-genome amplified neonatal dried blood spot DNA. *PLoS ONE* **2016**, *11*, e0153253. [CrossRef]
16. Berg, J.S.; Agrawal, P.B.; Bailey, D.B., Jr.; Beggs, A.H.; Brenner, S.E.; Brown, A.M.; Cakici, J.A.; Ceyhan-Birsoy, O.; Chan, K.; Chen, F.; et al. Newborn sequencing in genomic medicine and public health. *Pediatrics* **2017**, *139*, e20162252. [CrossRef] [PubMed]
17. Landau, Y.E.; Lichter-Konecki, U.; Levy, H.L. Genomics in newborn screening. *J. Pediatr.* **2014**, *164*, 14–19. [CrossRef] [PubMed]
18. van Campen, J.C.; Sollars, E.S.A.; Thomas, R.C.; Bartlett, C.M.; Milano, A.; Parker, M.D.; Dawe, J.; Winship, P.R.; Peck, G.; Grafham, D.; et al. Next generation sequencing in newborn screening in the United Kingdom National Health Service. *Int. J. Neonatal Screen.* **2019**, *5*, 40. [CrossRef] [PubMed]
19. Levy, H.L. Newborn screening: The genomics challenge. *Mol. Genet. Genom. Med.* **2014**, *2*, 81–84. [CrossRef] [PubMed]
20. Rajabi, F.; Levy, H.L. Expansion and implications of newborn screening. *Curr. Genet. Med. Rep.* **2015**, *3*, 110–117. [CrossRef]
21. Johnston, J.; Lantos, J.D.; Goldenberg, A.; Chen, F.; Parens, E.; Koenig, B.A. Sequencing newborns: A call for nuanced use of genomic technologies. *Hastings Center Rep.* **2018**, *48*, 1–49. [CrossRef] [PubMed]

International Journal of
Neonatal Screening

MDPI

Commentary

Ethical Issues Surrounding Newborn Screening

R. Rodney Howell

Department of Pediatrics, The Hussman Institute for Human Genomics and Genetics,
Miller School of Medicine, University of Miami, Coral Gables, FL 33146, USA; rhowell@miami.edu

Abstract: It would be difficult to overestimate the importance of persistent, thoughtful parents and their importance in the development of treatments for their children's rare disorders. Almost a century ago in Norway, observant parents led a brilliant young physician-scientist to his discovery of the underlying cause of their children's profound developmental delay—i.e., phenylketonuria, or PKU. Decades later, in a recovering war-ravaged Britain, an equally persistent mother pressed the scientists at Birmingham Children's Hospital to find a way to treat her seriously damaged daughter, Sheila, who suffered from PKU. Living on the financial edge, this mother insisted that Bickel and colleagues develop such a diet, and she volunteered Sheila to be the patient in the trial. The scientists concluded that the low phenylalanine diet helped but needed to be started very early—so, newborn screening was born to permit the implementation of this. Many steps brought us to where we are today, but these courageous parents made it all begin.

Keywords: parental advocacy history; residual dried blood spots; newborn screening expansion; recommended uniform screening panel (RUSP); secretary's advisory committee of heritable disorders in newborns and children (ACHDNC)

Although many intricacies surround the ethical issues in newborn screening, it is interesting from my perspective to have seen the evolution from no discussion of ethical issues to many discussions taking place in 2020 and consider the basis of this change.

It has been a century since an observant young mother in Norway, Borgny Egeland, and her dentist husband, Harry, were very concerned about the developmental delay of their 3-year-old daughter. Soon, a son was born who showed similar severe delay. They recognized a strange odor, and felt this odor represented a chemical abnormality in these children. Ms. Egeland sought out a professor who had taught Harry in dental school, the physician Asbjørn Følling, who had an interest in ketosis. Strongly aided by Ms. Egeland's extensive urine collection, Følling was able to isolate an unusual compound which was responsible for the striking evanescent green color with ferric chloride, a compound routinely used to detect ketones in urine. He laboriously but rapidly determined that the unusual compound was phenylpyruvic acid, and he determined that the children had very high concentrations of phenylalanine, an essential amino acid, in the blood. A quick survey of institutions housing developmentally delayed children by Følling determined that a portion of profoundly delayed children had similar chemical abnormalities, and it appeared to be inherited in an autosomal recessive fashion. Enormous excitement surrounded the discovery of a chemical abnormality which caused this profound delay. It was immediately considered that if the elevated phenylalanine was causing the delay, removing this essential amino acid should be beneficial.

Følling's remarkable discovery was published in 1934 [1], and in the ensuing years various attempts were made to modify the diet but nothing organized or effective was soon recognized. The Second World War was moving rapidly across Europe so biomedical research was greatly slowed. Much later, in the 1950s, Horst Bickel, a German Physician Scientist working in England, carried out a remarkable effort to treat a young child with classic phenylketonuria with a modified casein hydrolysate diet rendered low in phenylalanine [2]. Fortunately, Louis Woolf, working with a London drug house on special diets for war survivors, provided information to Bickel as to how to prepare such a diet (Dr. Woolf, retired in British Columbia, Canada, has recently celebrated his 100th birthday and has been widely recognized for his contributions in this area) [3]. Although the Bickel study showed strong improvement of the treated young child, it was thought that one would have to begin very early in order to get the best results.

The need to begin the lower phenylalanine diet very early brought Robert Guthrie on board, and he developed a simple but effective screening test, suitable for testing the entire population of newborns to identify babies with elevated phenylalanine—and so, newborn screening was born. Although there were many things to be learned, the identification and treatment of apparently healthy newborn infants with dramatic elevations of blood phenylalanine concentrations in the newborn period was clearly effective. The excitement was widespread and newborn screening was rather quickly begun across the entire United States. The ability to prevent severe developmental delay with a special diet was remarkable, and certainly at that time, there were no substantial voices opposing this remarkable new effort. This dramatic discovery resulted in national excitement with widespread publication. Our President of the United States at the time, President John F. Kennedy, keenly interested and involved in developmental delay because of his sister Rosemary, invited Asbjørn Følling to the White House where he was presented with a Joseph P. Kennedy, Jr. Foundation Award. Of course, there was the rare voice that cautioned that infants would be harmed or even killed. I was personally involved in treating children with this special diet very early in newborn screening. We would monitor blood phenylalanine concentrations carefully, and at times would find treated children slowed in growth, and/or who developed anemia, and we would increase phenylalanine in the diet and reverse this problem. It was miraculous to see children with essentially normal abilities (and progressively getting better as we learned more about the diet) when we had untreated children we were seeing in our clinic with profound developmental delays. A comprehensive review by medical historians found little evidence of death or disability that resulted from the inappropriate treatment of well children who were falsely identified by early newborn screening programs [4].

The dramatic effects in treating phenylketonuria (PKU) was not accompanied with any substantial discussion of ethical issues surrounding newborn screening. Over the ensuing 50 years, newborn screening has expanded greatly. The Secretary's Advisory Committee of Heritable Disorders in Newborns and Children (SACHDNC) was formed by federal legislation and signed into law by President Bush in 2007 and requires (using evidence-based guidelines) what should be on the recommended uniform panel across all states. This Committee's recommendations have extensively changed the face of inborn errors of metabolism as well as other conditions detected in the newborn period [5]. The establishment of the Recommended Uniform Panel and its adoption widely has, unfortunately, developed programs with low positive predictive values in some states, meaning that there was a dramatic increase in false-positive newborn screening results. While dealing with the many false-positive results of complex disorders, there has been increased interest in informed consent for all of newborn screening. At the same time, information provided to parents about newborn screening has been variable and provided at times of great stress during delivery of a baby, and so is usually not retained.

Although the residual dried blood spots (DBSs) from newborn screening have long been retained in many (most) states for laboratory quality control and for establishing new tests recommended by federal and state advisory panels, this has become a most contentious issue. I think that this derives from two reasons: the families were not advised that these spots were being retained for the purposes mentioned, and a misunderstanding of what can be achieved with such spots. Another major issue has developed when some became aware that the dried blood spots contained DNA, which caused serious concern among some. Protestors, I think, felt that a laboratory can identify a person from the DNA in the dried spot, which for practical purposes cannot be performed, and would serve no purpose if it could [6].

This author does not think that any competent parent, who understands inheritance would ever deny newborn screening for their infant. A common comment that screening is denied because nobody in the family has a genetic disease shows a serious lack of understanding. I do think that if the residual dried blood spots are to be used for identifiable research, the parents must be asked for permission to do so. I also think that very hard work to provide the best possible information to parents about newborn screening will go a long way to help parents understand the process, and feel comfortable that the best is being offered for their infant. The conditions that are being studied to become a part of the recommended uniform screening panel should be carefully studied with the best information available ensuring that the condition has a reliable test and an effective treatment. It is also important to understand the clinical course of a disorder, but at the same time be fully aware that one never knows the spectrum of any human disorder until one carries out screening on the apparently healthy unselected population. We have regularly seen the dramatic changes in our understanding of a disease once we have begun population-based newborn screening.

How informed consent is employed in newborn screening has been written about since the very earliest days of newborn screening in the United States [7,8]. The work of Faden cited here is widely discussed in the Bush-Bodamer manuscript in this Special Issue. My personal attitude about newborn screening is that there should be excellent material presented to all parents (and guardians) in an effort to convey understanding about the process overall. In this environment, I do not think that newborn screening for conditions recommended by the ACHDNC should require informed consent. Any condition for which screening is performed which does not meet these criteria I think should require full informed consent.

The widespread availability of whole-genome and whole-exon sequencing in clinical practice and the continuing significant decrease in cost of sequencing have raised the question of whether traditional metabolic newborn screening might be replaced by genome sequencing [9]. It has been clearly shown that DNA amplified from both old and new dried blood spots performs as well as their whole-blood reference samples with regard to error rates, indicating that DBSs are excellent sources of DNA for next-generation sequencing studies of disease [10]. Such studies have led to the widespread use of DBSs for second-tier confirmatory targeted next-generation sequencing.

Recent outstanding therapies for Duchenne Muscular Dystrophy (DMD) will likely result in this condition being nominated in the near future for inclusion on the Recommended Uniform Panel for newborn screening in the United States [9]. Two pilot newborn screening programs for this condition are already the subject of state-wide research programs. Interestingly, the current FDA approved drugs for DMD are mutation specific, meaning that the specific mutation must be known before treatment can begin. Therefore, whole-genome sequencing should logically follow when an infant has an initially positive newborn screening test. This could be the first major use of widespread sequencing, albeit secondary, in the NBS lab.

There is an enormous difference between the falling cost of genome sequencing and of mass spectroscopy. This will be an enormous impediment in the foreseeable future as far as using whole-genome and whole-exon sequencing as the primary newborn screening tools, but this may change rather quickly.

A most difficult situation will be the enormous issues with obtaining fully informed consent for broad sequencing of mostly healthy babies. Analyzing the genomic information of millions of healthy babies will present an enormous technical, as well as ethical, challenge for the foreseeable future. Recent studies have addressed some of the issues that arise when whole-exome/whole-genome sequencing is included in the newborn screening program. These authors point out that availability of genomic data require families to make decisions about information that may predict future events, with differing levels of certainly, ability to intervene, and may involve conditions that may not allow direct interventions among other challenges [11]. A diverse group of experts were brought together to consider these many challenges to the introduction of whole-genome sequencing into newborn screening [12,13]. We have not yet faced such an enormous challenge at a population level.

Funding: This research received no external funding.

Conflicts of Interest: The author declares no conflict of interest.

References

1. Følling, A. Excretion of phenylpyruvic acid in urine as a metabolic anomaly in connection with imbecility. *Nord. Med. Tidskr.* **1934**, *8*, 1054–1059.
2. Bickel, H.; Gerrard, J.; Hickmann, E.M. The influence of Phenylalanine Intake on the Chemistry and Behaviour of Phenylketonuric Child. *Acta Paediatr.* **1954**, *43*, 64–77. [CrossRef] [PubMed]
3. Howell, R.R.; Sinclair, G. A Visit with Dr. Louis Woolf, Recognizing his 100th Birthday and His Contributions to the Diagnosis and Treatment of Phenylketonuria. *Int. J. Neonatal Screen.* **2020**, *6*, 45. [CrossRef] [PubMed]
4. Brosco, J.P.; Seider, M.I.; Dunn, A.C. Universal newborn screening and adverse medical outcomes: A historical note. *Ment. Retard. Dev. Disabil. Res. Rev.* **2006**, *12*, 262–269. [CrossRef] [PubMed]
5. Kanungo, S.; Patel, D.R.; Neelakantan, M.; Ryali, B. Newborn screening and changing face of inborn errors of metabolism in the United States. *Ann. Transl. Med.* **2018**, *6*, 468. [CrossRef] [PubMed]
6. The government has your baby's DNA-CNN-Com. Available online: http://www.cnn.com/2010/HEALTH/02/04/baby.dna.government/index.html (accessed on 8 January 2021).
7. Faden, R.R.; Holtzman, N.A.; Chwalow, A.J. Parental rights, child welfare, and public health: The case of PKU screening. *Am. J. Public Health* **1982**, *12*, 1396–1400. [CrossRef] [PubMed]
8. Acuff, K.L.; Faden, R.R. A history of prenatal and newborn screening programs: Lessons for the future. *Analytic* **1991**, 59–93.
9. Reinstein, E. Challenges of using next generation sequencing in newborn screening. *Genet. Res.* **2015**, *97*, e21. [CrossRef] [PubMed]
10. Hollegaard, M.V.; Grauholm, J.; Nielsen, R.; Grove, J.; Mandrup, S.; Hougaard, D.M. Archived neonatal dried blood spot samples can be used for accurate whole genome and exome-targeted next-generation sequencing. *Mol. Genet. Metab.* **2013**, *110*, 65–72. [CrossRef] [PubMed]
11. Relizani, K.; Goyenvalle, A. The Use of Antisense Oligonucleotides for the Treatment of Duchenne Muscular Dystrophy. *Methods Mol. Biol.* **2018**, *1687*, 171–183. [PubMed]
12. Berg, J.S.; Agrawal, P.B.; Bailey, D.B.; Beggs, A.H.; Brenner, S.E.; Brower, A.M.; Cakici, J.A.; Ceyhan-Birsoy, O.; Chan, K.; Chen, F.; et al. Newborn Sequencing in Genomic Medicine and Public Health. *Pediatrics* **2017**, *139*, e20162252. [CrossRef] [PubMed]
13. Goldenberg, A.J.; Lloyd-Puryear, M.; Brosco, J.P.; Therrell, B.; Bush, L.; Berry, S.; Brower, A.; Bonhomme, N.; Bowdish, B.; Chrysler, D.; et al. Including ELSI research questions in newborn screening pilot studies. *Genet. Med.* **2019**, *21*, 525–533. [CrossRef] [PubMed]

International Journal of
Neonatal Screening

MDPI

Commentary

Expanded Newborn Screening and Genomic Sequencing in Latin America and the Resulting Social Justice and Ethical Considerations

Juan F. Cabello [1,2], Fernando Novoa [2], Hanalise V. Huff [3] and Marta Colombo [1,2,*]

1 Instituto de Nutrición y Tecnología de los Alimentos (INTA), University of Chile, Santiago 7830489, Chile; jfcabello@gmail.com
2 Pediatric Neurology Fellowship Program, University of Valparaíso, Valparaiso 2341131, Chile
3 Boston Children's Hospital, Harvard Medical School, Boston, MA 02115, USA; hanalise.huff@childrens.harvard.edu
* Correspondence: til@vtr.net

Abstract: Newborn screening (NBS) has widely been utilized in developed countries as a cost-effective public health strategy that reduces morbidity and mortality. Developing countries, however, are new to the NBS scene and have their own unique challenges, both in instituting the program as well as effectively acting on the results. NBS offers numerous ethical issues on a global scale, however, here we argue that there are unique ethical issues surrounding the development and expansion of newborn screening in Latin America given its highly heterogenous population. Once a NBS program is effectively instated, ethical considerations continue when pursuing expansion of screening to include further conditions. While Latin America grapples with the ethics of expanded newborn screening (ENBS), some developed countries discuss utility of genomic sequencing technologies in the newborn population. When the ability to detect further pathology is expanded, one must know what to do with this information. As rare diseases are identified either on ENBS or via genome sequencing, access to treatments for these rare diseases can be a real challenge. If we consider newborn screening as a global initiative, then we need more than a deontology approach to analyze these challenges; we need an approach that considers the unique characteristics of each territory and tremendous heterogeneity that exists prior to the implementation of these programs. As genomic technology advances further in the developed world, while some developing countries still lack even basic newborn screening, there is a further widening of the gap in global health disparities. The question is posed as to who has responsibility for these newborns' lives on an international level. Without an approach towards newborn screening that accounts for the diverse global population, we believe optimal outcomes for newborns and families across the world will not be achieved.

Keywords: ethics; Chile; Latin America; newborn genome sequencing; newborn sequencing

1. Introduction

Newborn screening (NBS) is a widely used public health strategy that has demonstrated high-cost effectiveness by reducing morbidity and mortality [1,2]. By focusing on diagnosis in the newborn period, there is a goal of initiating therapeutic intervention prior to irreversible damage, thereby dramatically improving outcomes and reducing the burden of devastating diseases. While the initiation of lifelong therapies including pharmaceuticals and special diets can be very costly on a society, it has been shown that it is in fact a greater financial burden on society for this individual to have immense neurologic deficits and the inability to be a productive member of society.

While some developed countries have expansive NBS programs and some programs have proposed newborn genome sequencing as a possibility in the future [2], some developing countries grapple with the institution of the initial NBS program. While there is a relationship between level of economic development of a country and the efficiency of NBS implementation, the fact that this strategy permits more efficient public resource usage has led to increased interest of lower income countries to accelerate their implementation. Latin America joined the NBS discussion 20 to 30 years after pioneer countries, allowing more informed decisions when choosing the technology and the list of conditions to include. Here we review the process by which Chile developed its NBS program and comment on the programs and lack thereof utilized by other Latin American countries.

The institution of newborn diagnostics poses various ethical dilemmas, and it is argued that the ethical challenges within Latin America are different than those of the NBS pioneer countries. When compared to the NBS pioneer countries, Latin American countries have important health system, political and cultural differences that may impact the utilization as well as costs and benefits of expanded newborn screening and genomic technologies. Latin American countries may differ in their approach to patient autonomy, access to pharmaceuticals, distribution of resources, and access to specialists and programs that ensure the treatment of those diagnosed in the screen. These important differences may in fact alter the cost–benefit ratio of the institution of NBS and genomic programs in certain contexts.

The ethical struggles often do not end with disease identification. The diagnosis of rare diseases presents a unique challenge for countries that lack infrastructure to research them and financial capability to fund the often highly-expensive treatment for their citizens. We argue the importance of considering the Latin American perspective as the developed world moves towards further advancement in the form of expanded newborn screening (ENBS) and integration of genomic technologies into common practice.

2. Institution of NBS Programs

2.1. Chile

According to data on child mortality, life expectancy and per capita income, Chile is among the countries with the best macroeconomic and health indicators within Latin America [3,4]. Despite this, there was a delay of more than 30 years in development of a newborn screen program following countries, such as the United States. This delay stemmed largely from skepticism of Chilean authorities regarding the existence of these seemingly rare diseases. In the 1980s, a group of health professionals published the utility of early treatment in patients with phenylketonuria (PKU) and congenital hypothyroidism (CHT). This NBS program was finally started in Chile in collaboration with the pioneers of the United States NBS program, such as Dr. Robert Guthrie, who personally trained the Chilean laboratory team in the implementation of NBS techniques.

In 1989, the National Institute for Nutrition and Food Technology (INTA), in conjunction with the Santiago Western Health Service, initiated a pilot NBS program of PKU and CHT which covered 20% of the country's newborn population, which is 230,000 live newborns every year [5]. At that time, convincing the authorities to start a NBS program was not easy given Chile had just recently defeated primary malnutrition as the main cause of infant mortality. Data were published establishing the prevalence of PKU and CHT in Chile to be 1:14,640 and 1:2000, respectively. This data enabled a favorable cost–benefit ratio to be established, further validating the utility of the NBS implementation as a national program. In 1992, Chile's Ministry of Health ruled on the start of the NBS program for PKU and CHT, which was implemented in a step-wise fashion until all 15 regions of the country were covered. In 1998 the program managed to cover the entire national territory. To this day, this program has achieved the detection of more than 3000 patients with CHT and 500 with PKU within Chile. Treatment coverage with special food is lifelong, and a team of highly specialized professionals is available to monitor them within a centralized program that provides regular follow-up and has proven excellent outcomes [6].

An ENBS pilot program is underway currently to increase the number of pathologies from 2 to 26 conditions, thereby extending the benefit to a significant number of newborns. All 26 conditions included in the pilot ENBS are treatable via therapeutics or special diet. The pilot program was introduced in a step-wise fashion and is currently in phase one of four. Phase one includes newborns of one large center to ensure follow-up. As it currently stands, these 26 conditions are identified later in life clinically once they have already caused irreversible neurologic sequelae. By identifying the conditions at the newborn stage and preventing the clinical effects of the disease, we are not only reducing disease burden and improving quality of lives of patients and families, but also reducing public health care expenditures. Public funding already exists for the treatment of these 26 diseases once identified clinically, however, by identifying the pathology via ENBS prior to symptoms, the public funding for lifelong therapeutics is accessed and the neurologically intact individual can contribute productively to society.

Chile has benefited immensely thus far from the NBS from a morbidity and mortality perspective as well as a cost-effectiveness perspective. The country is excitedly optimistic that the ENBS will provide further benefits for individuals, families and the health care system as a whole. As infrastructure for this addition to the newborn screening routine is solidified, there will likely be natural progression towards further advanced technologies such as genomic screening; however, there is no plan to integrate these advanced and comparatively expensive technologies at a universal, publicly-funded level at this time.

2.2. Latin America

Latin America is composed of countries that differ dramatically economically, culturally and politically, and thus, the region cannot be viewed as one homogenous entity. Within Latin America to this day, there are countries that have child mortality figures above 60 per 1000 live newborns, and poverty levels of about 40% [3,4]. In 2007, it was reported that less than 50% of newborns in the region were screened for some pathology [7]. Uruguay, Costa Rica, Cuba and Chile are noted for their establishment of NBS programs and for entering into ENBS [8]. Countries such as Brazil, Mexico and Argentina face the challenges of extreme heterogeneity between populations within each country. In Brazil, for example, regions deep in the Amazon struggle with providing basic NBS through public funding for newborns whereas in the wealthy aspects of Rio, families can pay out of pocket for genomic sequencing. Given the heterogeneities of the populations of these regions, there are often significant inequities in access to NBS and ENBS based on class system related health disparities. Other smaller countries within Latin America have unstable economies and government systems and therefore have no reported national screening programs.

3. Ethical Considerations of NBS and Incorporation of Genomic Technologies

3.1. Chile and Latin America

Implementation of a NBS program in a country with high levels of poverty, child mortality and primary malnutrition is completely different than in one with greater levels of economic and political stability and existing public health funding programs. Resource distribution becomes a limiting factor in the former. A country that is still struggling with childhood death due to malnutrition is less likely to be focused on newborn screening. Governments often opt for curative and non-preventive health initiatives, thereby neglecting preventive initiatives such as the NBS. The political and social stability of the country has a direct effect on the possibility of an NBS expansion as well as advancement of other central issues to health care development. A country requires the infrastructure to be able to process and distribute results once collected as well as a program set up to act on the results [9]. Diagnosis of PKU, for example, offers little benefit if there is no support and education system for families to perform diet changes essential to change the child's outcome. While some will discuss whether to initiate NBS for CHT, PKU or hemoglobinopathies in the first place, others will be discussing whether to expand the screening to 20 or 30 conditions, and others yet may discuss whether to incorporate genomics. The evidence of success demonstrated by the Chilean NBS and now ENBS pilot program will likely serve as both a model and inspiration for other Latin American countries going forward.

The emergence of the NBS within Latin America highlights the important role of the health team as patient and human rights advocates. A large part of the success of the Chilean program lies in the ability of the health care providers to demonstrate the burden of the disease through data and prove the cost effectiveness of the program's institution. It is, therefore, of utmost importance to positively influence local governments to implement and refine these public programs for the sake of our patients and their families. The role of patient advocate challenges us to be the voice of those who are not yet born, as well as that of a society that seeks equity of basic social rights such as health care.

Regional initiatives such as those within Latin America are essential as they encourage collaboration and assistance among countries of differing levels of cultural, political and economic stability. As physicians, we all aim to provide the best care and treatment for all of our patients and this care should not differ based on national origin. We argue that these international efforts should be coordinated by scientific societies and sustained by international collaborations. The exchange of experiences allows us to learn from each other and work together to save as many newborns from preventable multisystemic sequelae as possible, as we are all, ultimately, one global humanity.

3.2. The United States and Developed Countries

As technology advances quickly and there is a barrage of new diagnostic information available to providers, developed countries face ethical challenges regarding how to apply this new technology. Within the realm of newborn diagnosis, genomic sequencing has been proposed for use as an alternative, as a supplement and as a potential replacement of current standard NBS in some developed countries. In the United States, for example, a study in California compared whole exome sequencing (WES) to traditional NBS by tandem mass spectrometry (MS/MS) to determine whether WES could replace the traditional method. It was found that sensitivity and specificity of WES was in fact lower than the MS/MS method but there was possible utility of WES as a second tier [10]. In Norway, a study looked at the utility of Next Generation Sequencing (NGS) as a second tier to supplement NBS and showed benefit [11]. Pilot programs in the United States at several different sites used various genomic sequencing technologies to screen for conditions beyond the traditional NBS and looked at the utility both in populations of sick newborns and in those that are healthy [12].

Various ethical issues arise with these proposed new programs, such as the dilemma of how to communicate the genomic results to families and what to do with this information especially in the case of variants of unknown significance [13]. Further ethical discussion of these genomic technologies is beyond the scope of this paper. What we propose, however, as a relevant ethical dilemma is the advancement and implementation of these technologies in certain countries while basic screening in other countries has yet to be achieved. The use of genomic technologies expands beyond the goal of just decreasing infant morbidity and mortality and has the potential to further expand health disparities in different social and racial groups due to inequity in access to these techniques. We believe improving social and racial inequities through universal coverage programs emerges as a priority [14].

3.3. Global Ethical Considerations

Globally, the challenges are even greater. From an ethical approach, we might consider it fair to assume that if a human being is born in a developed country, then he or she will have mandatory screening of more than 40 different conditions, with some employing genomic technologies, and be given treatment that can both save his or her life and avoid disabling neurological sequelae. On the other hand, if this same human being is born in a country of less fortunate economic circumstances, the child may fall victim to consequences such as disability or even death. Despite scientific breakthroughs allowing diagnosis and treatment of now preventable metabolic illnesses, newborns still die globally based solely on the country they are born into. The dilemma of who the weight of responsibility of a preventable death should lie on is a great one. Should the wellbeing of this child be the responsibility of the parents, the state where this child is born or is it the responsibility of humanity as a whole? We argue that the global public health community should address as many newborns as it can to lobby for ENBS across the globe to reduce global morbidity and mortality due to preventable outcomes.

The new genomic technologies pose an important financial ethical dilemma that may perpetuate global inequities in newborn outcomes globally. In countries like the United States, some health insurance companies cover the costs of novel diagnostic techniques. Given economic and political circumstances, many Latin American countries are unable to tap into this technology solely for this reason. It can be argued that inequity in access to health is not just a local challenge but a global problem. If "global economies" are already being raised as initiatives to reduce these inequities, we argue that prioritizing NBS implementation globally should be one of the first points addressed.

3.4. Ethical Considerations When Approaching Rare Diseases

The ethical dilemmas of newborn pathology do not end with diagnosis. Upon diagnosis, the next important dilemma is setting the patient and family up with the best therapeutic strategy, which in some cases, may be quite costly. The source of funding for these therapeutic strategies is another ethical challenge that disproportionately effects developing countries. When the disease diagnosed is considered a rare disease, there is even less chance of a financially feasible therapy.

Many years have passed since governments have become aware of the characteristics and situation of patients with rare diseases yet many still die or live in very poor conditions due to lack of diagnosis and lack of treatment access. From an ethical point of view, these patients pose a complex dilemma of justice in which it is necessary to harmonize the rights of each individual to medical assistance and access to validated treatments with the rights of other patients with different conditions that also require high-cost treatments in resource-limited settings. In addition, it is necessary to make a thorough analysis of the efficacy and cost–benefit ratio of the different therapeutic alternatives available if a condition is identified through newborn screening with or without sequencing. One aspect that illustrates the difficulties that exist in the field of justice in this area, is the fact that drugs to treat this type of disease should it be detected through NBS technologies have had less development and production because they are not economically profitable for researchers especially in resource-limited settings.

For this same reason, there is a lack of motivation in researching drugs for very rare diseases, which is why they are known as "orphan drugs." The concept of "orphan drugs" originated in the 1980s with culmination in the Orphan Drug Act devised in the United States in 1982 [15]. This situation requires states to offer incentives to stimulate this area of research. Currently, there is limited availability of drugs but a high need resulting in an inability to provide optimal care to all patients. The balance of financial commitment to development of drugs for rare diseases identified through newborn screens with the financial and moral burden of the suffering of these untreated children with rare diseases is an important ethical conundrum. It is necessary also to rationalize their use and establish criteria to decide whether all those carriers of rare diseases detected through genetic technology deserve treatment or whether only those which will achieve a relevant benefit in quality of life and survival should be treated.

4. Discussion

In the lottery of nature, some persons are born equipped with special talents that facilitate their development while others are born with important deficiencies that will impede their ability to survive and thrive if they do not receive adequate treatment after correct diagnosis. Among these individuals are those with so-called rare diseases. These individuals, if not correctly diagnosed in the newborn period, will go on to have significant morbidity and mortality and result in a significant burden on families as well as society as a whole. With NBS, and particularly with genome-based technologies, there is the ability to now identify and treat many rare diseases prior to symptoms and therefore prior to lasting neurologic damage. It has been demonstrated through cost–benefit analysis that despite the large expenses of the lifelong therapies needed for these identified individuals, the overall cost is less than the financial burden alone of a neurologically devastated member of society, not to mention the overall benefit to the individual, their family and the community.

With this new technology, however, comes new ethical implications based in global inequities in access to both the diagnostic techniques as well as the therapeutic strategies. Here we highlight the wide spectrum of access to newborn diagnostic technologies depending on country of origin and socioeconomic status. Where countries in the developed world grapple with the new ethical dilemmas of introducing more thorough and expensive tests, such as genomic sequencing which can sometimes provide an excess of information with absence of treatment options, other countries struggle to impose basic NBS programs.

From the point of view of currently accepted ethical principles, it is a matter of deciding whether NBS for every newborn regardless of country origin is a matter of fairness (principle of first order) or a matter of charity (principle of second order). It is necessary to bear in mind that the decisions for the benefit of each patient always includes the global care of the patient and family, with or without genome-based technologies.

Rare diseases are unique in that while they are less frequent than other diseases, they present a burden of disease much higher than that of other more frequent diseases and secondary to this, require such costly treatments that patients cannot assume the financial burden individually. In the past, access to health was mainly assumed on an individual basis. With the progress of society, the previously unrelated realms of politics and health were united, forming health policies that allowed more equal access for people to adequately treat their diseases. As a result, it can be argued therefore, that this financial burden should be a function and responsibility of the State [16].

It can be argued that the institution of NBS in many countries was a way to improve equity within a society by allowing every newborn to have access to screening and therefore early identification and treatment of potentially devastating diseases, thereby preventing the negative effects of the disease regardless of socioeconomic status. Unfortunately, as new diagnostic technologies arise, such as the expansion of the NBS as well as genome sequencing, inequities both within countries and between the developed and developing world can in fact be increased. Technology has increased to the point that some newborns, when born into wealthy families within wealthy societies, can have a barrage of tests done often with information with unknown significance, whereas a similar newborn when born into a less financially fortunate circumstance would be unable to even have basic screening for treatable diseases. Though medical advances in diagnostic technology is important and essential for overall global progress, it is important to always consider the ethical implications of these advances and the possibilities, as in the case of ENBS and genomics, the perpetuation of global inequities.

5. Conclusions

The NBS is a tool that for decades has been shown to be cost effective in preventing mortality and morbidity, thus achieving health goals across the world. By identifying treatable diseases before they have produced their devastating and permanent effects, one not only reduces the overall cost on society of supporting a neurologically devastated child possibly into adulthood, but also provides an immense improvement in quality of life for the individual, their family and the community. In an ideal world, all countries, regardless of economic status, would have access to this vital program. This, however, is not the case, resulting in global inequities in access to lifesaving diagnostics and therapeutics. A primary goal of NBS and ENBS is to identify only diseases for which there is treatment and where a measurable impact can be made in cost to quality of life by early identification and treatment. Genomic sequencing, while sometimes used in a targeted manner or as a confirmatory test or second tier, can other times identify diseases and unknown mutations for which a treatment is lacking. Exploring the utility of newborn genomic screening technologies in certain countries while other countries lack the capability of identifying treatable diseases such as PKU and CHT perpetuates global inequities in health outcomes.

We encourage the global medical community to look at the ethical issues associated with NBS, ENBS and genomics from a perspective outside the developed world. We suggest working towards a world where all countries regardless of economic status can provide basic NBS with access to therapeutics upon diagnosis prior to engaging in further diagnostic advancements which perpetuates heath inequities globally. As we are all one global humanity, we believe we must all work together to increase access to care and improve health outcomes for all newborns regardless of origin.

Author Contributions: Conceptualization of original idea by J.F.C., F.N., H.V.H. and M.C.; writing of original draft as well as reviewing and editing of final draft by J.F.C. and H.V.H. Final draft was read and approved by all authors. All authors have read and agreed to the published version of the manuscript.

Funding: This research received no external funding.

Conflicts of Interest: The authors declare no conflict of interest.

References

1. Centers for Disease Control and Prevention. *Ten Great Public Health Achievements—United States, 2001–2010*; Morbidity and Mortality Weekly Report (MMWR); Centers for Disease Control and Prevention: Atlanta, GA, USA, 2011; Volume 60, pp. 619–623.
2. Urv, T.K.; Parisi, M.A. Newborn Screening: Beyond the Spot. *Adv. Exp. Med. Biol.* **2017**, *1031*, 323–346. [PubMed]
3. Preliminary Overview of the Economies of Latin America and the Caribbean. Available online: https://repositorio.cepal.org/bitstream/handle/11362/45001/129/S1901096_en.pdf (accessed on 21 June 2020).
4. World Health Statistics 2020. Available online: https://apps.who.int/iris/bitstream/handle/10665/332070/9789240005105-eng.pdf (accessed on 21 June 2020).
5. Colombo, M.; Troncoso, L.; Raimann, E.; Perales, C.G.; Barros, T.; Cornejo, V. Diagnóstico de Fenilquetonuria en Chile. *Rev. Chil. Pediatr.* **1988**, *59*, 235–239. [CrossRef] [PubMed]
6. Cornejo, V.; Raimann, E.; Cabello, J.F.; Valiente, A.; Becerra, C.; Opazo, M.; Colombo, M. Past, present and future of newborn screening in Chile. *J. Inherit. Metab. Dis.* **2010**, *33* (Suppl. 3), S301–S306. [CrossRef] [PubMed]
7. Borrajo, G.J. Newborn screening in Latin America at the beginning of the 21st century. *J. Inherit. Metab. Dis.* **2007**, *30*, 466–481. [CrossRef] [PubMed]
8. Therrell, B.L.; Padilla, C.D.; Loeber, J.G.; Kneisser, I.; Saadallah, A.; Borrajo, G.J.; Adams, J. Current status of newborn screening worldwide: 2015. *Semin. Perinatol.* **2015**, *39*, 171–187. [CrossRef] [PubMed]
9. Burgard, P.; Rupp, K.; Lindner, M.; Haege, G.; Rigter, T.; Weinreich, S.S.; Loeber, J.G.; Taruscio, D.; Vittozzi, L.; Cornel, M.C.; et al. Newborn screening programmes in Europe; arguments and efforts regarding harmonization. Part 2—From screening laboratory results to treatment, follow-up and quality assurance. *J. Inherit. Metab. Dis.* **2012**, *35*, 613–625. [CrossRef] [PubMed]
10. Adhikari, A.N.; Gallagher, R.C.; Wang, Y.; Currier, R.; Amatuni, G.; Bassaganyas, L.; Chen, F.; Kundu, K.; Kvale, M.; Mooney, S.D.; et al. The role of exome sequencing in newborn screening for inborn errors of metabolism. *Nat Med.* **2020**, *26*, 1392–1397. [CrossRef] [PubMed]
11. Tangeraas, T.; Sæves, I.; Klingenberg, C.; Jørgensen, J.; Kristensen, E.; Gunnarsdottir, G.; Hansen, E.V.; Strand, J.; Lundman, E.; Ferdinandusse, S.; et al. Performance of Expanded Newborn Screening in Norway Supported by Post-Analytical Bioinformatics Tools and Rapid Second-Tier DNA Analyses. *Int. J. Neonatal Screen.* **2020**, *6*, 51. [CrossRef] [PubMed]
12. Berg, J.S.; Agrawal, P.B.; Bailey, D.B., Jr.; Beggs, A.H.; Brenner, S.E.; Brower, A.M.; Cakici, J.A.; Ceyhan-Birsoy, O.; Chan, K.; Chen, F.; et al. Newborn Sequencing in Genomic Medicine and Public Health. *Pediatrics* **2017**, *139*, e20162252. [CrossRef] [PubMed]
13. Tarini, B.A.; Goldenberg, A.J. Ethical issues with newborn screening in the genomics era. *Annu Rev. Genomics Hum. Genet.* **2012**, *13*, 381–393. [CrossRef] [PubMed]

14. Sohn, H.; Timmermans, S. Inequities in newborn screening: Race and the role of medicaid. *SSM Popul. Health* **2019**, *9*, 100496. [CrossRef] [PubMed]
15. Haffner, M.E. History of Orphan Drug Regulation-United States and Beyond. *Clin. Pharmacol. Ther.* **2016**, *100*, 342–343. [CrossRef] [PubMed]
16. Closing the Gap in a Generation: Health Equity Taking Action on the Causes of the Causes, The Commission on Social Determinants of Health Draft. Final Report. December 2007. Available online: https://www.who.int/social_determinants/final_report/csdh_finalreport_2008.pdf (accessed on 7 July 2020).

International Journal of
Neonatal Screening

MDPI

Commentary

Ethical Considerations for Equitable Access to Genomic Sequencing for Critically Ill Neonates in the United States

Kristen P. Fishler [1,*], Joshua C. Euteneuer [2] and Luca Brunelli [3]

1 Munroe-Meyer Institute for Genetics and Rehabilitation, University of Nebraska Medical Center, Omaha, NE 68198, USA
2 Methodist Women's Hospital, Omaha, NE 68022, USA; joshua.euteneuer@nmhs.org
3 Division of Neonatology, University of Utah School of Medicine, Salt Lake City, UT 84132, USA; luca.brunelli@hsc.utah.edu
* Correspondence: kristen.fishler@unmc.edu

Abstract: Rare diseases impact all socio-economic, geographic, and racial groups indiscriminately. Newborn screening (NBS) is an exemplary international public health initiative that identifies infants with rare conditions early in life to reduce morbidity and mortality. NBS theoretically promotes equity through universal access, regardless of financial ability. There is however heterogeneity in access to newborn screening and conditions that are screened throughout the world. In the United States and some other developed countries, NBS is provided to all babies, subsidized by the local or federal government. Although NBS is an equitable test, infants admitted to neonatal intensive care units (NICUs) may not receive similar benefits to healthier infants. Newborns in the NICU may receive delayed and/or multiple newborn screens due to known limitations in interpreting the results with prematurity, total parenteral nutrition, blood transfusions, infection, and life support. Thus, genomic technologies might be needed in addition to NBS for equitable care of this vulnerable population. Whole exome (WES) and genome sequencing (WGS) have been recently studied in critically ill newborns across the world and have shown promising results in shortening diagnostic odysseys and providing clinical utility. However, in certain circumstances several barriers might limit access to these tests. Here, we discuss some of the existing barriers to genomic sequencing in NICUs in the United States, explore the ethical implications related to low access, consider ways to increase access to genomic testing, and offer some suggestions for future research in these areas.

Keywords: ethics; diagnostic odyssey; newborn genomic sequencing; NICU; health disparities; equity; justice

1. Introduction

In the United States and across the globe, newborn screening (NBS) is a successful public health program to identify infants with rare genetic conditions early in life with the goal of reducing morbidity and mortality. In this way, newborn screening programs promote equity and protect vulnerable infants, regardless of the financial abilities of the family. However, there is heterogeneity in access to newborn screening as well as the conditions that are screened throughout the world [1]. Some developing countries have yet to initiate a newborn screening program due to limited infrastructure to conduct research and/or financial capability to fund treatments, widening global equity gaps [2]. In the United States and some other developed countries, NBS is provided to all babies, subsidized by the local or federal government. Rare diseases impact all socio-economic, geographic, and racial groups indiscriminately, with NBS providing an opportunity to promote equity within and across these groups.

The United States is one of the countries in which the newborn screening program is supported through national recommendations for conditions which should be screened [1]. Although NBS is an equitable test in healthy newborns, there are instances in the United

States in which some infants do not receive the same benefit. For example, infants admitted to a neonatal intensive care unit (NICU) shortly after birth may receive delayed results and/or require multiple newborn screens due to known limitations in interpreting the results in infants who are premature, receive total parenteral nutrition, have a current infection, have received a blood transfusion, require life support, etc. [3]. Thus, the most vulnerable infants with higher risks of testing positive on newborn screening may be disadvantaged compared to healthy infants. In addition, the limited testing on NBS may not be sufficient to diagnose the cause of disease in critically ill infants with multiple congenital anomalies and/or other causes of morbidity and mortality. These considerations suggest that approaches such as genomic technologies might be needed in the vulnerable NICU population in addition to NBS.

Whole exome (WES) and genome sequencing (WGS) have been recently studied in critically ill newborns in NICUs across the world, with investigations into the clinical utility, cost effectiveness, diagnostic utility, etc. More than 20 clinical trials have been performed, with more currently planned [4]. In critically ill newborns, genomic sequencing has well established diagnostic yield and potential clinical utility [5–9]. In the NICU, the diagnostic yield of these next-generation sequencing tests is between 21% and 58% [9–17]. Changes to medical management have been reported in 28–32% of infants with diagnoses [9,17,18]. Other studies have suggested that genomic sequencing might reduce downstream healthcare costs by facilitating targeted and preventative medical care and avoiding costly, unnecessary procedures [18–21]. As a result of these studies, genomic sequencing is beginning to be covered by some insurance companies. These studies also suggest that clinical teams are in an ideal position to decide which babies should be offered these tests. However, for some cases, other barriers might limit access to these tests in the NICU.

Barriers to the implementation of genomic sequencing in the NICU include additional educational needs of non-genetics providers, clarification of professional roles for neonatal and genetics providers, lack of efficient workflows to manage logistics, concerns regarding the complexity of the information that could be learned from the test, insurance coverage, and geographic and financial access [22,23]. This commentary aims to review barriers that may impact access to genomic sequencing in the NICU, discuss the ethical implications of potential barriers to genomic testing, explore ways in which access to testing might be enhanced, and offer suggestions for future research in these areas.

2. Factors Impacting the Variability in Access to Genomic Sequencing

2.1. Insurance Approval Requirements

Currently in United States NICUs, genetic testing may be paid for by any one or a combination of the following parties: hospital, neonate's family, private funding, community funding, insurance payer, and/or government sources. In an inpatient setting, this testing often goes through institutional billing, where the bill is generated by the institution and becomes part of daily NICU charges. Costs that are not covered by the payer are paid through a combination of the hospital and patient. The variability in these costs is largely moderated by hospital policy regarding balance billing, the patient's insurance plan, and demonstrated financial abilities of the patient. One common criticism of implementing genomic testing as part of a newborn screening program is the high cost. These are valuable concerns, but the cost of genomic testing has continued to decline since its implementation into clinical care and may be cost-effective in managing infants in high acuity NICU settings [8,9]. Currently, since genomic technologies are not typically embedded into federal or state programs, each hospital manages their financial risk related to implementation of this testing in different ways. Many hospitals have checks and balances in place to protect financial loss, such as committee review of medical necessity or prior-authorization requirements for genetic testing. Prior reports have noted prior-authorization to be a pressing barrier to implementing WES, highlighting the tension between widespread implementation and equitable access [24]. Therein lies a tension between financial protection of an organization at the cost of providing equitable care for all neonates in this setting.

In some NICUs, insurance approval is required prior to initiating genetic testing. Even for patients with similar phenotypes, insurance coverage may differ based on the payer, as reimbursement policies for genetic testing are not well-established [23]. In one study of over 1000 people of varying races/ethnicities, blacks were significantly more likely to be insured through Medicaid/Medicare than non-Hispanic whites, which may decrease access to genetic testing if dependent upon insurance approval [25]. In our experience, public payers, such as Medicaid, typically lag behind private insurers in providing approval for medically indicated genetic testing. In this way, instituting insurance approval requirements during an inpatient stay might increase health disparities. Although genome sequencing in high acuity NICUs has been demonstrated to provide more diagnoses, and possibly improve clinical outcomes, insurance denials remain common [19].

To further explore the potential relevance of these considerations, we reviewed 256 infants <120 days old admitted to a single Level IV NICU during a time in which the hospital required insurance approval prior to completing inpatient genetic testing. IRB approval was obtained for this review. During a 6-month period in 2017, 50 infants were eligible for genomic sequencing based on specific criteria [26]. These criteria were similar to those commonly used in a NICU setting for determining clinical trial inclusion for rapid WES and/or WGS [11,12,14–16,26]. At that time, few insurance companies were approving clinical WES for inpatients and no insurance company was approving clinical WGS [27]. Most infants (45/50) received genetics consults in the NICU. However, only 22% (11/50) received WES/WGS. Of the 39 neonates who did not, 30 received FISH and/or chromosomal microarray (CMA) with or without single gene or gene panel testing, 3 received only a single gene or gene panel testing, and 6 did not receive any genetic. Among those who did not get tested, one family declined testing, and two cases who were consulted by genetics did not receive any testing recommendation (Figure 1). Is it possible that the need for insurance pre-approval played a role in explaining why there were relatively few patients who received WES/WGS? Regardless of the answer, should genetic testing for acutely ill infants be limited by insurance pre-approval? Does this approach ensure equitable access to a rapid genetic diagnosis?

Of the infants who received WES/WGS, five were diagnosed, resulting in a 45% diagnostic yield. FISH and/or CMA were used in 60% (30/50) of neonates and diagnosed 2, resulting in a 7% (2/30) diagnostic yield (Figure 2). Thus, although the utilization of WES/WGS was low, it accounted for most of the genetic diagnoses.

None of the diagnoses that were made are currently on the recommended uniform screening panel (RUSP) and would have been missed by NBS alone (Figure 3).

2.2. Hospital Review/Approval Committees

For hospitals where insurance approval requirements may not exist, some have developed internal review/approval committees. These committees may be led by local genetics specialists/other experts to evaluate which inpatients may be best suited to receive genomic sequencing based on certain criteria. Common criteria include assessment of phenotype and likelihood of changes to clinical management. These committees are designed to facilitate genomic sequencing by approving testing for the sickest infants at the institutional level, curbing insurance approval and minimizing financial loss. With this model, infants who are most likely to receive testing are those that are perceived by the local committees and/or particular individuals as having the highest likelihood of having a genetic condition and/or changing medical management. Committee approval may allow for testing beyond what the neonate's payer would cover compared to going through insurance alone. However, other neonates with similarly complex symptoms that are less well understood may not be granted similar access to testing if a change of management is less likely or perceived as less necessary, based on current knowledge about these conditions. It is known that requiring a suspicion of a genetic disorder as their reason for admission will miss about half of patients with a genetic etiology [6,18,23]. Given the vast evolution of our knowledge and technology in detecting rare genetic conditions, should we limit testing to those with a subjectively "higher risk" than other neonates judged by local experts to be at "lower risk" for genetic disease? Are we facilitating equity for infants who may also have an underlying genetic etiology, but whose phenotype has not been studied as extensively or is not as recognizable?

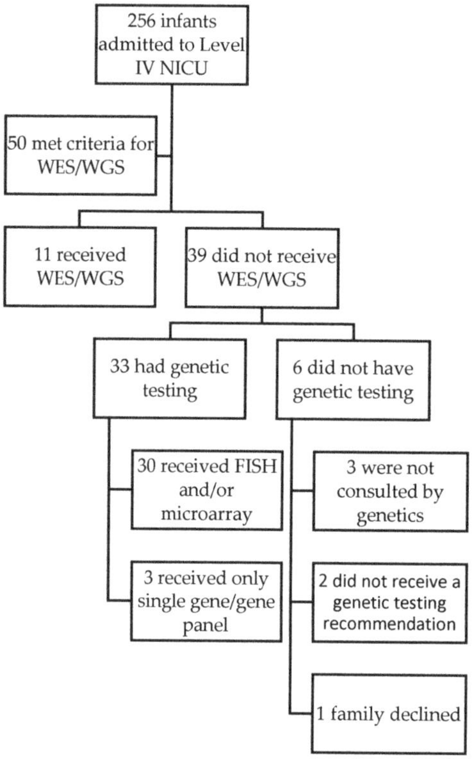

Figure 1. Uptake of WES/WGS. 50 neonates met criteria for WES/WGS. However, only 22% (11/50) received it within the study timeframe. Of the 39 who did not receive WES/WGS, only 1 family declined genetic testing. Of the remaining 39, six received no genetic testing and 33 received other genetic testing that did not include WES/WGS.

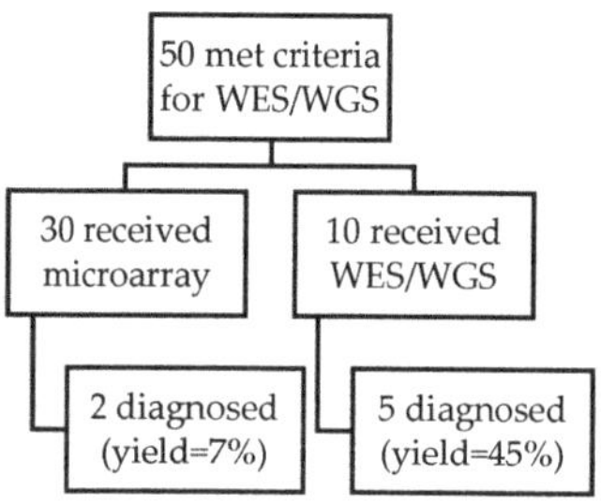

Figure 2. Although more neonates had FISH and/or microarray testing than WES/WGS in our cohort, the yield of microarray was much lower. The yield of microarray was 7% and the yield of WES/WGS was 45%.

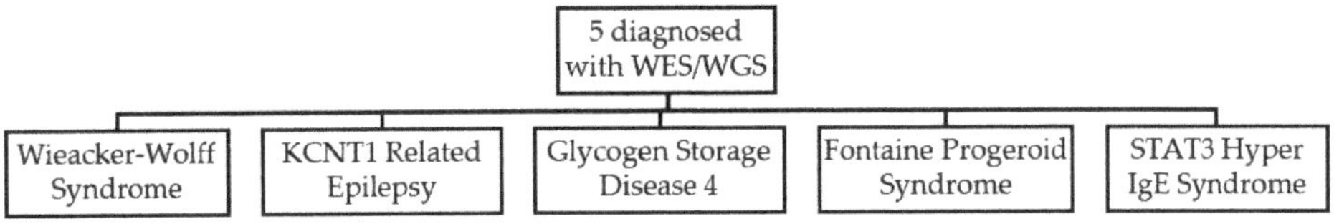

Figure 3. None of the conditions that were diagnosed by WES/WGS are on the RUSP.

2.3. *Inconsistent Definitions of "Change of Management" Impacts Insurance Coverage Policies*

What is defined by "change of management" is not standardized across clinical trials/studies exploring the impact of WES/WGS. Previously published definitions of this term have included recommendations for additional testing, specialty consultation, specific medical and/or surgical treatment, change in recurrence counseling, transfer of care, and/or redirection of care [10,13,14]. However, these outcomes may not align with insurance payers' perspectives on what would be an "acceptable" change of management to warrant insurance coverage. A study by Trosman et al. surveyed and interviewed executives from 14 different insurance payers to learn more about their perspectives on insurance coverage for exome sequencing [28]. Most participants agreed that the impact on patient care/clinical management was most important when considering coverage. However, all participants agreed that reproductive risk information or knowledge that could impact diagnosis in other family members was not enough for coverage on its own. Additional discussion between clinical and payer stakeholders is warranted to determine whether including reproductive/genetic counseling outcomes as a "change of management" might be appropriate. Harmonizing what outcomes should be defined by the term "change of management" between research studies and insurance payers is necessary so that the available evidence regarding this variable aligns with what is most likely to provide evidence of medical necessity. Additionally, payers ought to be more transparent about what evidence/criteria they use to make approval decisions about next-generation sequencing and what pieces of evidence are most likely to influence claim decisions. This will allow for meta-analysis and meaningful appeals to alter payer denial patterns and/or revisions to insurance policy.

3. Ethical Implications for Barriers to Genomic Sequencing

3.1. *Legal Implications*

Underlying newborn medical care (and healthcare overall) is a moral obligation to protect children, especially vulnerable newborns, who are unable to protect themselves, regardless of economic considerations. In many countries, this extends to larger legal obligations. Some NICUs are nested within children's hospitals that are tax exempt, non-profit organizations. US law of tax-exempt entities suggests that these organizations need to provide care regardless of the ability of families to pay and/or of insurance coverage.

Barriers such as requirements for insurance prior-authorization have been shown to alter physician prescribing patterns towards being more conservative [29]. Therefore, it is possible that a geneticist's desire to recommend testing may be confounded by their prior awareness/experience of being unable to obtain coverage for WES/WGS with the neonate's payer, especially if prior peer-to-peer and/or appeals have not altered denial decisions for similarly complex situations in the past. Under-recommendation of genomic sequencing due to prior experience in navigating payer decisions may lead to genomic malpractice suits. These suits may be pursued by neonates' families in situations where a genetic test with known clinical utility was not offered by the clinical team. This genetic information may have clarified recurrence risk. Wrongful conception was upheld in court for a family who had two children with Fragile X, when they were not made aware that their first child had this condition ("Molloy v. Meier," 2003). Thus, the absence of a genetic diagnosis may potentially lead to future wrongful conception claims for physicians who did not recommend medically indicated testing. It has also been postulated that insurers may be liable if a clinically appropriate test recommended by the clinical team was denied by the insurer [30]. This highlights the importance of insurance companies staying abreast of current literature regarding the clinical utility of genomic testing.

3.2. Psychosocial Implications for Parents and Providers

Inequitable access to genomic sequencing impacts not only the provision of medical services, but can also lead to parental and provider moral distress. Parents of children with undiagnosed diseases are known to experience emotions such as anxiety, depression, uncertainty, anger, powerlessness, frustration, and denial [31–34]. One study identified this prevalence to be 40%, with parents with older children and longer duration of illness having lower depressive and anxious symptoms and better coping self-efficacy [33]. An additional qualitative study interviewing parents of children with undiagnosed disease regarding coping with the diagnostic processes identified that it was an important piece of the coping process to know that everything possible had been done for their child. They also discussed a personal responsibility to follow-up with doctors, read the medical literature, ask for second opinions, and seek alternative treatment options. This was motivated by a fear for the possibility of realizing in the future that they failed their child if they did not access something that could have helped them [31]. Thus, unequitable distribution of genomic tests may contribute further to this fear and facilitate challenges to parental coping throughout the diagnostic process.

From the parental perspective, waiting for a medically indicated test is not common for other tests ordered in the NICU. For example, imaging and surgery can be done without insurance or hospital approval. These interventions cost thousands of healthcare dollars, may at times have similarly uncertain outcomes, and may have clinical utility that is not well-understood. Thus, when genetics specialists believe that a genetic test is needed for diagnostic purposes with hopes to end the diagnostic odyssey, it is likely distressing for both medical providers and families to wait, albeit genetic tests are much cheaper than other medical interventions that are done routinely without insurance approval. For most parents who participated in a qualitative study, when their expectations about their child's care were not met, such as finding a diagnosis or accessing diagnostic tools/treatment, they experienced serious frustration and distrust, increasing their feeling of powerlessness [31]. In addition to considering the impact of not having a diagnosis on families' coping, these emotions can also impact the patient-provider relationship.

Moral distress has been noted to have a higher prevalence in palliative, emergency, intensive, and pediatric providers. In one study, the leading causes of moral distress included lack of resources, lack of administrative action, providing false hope, and excessive documentation that interferes with patient care [35]. More recently, it has also been reported amongst genetics specialists who see patients in an inpatient setting [36–38]. Specifically, one recent qualitative study found that a common source of moral distress for genetics providers was related to lack of/poor insurance coverage for clinically indicated genetic testing for their patients [37]. In our experience, it is distressing to providers who have recommended a genetic test to not be able to utilize the results as part of inpatient medical management and counseling, when suspicion for a genetic etiology is high. A prior study of NICU nurses identified that moral distress related to the hospital ethical climate was a significant factor for them to consider leaving their institution [39]. This finding is concerning for genetics providers who already report high levels of distress and burnout and see a reduction in medical trainees pursuing the field. However, this phenomenon has not been studied for genetics professionals in the NICU as well as whether the presence of barriers to genetic testing contributes to the 'hospital ethical climate' or moral distress,

4. Considerations to Promote Access to Genomic Sequencing

4.1. Standardized Approval of Genomic Sequencing for All Neonates with Phenotype Known to Have High Yield

One approach to facilitate access to genomic testing on a population-based scale for infants in a Level IV NICU is to consider the standardized approval of genomic sequencing for neonates who are known to have the highest chance of benefit, regardless of financial status and/or insurance policy. Providing WES as a first-tier test for all infants meeting similar inclusion/exclusion criteria may prove beneficial, as has recently been suggested for individuals with neurodevelopmental delays [40]. Currently, data has shown patients with seizures and/or neurodevelopmental phenotypes to have a high yield with WES, affecting management 41–48% of the time [24,41]. Additionally, patients with inborn errors of metabolism have been reported to have yields as high as 68% with WES technology [42]. Another study identified at least a 25% yield for patients who received WES with phenotypes associated with muscular dystrophies/myopathies, dermatologic conditions, multiple congenital anomalies, skeletal dysplasias, hypotonia, cardiac disease, metabolic disorders, hematologic conditions, seizures, and others [43]. These presentations are common in a Level IV NICU setting. Providing access to genomic testing for neonates with these characteristics, regardless of their financial and/or insurance status, would promote equity [8]. Even broader approaches, such as offering genomic sequencing for all neonates in a Level IV NICU may identify additional infants with conditions that are relatively rare but may alter medical management for that child or other children in the future.

4.2. Creative Technological Solutions to Extend Genetic Evaluation to Areas without Genetics Experts

Genetic disease is common in infants admitted to any NICU and is likely enriched in Level IV NICU's. However, Level III NICUs admit infants with genetic disease including aneuploidy, sexual differences of development, encephalopathy, hypotonia, hyperinsulinism, milder forms of known genetic conditions that we may not currently understand, and/or rarer and milder genetic conditions not requiring admission to a Level IV NICU. Thus, for any NICU without direct access to genetics expertise, it would be reasonable to pursue creative technological solutions to enable genetic evaluation. There are opportunities for mobile application development, interactive education modules for neonatal trainees and providers, and decision support tools for neonatal providers. These efforts ought to occur in collaboration with genetics experts including board-certified geneticists and genetic counselors.

5. Opportunities for Future Research

- Measure the short- and long-term healthcare outcomes for critically ill neonates, stratified by phenotype, who did and did not receive genomic sequencing while in the NICU.
- Characterize social indicators that may predict health disparities regarding access to genomic sequencing.
- Evaluate the criteria used to make decisions about which patients can access genomic sequencing within hospital-based committee structures.
- Explore whether prior-authorization and/or hospital-based committee approval for genomic sequencing in the inpatient setting contributes to the perceived 'hospital ethical climate' and/or moral distress for genetics specialists and other neonatal providers.
- Explore the parental experience of navigating prior authorization, hospital-based committee approval, and/or other barriers to genomic sequencing in the NICU to better understand their psychosocial impact. Although prior research identified psychosocial distress in parents of undiagnosed children, few studies have occurred in parents of newborns who are still in the hospital.

- Development and implementation of mobile applications and/or decision support tools for neonatal providers to extend genetics evaluation to NICUs in geographic areas where this access does not exist or is limited.
- Development and implementation of interactive education modules for neonatal trainees and/or current neonatal providers to support their decision making, triage, and advocacy for access to genomic sequencing for their patients.

6. Conclusions

Newborn screening is a successful public health program implemented in numerous countries across the world for the early identification of infants with rare genetic disease to prevent morbidity and mortality. However, in the United States, neonates in a NICU are unlikely to receive optimal benefit from this screen compared to healthy infants. Thus, neonates admitted to a NICU setting would likely benefit from wider screening, to include consideration of genomic sequencing. In lieu of this testing being offered as part of federal or state efforts, we suspect that several barriers and social forces impact access to genetic testing in NICUs of varying sizes and levels across the United States. Our review considers the potential barriers that might stand in the way of equitable assessment of vulnerable infants in a setting that is known to exacerbate health disparities. There may be opportunities for hospitals to lower risks and cost while fostering beneficence for neonates by routinely facilitating genomic testing for infants with certain phenotypes with high yield such as neurodevelopmental conditions including seizures, muscular dystrophies/myopathies, dermatologic conditions, multiple congenital anomalies, skeletal dysplasias, hypotonia, cardiac disease, metabolic disorders, and hematologic conditions. Further, this may suggest an opportunity for payers to partner with hospitals and NICU/genetics experts to foster standardized approval practices for infants with complex healthcare needs. The tension between financial risks and beneficence must be addressed before considering the widespread implementation of genomic testing in this population to promote equitable care for the most vulnerable and acutely ill infants in the United States and across the globe.

Author Contributions: Conceptualization, K.P.F., J.C.E. and L.B.; methodology, K.P.F. and J.C.E. and L.B.; formal analysis, K.P.F. and L.B.; writing—original draft preparation, K.P.F.; writing—review and editing, K.P.F., J.C.E. and L.B.; supervision, L.B. All authors have read and agreed to the published version of the manuscript.

Funding: This research received no external funding.

Institutional Review Board Statement: The study was conducted according to the guidelines of the Declaration of Helsinki, and approved by the Institutional Review Board of the University of Nebraska Medical Center (protocol 0718-19-EP, approved 10/4/2019).

Informed Consent Statement: Patient consent was waived due to the research not being able to be practicably carried out due to the nature of medical record review without the waiver or alteration of consent under the provisions of 45 CFR 46.116(e) or (f) and HIPAA Privacy Rule (as applicable).

Data Availability Statement: The data presented in this study are available within the text of this article.

Acknowledgments: The authors thank Denise Hoover, for her support in obtaining IRB approval, Sasha Kapil for her work in curating the initial data set, and Kimberly Widmeyer for her thoughtful review of the paper prior to submission.

Conflicts of Interest: The authors declare no conflict of interest.

References

1. Therrell, B.L.; Padilla, C.D.; Loeber, J.G.; Kneisser, I.; Saadallah, A.; Borrajo, G.J.; Adams, J. Current status of newborn screening worldwide: 2015. *Semin. Perinatol.* **2015**, *39*, 171–187. [CrossRef] [PubMed]
2. Cabello, J.F.; Novoa, F.; Huff, H.V.; Colombo, M. Expanded Newborn Screening and Genomic Sequencing in Latin America and the Resulting Social Justice and Ethical Considerations. *Int. J. Neonatal Screen.* **2021**, *7*, 6. [CrossRef] [PubMed]

3. Fabie, N.A.V.; Pappas, K.B.; Feldman, G.L. The Current State of Newborn Screening in the United States. *Pediatr. Clin. N. Am.* **2019**, *66*, 369–386. [CrossRef] [PubMed]
4. Stark, Z.; Ellard, S. Rapid genomic testing for critically ill children: Time to become standard of care? *Eur. J. Hum. Genet.* **2021**, 1–8. [CrossRef]
5. Stark, Z.; Tan, T.Y.; Chong, B.; Brett, G.R.; Yap, P.; Walsh, M.; Yeung, A.; Peters, H.; Mordaunt, D.; Cowie, S.; et al. A prospective evaluation of whole-exome sequencing as a first-tier molecular test in infants with suspected monogenic disorders. *Genet. Med.* **2016**, *18*, 1090–1096. [CrossRef] [PubMed]
6. Kingsmore, S.F.; Cakici, J.A.; Clark, M.M.; Gaughran, M.; Feddock, M.; Batalov, S.; Bainbridge, M.N.; Carroll, J.; Caylor, S.A.; Clarke, C.; et al. A Randomized, Controlled Trial of the Analytic and Diagnostic Performance of Singleton and Trio, Rapid Genome and Exome Sequencing in Ill Infants. *Am. J. Hum. Genet.* **2019**, *105*, 719–733. [CrossRef]
7. Clark, M.M.; Hildreth, A.; Batalov, S.; Ding, Y.; Chowdhury, S.; Watkins, K.; Ellsworth, K.; Camp, B.; Kint, C.I.; Yacoubian, C.; et al. Diagnosis of genetic diseases in seriously ill children by rapid whole-genome sequencing and automated phenotyping and interpretation. *Sci. Transl. Med.* **2019**, *11*, eaat6177. [CrossRef]
8. Farnaes, L.; Hildreth, A.; Sweeney, N.M.; Clark, M.M.; Chowdhury, S.; Nahas, S.; Cakici, J.A.; Benson, W.; Kaplan, R.H.; Kronick, R.; et al. Rapid whole-genome sequencing decreases infant morbidity and cost of hospitalization. *NPJ Genom. Med.* **2018**, *3*, 1–8. [CrossRef]
9. Dimmock, D.; Caylor, S.; Waldman, B.; Benson, W.; Ashburner, C.; Carmichael, J.L.; Carroll, J.; Cham, E.; Chowdhury, S.; Cleary, J.; et al. Project Baby Bear: Rapid precision care incorporating rWGS in 5 California children's hospitals demonstrates improved clinical outcomes and reduced costs of care. *Am. J. Hum. Genet.* **2021**, *108*, 1231–1238. [CrossRef]
10. Brunelli, L.; Jenkins, S.M.; Gudgeon, J.M.; Bleyl, S.B.; Miller, C.E.; Tvrdik, T.; Dames, S.A.; Ostrander, B.; Daboub, J.A.F.; Zielinski, B.A.; et al. Targeted gene panel sequencing for the rapid diagnosis of acutely ill infants. *Mol. Genet. Genom. Med.* **2019**, *7*, e00796. [CrossRef]
11. Daoud, H.; Luco, S.M.; Li, R.; Bareke, E.; Beaulieu, C.; Jarinova, O.; Carson, N.; Nikkel, S.M.; Graham, G.E.; Richer, J.; et al. Next-generation sequencing for diagnosis of rare diseases in the neonatal intensive care unit. *Can. Med. Assoc. J.* **2016**, *188*, E254–E260. [CrossRef] [PubMed]
12. French, C.E.; Delon, I.; Dolling, H.; Sanchis-Juan, A.; Shamardina, O.; Mégy, K.; Raymond, F.L. Whole genome sequencing reveals that genetic conditions are frequent in intensively ill children. *Intensive Care Med.* **2019**, *45*, 627–636. [CrossRef] [PubMed]
13. Meng, L.; Pammi, M.; Saronwala, A.; Magoulas, P.; Ghazi, A.R.; Vetrini, F.; Lalani, S.R. Use of Exome Sequencing for Infants in Intensive Care Units: Ascertainment of Severe Single-Gene Disorders and Effect on Medical Management. *JAMA Pediatr.* **2017**, *171*, e173438. [CrossRef]
14. Petrikin, J.E.; Cakici, J.A.; Clark, M.M.; Willig, L.K.; Sweeney, N.M.; Farrow, E.G.; Saunders, C.J.; Thiffault, I.; Miller, N.A.; Zellmer, L.; et al. The NSIGHT1-randomized controlled trial: Rapid whole-genome sequencing for accelerated etiologic diagnosis in critically ill infants. *NPJ Genom. Med.* **2018**, *3*, 1–11. [CrossRef] [PubMed]
15. Willig, L.; Petrikin, J.E.; Smith, L.D.; Saunders, C.J.; Thiffault, I.; Miller, N.A.; Soden, S.E.; Cakici, J.; Herd, S.M.; Twist, G.; et al. Whole-genome sequencing for identification of Mendelian disorders in critically ill infants: A retrospective analysis of diagnostic and clinical findings. *Lancet Respir. Med.* **2015**, *3*, 377–387. [CrossRef]
16. Brunelli, L.; Mao, R.; Jenkins, S.M.; Bleyl, S.B.; Dames, S.A.; Miller, C.E.; Ostrander, B.; Tvrdik, T.; Andrews, S.; Flores, J.; et al. A rapid gene sequencing panel strategy to facilitate precision neonatal medicine. *Am. J. Med. Genet. Part A* **2017**, *173*, 1979–1982. [CrossRef] [PubMed]
17. Krantz, I.D.; Medne, L.; Weatherly, J.M.; Wild, K.T.; Biswas, S.; Devkota, B. Effect of Whole-Genome Sequencing on the Clinical Management of Acutely Ill Infants with Suspected Genetic Disease: A Randomized Clinical Trial. *JAMA Pediatr.* **2021**, *175*, 1218–1226.
18. Stark, Z.; Schofield, D.; Martyn, M.; Rynehart, L.; Shrestha, R.; Alam, K.; Lunke, S.; Tan, T.Y.; Gaff, C.L.; White, S.M. Does genomic sequencing early in the diagnostic trajectory make a difference? A follow-up study of clinical outcomes and cost-effectiveness. *Genet. Med.* **2019**, *21*, 173–180. [CrossRef]
19. Stark, Z.; Schofield, D.; Alam, K.; Wilson, W.; Mupfeki, N.; Macciocca, I.; Shrestha, R.; White, S.M.; Gaff, C. Prospective comparison of the cost-effectiveness of clinical whole-exome sequencing with that of usual care overwhelmingly supports early use and reimbursement. *Genet. Med.* **2017**, *19*, 867–874. [CrossRef]
20. Hayeems, R.Z.; Bhawra, J.; Tsiplova, K.; Meyn, M.S.; Monfared, N.; Bowdin, S.; Stavropoulos, D.J.; Marshall, C.R.; Basran, R.; Shuman, C.; et al. Care and cost consequences of pediatric whole genome sequencing compared to chromosome microarray. *Eur. J. Hum. Genet.* **2017**, *25*, 1303–1312. [CrossRef]
21. Swaggart, K.A.; Swarr, D.T.; Tolusso, L.K.; He, H.; Dawson, D.B.; Suhrie, K.R. Making a Genetic Diagnosis in a Level IV Neonatal Intensive Care Unit Population: Who, When, How, and at What Cost? *J. Pediatr.* **2019**, *213*, 211–217.e4. [CrossRef] [PubMed]
22. Franck, L.S.; Kriz, R.M.; Rego, S.; Garman, K.; Hobbs, C.; Dimmock, D. Implementing Rapid Whole-Genome Sequencing in Critical Care: A Qualitative Study of Facilitators and Barriers to New Technology Adoption. *J. Pediatr.* **2021**, *237*, 237–243.e2. [CrossRef] [PubMed]
23. Jooma, S.; Hahn, M.J.; Hindorff, L.A.; Bonham, V.L. Defining and Achieving Health Equity in Genomic Medicine. *Ethn. Dis.* **2019**, *29* (Suppl. 1), 173–178. [CrossRef] [PubMed]

24. Nolan, D.; Carlson, M. Whole exome sequencing in pediatric neurology patients: Clinical implications and estimated cost analysis. *J. Child Neurol.* **2016**, *31*, 887–894. [CrossRef]
25. Suther, S.; Kiros, G.-E. Barriers to the use of genetic testing: A study of racial and ethnic disparities. *Genet. Med.* **2009**, *11*, 655–662. [CrossRef]
26. Kapil, S.; Fishler, K.P.; Euteneuer, J.C.; Brunelli, L. Many newborns in level IV NICUs are eligible for rapid DNA sequencing. *Am. J. Med. Genet. Part A* **2018**, *179*, 280–284. [CrossRef]
27. Phillips, K.A.; Deverka, P.A.; Trosman, J.R.; Douglas, M.; Chambers, J.D.; Weldon, C.B.; Dervan, A.P. Payer coverage policies for multigene tests. *Nat. Biotechnol.* **2017**, *35*, 614–617. [CrossRef]
28. Trosman, J.R.; Weldon, C.B.; Slavotinek, A.; Norton, M.E.; Douglas, M.P.; Phillips, K.A. Perspectives of US private payers on insurance coverage for pediatric and prenatal exome sequencing: Results of a study from the Program in Prenatal and Pediatric Genomic Sequencing (P3EGS). *Genet. Med.* **2019**, *22*, 283–291. [CrossRef]
29. Kahan, N.R.; Chinitz, D.P.; Waitman, D.-A.; Kahan, E. When gatekeepers meet the sentinel: The impact of a prior authorization requirement for cefuroxime on the prescribing behaviour of community-based physicians. *Br. J. Clin. Pharmacol.* **2006**, *61*, 341–344. [CrossRef]
30. Marchant, G.L.R. Genomic malpractice: An emerging tide or gentle ripple? *Food Drug Law J.* **2018**, *73*, 1–37.
31. Graungaard, H.A.; Skov, L. Why do we need a diagnosis? A qualitative study of parents' experiences, coping and needs, when the newborn child is severely disabled. *Child Care Health Dev.* **2007**, *33*, 296–307. [CrossRef] [PubMed]
32. Lopes, M.T.; Koch, V.H.; Sarrubbi-Junior, V.; Gallo, P.R.; Carneiro-Sampaio, M. Difficulties in the diagnosis and treatment of rare diseases according to the perceptions of patients, relatives and health care professionals. *Clinics* **2018**, *73*, e68. [CrossRef] [PubMed]
33. McConkie-Rosell, A.; Hooper, S.R.; Pena, L.D.; Schoch, K.; Spillmann, R.C.; Jiang, Y.H.; Shashi, V. Psychosocial Profiles of Parents of Children with Undiagnosed Diseases: Managing Well or Just Managing? *J. Genet. Couns.* **2018**, *27*, 935–946. [CrossRef] [PubMed]
34. Madeo, A.C.; O'Brien, K.E.; Bernhardt, B.A.; Biesecker, B.B. Factors associated with perceived uncertainty among parents of children with undiagnosed medical conditions. *Am. J. Med. Genet. Part A* **2012**, *158A*, 1877–1884. [CrossRef]
35. Epstein, E.G.; Whitehead, P.B.; Prompahakul, C.; Thacker, L.R.; Hamric, A.B. Enhancing Understanding of Moral Distress: The Measure of Moral Distress for Health Care Professionals. *AJOB Empir. Bioeth.* **2019**, *10*, 113–124. [CrossRef]
36. Braithwaite, M. Nurse Burnout and Stress in the NICU. *Adv. Neonatal Care* **2008**, *8*, 343–347. [CrossRef]
37. Bernhardt, B.A.; Silver, R.; Rushton, C.H.; Micco, E.; Geller, G. What keeps you up at night? Genetics professionals' distressing experiences in patient care. *Genet. Med.* **2010**, *12*, 289–297. [CrossRef]
38. Wagner, C. Moral distress as a contributor to nurse burnout. *AJN Am. J. Nurs.* **2015**, *115*, 11. [CrossRef]
39. Barr, P. Moral Distress and Considering Leaving in NICU Nurses: Direct Effects and Indirect Effects Mediated by Burnout and the Hospital Ethical Climate. *Neonatology* **2020**, *117*, 646–649. [CrossRef]
40. Srivastava, S.; Love-Nichols, J.A.; Dies, K.A.; Ledbetter, D.H.; Martin, C.L.; Chung, W.K.; Firth, H.V.; Frazier, T.; Hansen, R.L.; Prock, L.; et al. Meta-analysis and multidisciplinary consensus statement: Exome sequencing is a first-tier clinical diagnostic test for individuals with neurodevelopmental disorders. *Genet. Med.* **2019**, *22*, 1731–1732. [CrossRef]
41. Srivastava, S.; Cohen, J.S.; Vernon, H.; Barañano, K.; McClellan, R.; Jamal, L.; Naidu, S.; Fatemi, A. Clinical whole exome sequencing in child neurology practice. *Ann. Neurol.* **2014**, *76*, 473–483. [CrossRef] [PubMed]
42. Tarailo-Graovac, M.; Shyr, C.; Ross, C.J.; Horvath, G.A.; Salvarinova, R.; Ye, X.C.; van Karnebeek, C.D. Exome sequencing and the management of neurometabolic disorders. *N. Engl. J. Med.* **2016**, *374*, 2246–2255. [CrossRef] [PubMed]
43. Retterer, K.; Juusola, J.; Cho, M.T.; Vitazka, P.; Millan, F.; Gibellini, F.; Vertino-Bell, A.; Smaoui, N.; Neidich, J.; Monaghan, K.G.; et al. Clinical application of whole-exome sequencing across clinical indications. *Genet. Med.* **2016**, *18*, 696–704. [CrossRef] [PubMed]

International Journal of
Neonatal Screening

MDPI

Commentary

The Burden and Benefits of Knowledge: Ethical Considerations Surrounding Population-Based Newborn Genome Screening for Hearing

Calli O. Mitchell [1], Greysha Rivera-Cruz [2], Matthew Hoi Kin Chau [3,4,5], Zirui Dong [3,4,5], Kwong Wai Choy [3,4,5,6], Jun Shen [7,8], Sami Amr [7,8,9], Anne B. S. Giersch [7,8] and Cynthia C. Morton [1,7,8,10,11,*]

1 Department of Obstetrics and Gynecology, Brigham and Women's Hospital, Boston, MA 02115, USA; comitchell@bwh.harvard.edu
2 Department of Pediatrics, Division of Genetics and Genomics, Boston Children's Hospital, Boston, MA 02115, USA; greysha.rivera-cruz@childrens.harvard.edu
3 Department of Obstetrics & Gynaecology, The Chinese University of Hong Kong, Hong Kong, China; matthewchau@cuhk.edu.hk (M.H.K.C.); elvisdong@cuhk.edu.hk (Z.D.); richardchoy@cuhk.edu.hk (K.W.C.)
4 Shenzhen Research Institute, The Chinese University of Hong Kong, Shenzhen 518172, China
5 Hong Kong Hub of Paediatric Excellence, The Chinese University of Hong Kong, Hong Kong, China
6 The Chinese University of Hong Kong-Baylor College of Medicine Joint Center for Medical Genetics, Hong Kong, China
7 Department of Pathology, Brigham and Women's Hospital, Boston, MA 02115, USA; jun.shen.98@gmail.com (J.S.); samr@bwh.harvard.edu (S.A.); agiersch@bwh.harvard.edu (A.B.S.G.)
8 Harvard Medical School, Boston, MA 02115, USA
9 Laboratory for Molecular Medicine, Partners Healthcare Personalized Medicine, Cambridge, MA 02139, USA
10 Broad Institute of MIT and Harvard, Cambridge, MA 02142, USA
11 Manchester Centre for Audiology and Deafness, School of Health Sciences, University of Manchester, Manchester M13 9PL, UK
* Correspondence: cmorton@bwh.harvard.edu

Abstract: Recent advances in genomic sequencing technologies have expanded practitioners' utilization of genetic information in a timely and efficient manner for an accurate diagnosis. With an ever-increasing resource of genomic data from progress in the interpretation of genome sequences, clinicians face decisions about how and when genomic information should be presented to families, and at what potential expense. Presently, there is limited knowledge or experience in establishing the value of implementing genome sequencing into newborn screening. Herein we provide insight into the complexities and the burden and benefits of knowledge resulting from genome sequencing of newborns.

Keywords: genome sequencing; newborn hearing screening; newborn screening; newborn genome sequencing; incidental findings; secondary findings; carrier status

1. Introduction

Since the 1960s, with initiation of the Guthrie card [1], newborn screening (NBS) has improved the lives of countless newborns and their families. The mandate of NBS is to identify treatable conditions in the newborn period that are not necessarily apparent at birth, but that could have life-long or fatal sequelae if untreated. A notable NBS advancement was the introduction of Newborn Hearing Screening (NBHS) in 1994 after endorsement by the Joint Committee on Infant Hearing [2]. This public health initiative makes possible early diagnosis and management for deaf and hard-of-hearing (DHH) babies, and better health outcomes for children and their families worldwide. Today, NBHS has been widely adopted in the United States with greater than 97% of newborns screened by one month of age [3].

Congenital deafness affects 1.7 of 1000 newborns [4] in the United States and is the most prevalent congenital sensory anomaly diagnosed in industrialized countries [5]. DHH is unparalleled in its heterogeneity with both genetic and environmental causes. With greater than 50% of congenital DHH having a genetic etiology, the importance of genetic testing in diagnosis and management of DHH individuals is paramount. Among genetic forms, both nonsyndromic and syndromic cases may result from variation in individual genes, and the same gene may be responsible for either dominant or recessive DHH. Over 400 types of syndromic DHH are recognized by the involvement of other organ systems in addition to the inner ear [6]. Nonsyndromic deafness is more prevalent than syndromic deafness and accounts for 70% of hereditary DHH [7].

2. Considering Health Outcomes for DHH Individuals

Given the auditory dominance of personal communication in the world, deafness has implications for an individual's well-being on all socioecological levels, disrupting interpersonal interactions, relationships in community settings, and with society at large [8]. Due to inheritance patterns and environmental causes of hearing loss, greater than 90% of DHH individuals are born to hearing parents [9] who likely have limited knowledge surrounding deafness. Many factors influence communication among children and adolescents, including the degree of hearing loss. Studies have shown that DHH individuals may experience barriers which impact educational attainment, the likelihood of future employment, future earnings, use of healthcare systems, and life expectancy [10]; thus, access for all to early diagnosis and interventions are crucial for DHH health outcomes.

Shearer and co-authors provide promising evidence that a genetic etiology for hearing loss can influence the treatment and management of a child's care [11]. In fact, research demonstrates the established benefits on speech performance after cochlear implantation of infants with *GJB2* or *SLC26A4* diagnoses [12,13]. The benefits of cochlear implantation for genetic etiologies including *OTOF*, *CACNA1D*, *CABP2*, *SLC17A8*, *DIAPH3*, *OPA1*, and *ROR1* have been illustrated [11]. Thus, a comprehensive approach to newborn hearing screening which includes genome sequencing (GS), physiologic hearing screening, and congenital cytomegalovirus (cCMV) testing [14] provides beneficence to DHH newborns and may influence development of future interventions or therapeutics.

3. Comprehensive Newborn Genome Sequencing: SEQuencing a Baby for an Optimal Outcome

SEQaBOO (SEQuencing a Baby for an Optimal Outcome), a research project initiated in Boston, Massachusetts [15], offers genome sequencing for newborns who are referred for diagnostic audiometry following physiologic screening. DHH is serving as a paradigm for integrating population-based genome screening into NBS at large. Recruitment is ongoing at three Harvard-affiliated hospitals: Brigham and Women's, Boston Children's, and Massachusetts Eye and Ear. SEQaBOO provides comprehensive genome sequencing and variant interpretation of DHH-associated genes, as well as optional (for parents only) ACMG secondary findings (SF) v 3.0 [16]. In collaboration with the Chinese University of Hong Kong, genome-wide copy number variant (CNV) analysis is assessed on all participants [17–19]. This analytic platform can also identify chromosomal aneuploidy, absence of heterozygosity, and chromosomal structural rearrangements including translocations. Through this method, balanced chromosomal translocations, sex chromosome aneuploidy, and pathogenic CNVs in genes associated with DHH have been detected. Such findings resulted in numerous protracted conversations surrounding the positive and negative ethical implications of disclosing incidental genomic findings from a research study that ultimately may not be related to the infant's DHH phenotype.

SEQaBOO has proven the feasibility of implementing comprehensive genome sequencing into NBHS to facilitate earlier intervention and treatment options for DHH individuals. Similar studies have demonstrated the importance of genetic screening in the newborn period as a mechanism to improve health outcomes for DHH individuals [20–25]. For example, newborns with a positive genetic finding may pass physiologic NBHS as frequently as 50% of the time yet are diagnosed as DHH later in childhood [15]. A population-based study of this capacity also has the potential to identify novel genomic variants contributing to DHH and other heritable disorders.

4. Ethical Dilemmas in Real Time

Given the comprehensive nature of SEQaBOO, various ethical dilemmas have arisen and are illustrative of the portending future of genomic medicine. Incidental findings from interpretation of the SEQaBOO genome analysis led to obtaining further Institutional Review Board (IRB) approval to inform families of unanticipated research results. IRB approval was given with the request pending assessment of "the need to know" as determined by medical geneticists on the SEQaBOO staff. Although the etiology of many babies' DHH has been determined, the incidental findings exemplify the complexity and ethical dilemmas that reporting genetic research results may have on the family of a newborn. In addition, such knowledge can be burdensome for the healthcare team, specifically primary care clinicians. These clinicians are responsible for requesting confirmatory testing of research results and may also have limited knowledge about genetic testing and interpretation.

5. Lessons Learned: Copy Number Variants and Contiguous Genes

In addition to single nucleotide variants (SNVs), many genes associated with DHH are characterized by well-known etiologic CNVs [26], making important the assessment of the genome sequence for such anomalies. For example, large deletions of both copies of stereocilin (*STRC*) can be etiologic in mild to moderate sensorineural deafness and are responsible for 5.4–16.1% of DHH diagnoses in mixed-ethnicity populations [27]. Due to a segmental duplication that leads to frequent non-allelic homologous recombination in the *STRC* locus on chromosome 15, contiguous deletions of *STRC* and *CATSPER2* genes [27,28] may occur resulting in Deafness Infertility Syndrome (DIS) in males. Informing a family of an infant's hearing impairment can be valuable for clinical management, but concomitant reporting of the possibility that a male child may have fertility problems in adulthood adds additional distress for the family. SEQaBOO investigators identified a male participant with contiguous deletions of *STRC* and *CATSPER2*. Due to the fact that SEQaBOO is a research study designed to identify genes associated with hearing (and potentially secondary findings as reported in ACMG SF v 3.0), SEQaBOO investigators debated whether to disclose the associated infertility phenotype in a male newborn as the fertility issue would be considered as an adult phenotype. In this case, a decision was made to disclose this finding to the family, in addition to the origin of the DHH, for two reasons: (1) DIS is a recognized heritable deafness syndrome including infertility in males, and (2) the contiguous *STRC/CATSPER2* deletion would be revealed to the family upon clinical validation of the research result.

As part of this research study, all pathogenic CNVs are scored based on the American College of Medical Genetics and Genomics recommendations for reporting pathogenicity of CNVs [29]. Added benefit is derived in reporting CNVs associated with DHH; however, given the complexity of interpretation for genome-wide CNV analysis, there are ethical implications that warrant consideration. For instance, many CNVs detected in this study are not likely to be pathogenic which leaves families without an etiology for their child's DHH, and may cause a psychosocial burden. Both positive and negative ethical implications arise when determining which CNVs should be reported to families. For example, determining a child's etiologic DHH diagnosis can influence the future care and management of the DHH, but identifying a variant associated with a later onset disorder can result in a significant burden for the family, clinicians, and healthcare system. These findings present the importance of developing guidelines for reporting CNVs identified in the newborn period as part of a research study, especially when clinical confirmation may be beyond available routine genetic testing. Another ethical aspect to consider is the benefit that reporting this information has for the child. Identifying a child's predisposition to fertility issues at birth can be the source of psychological distress and subject the child and family to additional stress throughout the child's life. Thus, it is imperative to respect the child's autonomy when complex ethical dilemmas arise; this is a challenge that will remain apparent as genomic sequencing technologies and access to such technologies improve, especially in population-based genomic NBS.

6. Lessons Learned: Variants of Uncertain Significance and Carrier Status

Genome sequencing can provide useful information that translates into a timely diagnosis, early intervention, and overall improvement of health outcomes. However, genome sequencing presents a level of uncertainty whenever indeterminate results are identified. Variants of uncertain significance (VUS) are genetic variants of uncertain pathogenic potential, as there is insufficient evidence to determine whether the variants cause the phenotype. When clinicians receive such genetic results, additional investigations, such as research and functional studies, clinical correlations, segregation analyses, and case-control statistics, are needed to elucidate or rule out pathogenicity. Further, as broader genetic testing approaches are implemented in medical care, the likelihood of obtaining uncertain results increases. Discussion of testing limitations and the type of genetic results should be included regularly during pre- and post-genetic counseling. Uncertain results may often have psychosocial implications for both patients and clinicians, especially when a VUS is present in a gene, or genes, related to the phenotype. However, as the clinical significance of a VUS is not well established, such variants should not be considered in decisions for clinical management or interventions.

Two potential paths are possible when disclosing VUSs. Some patients experience a positive view or hope that learning indeterminate results most likely indicates that a pathogenic or true diagnosis was not confirmed, whereas others may express adverse emotions, such as distress, frustration, guilt, and confusion as they lack understanding of what a VUS truly means for them or their clinical care [30]. Uncertain results also present ethical dilemmas as they may cause patient dissatisfaction, mistrust of genetic testing, the clinician or science, and uncertain clinical utility, thus complicating the counseling process.

Another source for uncertainty arises when sequencing the genome for DHH-associated genes, as it is not uncommon to identify individuals carrying a single pathogenic genetic variant in a gene associated with recessive DHH (i.e., the individual has a heterozygous variant only in one copy of a gene associated with recessive DHH). Given that up to 80% of DHH is inherited in a recessive pattern [6], there is potential benefit in reporting parental carrier status for the risk associated for future children, whereas reporting carrier status in a newborn provides limited benefit for the family and adds burden and concern. Thus, ethically reporting carrier status in an infant who will not be of reproductive age for over a decade provides minimal beneficence to the family and the child.

7. Lessons Learned: Chromosomal Structural Rearrangements

Previous studies highlight the importance of integrating the assessment of chromosome rearrangements involving DHH-related genes into comprehensive genome sequencing; several cases have been detected of a chromosomal translocation was found to disrupting a gene responsible for an individual's DHH diagnosis [31–35]. Chromosomal structural rearrangements may result in repositioning of segments of chromatin known as translocations, inversions, and duplications/deletions, among others. These events can result in balanced or unbalanced genomes. Balanced translocations are the most frequently reported chromosomal structural rearrangements, estimated at approximately one per 500 individuals [36]. A balanced chromosomal translocation may not involve copy number alterations or gene disruption and, most often, is not responsible for a clinical phenotype. In fact, most balanced translocation carriers are unaware of their chromosomal rearrangement. However, such a genetic alteration may be discovered during childbearing years as individuals with such rearrangements are at increased risk of producing unbalanced gametes. This typically presents with a history of infertility due to recurrent miscarriages, fetal death, or children born with congenital anomalies and/or physical–intellectual disabilities [37]. When a member of a couple harbors a balanced reciprocal translocation, the risk of having an affected child with congenital anomalies ranges from 6 to 12% [36,37]. Dong and co-authors present findings indicating that greater than 11% of couples with recurrent miscarriage are at risk to have a chromosomal abnormality [38]. Thus, balanced translocation information can be informative for reproductive planning and decisions. However, its association with DHH may be etiologic or not yet known.

With the aid of our comprehensive genome analysis tools, the SEQaBOO study has encountered two cases thus far of both an infant and one of their parents being a carrier of a balanced chromosome rearrangement. In one case, it was possible the rearrangement was etiologic for the child's DHH as a hearing-related gene was disrupted, and the carrier parent also had mild hearing loss. In the other case, the child ultimately passed their audiology exam and did not have DHH, and it appeared unlikely the translocation would cause a phenotype in the carrier (parent or child). The concern then became, not for the proband, but for the young parents who were (possibly unknowingly) at risk of having a child with an unbalanced chromosome complement. Furthermore, the proband would have the same reproductive risk as the parents when of reproductive age. A decision was made to disclose the finding of the translocations to both families, who were aware from an infertility work-up that a member of each couple harbored a rearrangement. Both newborns were conceived by in vitro fertilization (IVF), and no additional genetic testing was performed on the embryos. While reproductive decision making is not included in traditional Wilson–Junger screening criteria, newer criteria frameworks provide insight into the added benefits beyond the individual child, such as family interests, but without ignoring the best interests of the child [39].

8. Discussion

Advancements in technologies make possible the application of sequencing in newborns in a timely fashion. This enables interpretation of genetic variants as the molecular etiologies for the clinical phenotype of interest. However, fully informative interpretations of the pathogenicity of variants remains under development, and the possibility of unintended discovery of incidental findings is challenging [40]. The burden and benefits of knowledge obtained from comprehensive newborn sequencing warrants ongoing ethical discussions and prudent considerations.

Genome sequencing is now able to provide information about chromosomal structural rearrangements and occasionally offers clinical utility to identify the etiology of the disorder. It remains important to consider, when involving parents (trio) or single parents (duo), that such rearrangements can be informative for parents themselves, revealing an increased reproductive risk for the couple and biological relatives. Identification of incidental findings in newborns can affect future reproductive outcomes for the family and biological relatives and may be unrelated to the initial indication for genetic testing. In such cases, thoughtful and careful consideration of the utility and importance of reporting incidental findings on newborns for late-onset situations comes with a burden for both the family and clinicians.

The clinical and research team should be aware of some key elements when disclosing incidental findings to families involved in genomic NBS. It is important to contemplate and appreciate the level of distress and anxiety a family may experience when receiving results of incidental findings. This discussion is also impacted by the couple's level of understanding about genetic information, including different perspectives between the couple themselves. An additional level of complexity is related to the parent's actionability towards these results, as most disorders with late-onset penetrance would not pose immediate health implications. Physicians' and/or researchers' personal biases can impact the perception of genomic incidental results, and awareness of this possibility should be considered when deciding to report such results in the newborn period.

With increased utilization of genetic testing will come complexities of interpretation as researchers and clinicians work together to provide the best care for their research participants or patients. Boundaries need to be delineated with regards to genomic data that clinicians share with patients, especially if the genomic findings are identified as part of a research project.

Increasing access to genome sequencing presents a learning curve in which clinicians, patients, and the public will need to adapt to the ever-changing breadth of knowledge. It remains crucial for clinicians to establish the best practices for reporting genomic results to families to ensure patients' best understanding. Clinicians are ultimately responsible for communicating genomic results to their patients and should strive to deliver the knowledge in a compassionate manner, such that it reduces excessive distress yet is accurate. This is particularly relevant when it comes with the potential psychosocial complexities of presenting information regarding a newborn's reproductive future. That being said, it remains important to identify the genetic etiology for a child's DHH as it may impact management and treatment. However, the need for appropriate genetic counselling will continue to be essential, and experts in the field of genetics must be cognizant of placing the burden of knowledge onto primary care physicians and other specialists.

When considering population-based genome sequencing in the newborn period, equity and access to historically underrepresented populations will need to be carefully guarded as it opens another set of ethical issues. Future projects utilizing genomic NBS must first consider equity and diversity as a priority to provide access to advanced technologies for all families to prevent the further broadening of existing healthcare disparities. Although genome sequencing has become more accessible and more cost effective, limitations persist. For example, the interpretation of genomic results is complicated by the lack of diverse genetic ancestry reference data. Equitable access to genomic technologies is important, as access to these technologies is frequently limited by economic factors as well as additional social determinants of health. Other considerations must be kept in mind when proposing equitable population-based NBS, such as follow-up medical care, further genetic testing, and insurance coverage. Increasing knowledge of the genome and its workings brings the benefit of better health outcomes but is not without additional burden as healthcare systems cautiously learn their way forward.

9. Conclusions

Advances in sequencing technologies and analytic pipelines facilitate new discoveries. Limited studies of this nature have made possible identification of unexpected findings in newborn genome sequencing. Researchers and clinicians must work together to establish optimal practices for reporting such information to families. Overall, the benefits of genome sequencing in the newborn period are reflected in advancements in newborn screening technologies. Various considerations with public trust in genomic science will facilitate large-scale implementation.

Author Contributions: C.O.M., G.R.-C., and C.C.M. wrote the paper with input and edits from all authors. All authors have read and agreed to the published version of the manuscript.

Funding: This research is supported by the National Institutes of Deafness and Other Communication Disorders, National Institutes of Health (DC015052) and supported by the NIHR Manchester Biomedical Research Centre. We are grateful for a philanthropic donation to Brigham and Women's Hospital for supporting this research.

Institutional Review Board Statement: The study was approved by the Massachusetts General Brigham Institutional Review Board (Protocol # 2017P000870 11/20/2017).

Informed Consent Statement: Written informed consent was obtained from the biological mother and biological father (when applicable) for all subjects involved in the study.

Acknowledgments: The authors appreciate the participation of families in the SEQaBOO study. G.R.-C. is supported by NIGMS T32 GM007748.

Conflicts of Interest: The authors declare no conflict of interest.

References

1. Levy, H.L. Robert guthrie and the trials and tribulations of newborn screening. *Int. J. Neonatal Screen.* **2021**, *7*, 5. [CrossRef] [PubMed]
2. Joint Committee on Infant Hearing (JCIH). Position Statement 1994. *Pediatrics* **1995**, *95*, 152–156. Available online: http://www.jcih.org/JCIH1994.pdf (accessed on 4 February 2022). [CrossRef]
3. 2018 Summary of National CDC EHDI Data | Annual Data EHDI Program | CDC. Available online: https://www.cdc.gov/ncbddd/hearingloss/2018-data/01-data-summary.html (accessed on 4 February 2022).
4. US Centers for Disease Control and Prevention. 2018 Summary of Diagnostics among Infants Not Passing Hearing Screening. Available online: https://www.cdc.gov/ncbddd/hearingloss/2018-data/06-diagnostics.html (accessed on 4 February 2022).
5. Thorpe, R.K.; Smith, R.J.H. Future directions for screening and treatment in congenital hearing loss. *Precis. Clin. Med.* **2020**, *3*, 175–186. [CrossRef] [PubMed]
6. Shearer, A.E.; Hildebrand, M.S.; Smith, R.J. Hereditary Hearing Loss and Deafness Overview. GeneReviews®. 2017; pp. 1–27. Available online: http://www.ncbi.nlm.nih.gov/pubmed/20301607 (accessed on 4 February 2022).
7. Chang, K.W. Genetics of Hearing Loss-Nonsyndromic. *Otolaryngol. Clin. N. Am.* **2015**, *48*, 1063–1072. [CrossRef] [PubMed]
8. Smith, S.R.; Chin, N.P. Social Determinants of Health in Deaf Communities. In *Public Health-Social and Behavioral Health*; IntechOpen: London, UK, 2012; pp. 449–460.
9. Hall, W.C.; Smith, S.R.; Sutter, E.J.; Dewindt, L.A.; Dye, T.D. Considering parental hearing status as a social determinant of deaf population health: Insights from experiences of the 'dinner table syndrome'. *PLoS ONE* **2018**, *13*, e0202169. [CrossRef]
10. Smith, R.J.H.; Bale, J.F.; White, K.R. Sensorineural hearing loss in children. *Lancet* **2005**, *365*, 879–890. [CrossRef]
11. Shearer, A.E.; Hansen, M.R. Auditory synaptopathy, auditory neuropathy, and cochlear implantation. *Laryngoscope Investig. Otolaryngol.* **2019**, *4*, 429–440. [CrossRef]
12. Green, G.E.; Scott, D.A.; McDonald, J.M.; Teagle, H.F.; Tomblin, B.J.; Spencer, L.J.; Woodworth, G.G.; Knutson, J.F.; Gantz, B.J.; Sheffield, V.C.; et al. Performance of cochlear implant recipients with GJB2-related deafness. *Am. J. Med. Genet.* **2002**, *109*, 167–170. [CrossRef]
13. Yan, Y.J.; Li, Y.; Yang, T.; Huang, Q.; Wu, H. The effect of GJB2 and SLC26A4 gene mutations on rehabilitative outcomes in pediatric cochlear implant patients. *Eur. Arch. Oto-Rhino-Laryngol.* **2013**, *270*, 2865–2870. [CrossRef]
14. Shearer, A.E.; Shen, J.; Amr, S.; Morton, C.C.; Smith, R.J. A proposal for comprehensive newborn hearing screening to improve identification of deaf and hard-of-hearing children. *Genet. Med.* **2019**, *21*, 2614–2630. [CrossRef]
15. Mitchell, C.O.; Morton, C.C. Genetics of Childhood Hearing Loss. *Otolaryngol. Clin. N. Am.* **2021**, *54*, 1081–1092. [CrossRef] [PubMed]
16. Miller, D.T.; Lee, K.; Chung, W.K.; Gordon, A.S.; Herman, G.E.; Klein, T.E.; Stewart, D.R.; Amendola, L.M.; Adelman, K.; Bale, S.J.; et al. ACMG SF v3.0 list for reporting of secondary findings in clinical exome and genome sequencing: A policy statement of the American College of Medical Genetics and Genomics (ACMG). *Genet. Med.* **2021**, *23*, 1381–1390. [CrossRef] [PubMed]
17. Chau, M.H.K.; Wang, H.; Lai, Y.; Zhang, Y.; Xu, F.; Tang, Y.; Wang, Y.; Chen, Z.; Leung, T.Y.; Chung, J.; et al. Low-pass genome sequencing: A validated method in clinical cytogenetics. *Qual. Life Res.* **2020**, *139*, 1403–1415. [CrossRef]
18. Dong, Z.; Wang, H.; Chen, H.; Jiang, H.; Yuan, J.; Yang, Z.; Wang, W.-J.; Xu, F.; Guo, X.; Cao, Y.; et al. Identification of balanced chromosomal rearrangements previously unknown among participants in the 1000 Genomes Project: Implications for interpretation of structural variation in genomes and the future of clinical cytogenetics. *Genet. Med.* **2018**, *20*, 697–707. [CrossRef] [PubMed]
19. Wang, H.; Dong, Z.; Zhang, R.; Chau, M.H.K.; Yang, Z.; Tsang, K.Y.C.; Wong, H.K.; Gui, B.; Meng, Z.; Xiao, K.; et al. Low-pass genome sequencing versus chromosomal microarray analysis: Implementation in prenatal diagnosis. *Genet. Med.* **2020**, *22*, 500–510. [CrossRef] [PubMed]
20. Dai, P.; Huang, L.-H.; Wang, G.-J.; Gao, X.; Qu, C.-Y.; Chen, X.-W.; Ma, F.-R.; Zhang, J.; Xing, W.-L.; Xi, S.-Y.; et al. Concurrent Hearing and Genetic Screening of 180,469 Neonates with Follow-up in Beijing, China. *Am. J. Hum. Genet.* **2019**, *105*, 803–812. [CrossRef] [PubMed]
21. Wang, Q.; Xiang, J.; Sun, J.; Yang, Y.; Guan, J.; Wang, D.; Song, C.; Guo, L.; Wang, H.; Chen, Y.; et al. Nationwide population genetic screening improves outcomes of newborn screening for hearing loss in China. *Genet. Med.* **2019**, *21*, 2231–2238. [CrossRef]
22. Wu, C.-C.; Tsai, C.-H.; Hung, C.-C.; Lin, Y.-H.; Lin, Y.-H.; Huang, F.-L.; Tsao, P.-N.; Su, Y.-N.; Lee, Y.L.; Hsieh, W.-S.; et al. Newborn genetic screening for hearing impairment: A population-based longitudinal study. *Genet. Med.* **2017**, *19*, 6–12. [CrossRef]
23. Minami, S.B.; Mutai, H.; Nakano, A.; Arimoto, Y.; Taiji, H.; Morimoto, N.; Sakata, H.; Adachi, N.; Masuda, S.; Sakamoto, H.; et al. GJB2-associated hearing loss undetected by hearing screening of newborns. *Gene* **2013**, *532*, 41–45. [CrossRef]
24. Guo, L.; Xiang, J.; Sun, L.; Yan, X.; Yang, J.; Wu, H.; Guo, K.; Peng, J.; Xie, X.; Yin, Y.; et al. Concurrent hearing and genetic screening in a general newborn population. *Hum. Genet.* **2020**, *139*, 521–530. [CrossRef]
25. Downie, L.; Halliday, J.; Burt, R.; Lunke, S.; Lynch, E.; Martyn, M.; Poulakis, Z.; Gaff, C.; Sung, V.; Wake, M.; et al. Exome sequencing in infants with congenital hearing impairment: A population-based cohort study. *Eur. J. Hum. Genet.* **2020**, *28*, 587–596. [CrossRef] [PubMed]

26. Shearer, A.E.; Kolbe, D.L.; Azaiez, H.; Sloan, C.M.; Frees, K.L.; E Weaver, A.; Clark, E.T.; Nishimura, C.J.; Black-Ziegelbein, E.A.; Smith, R.J.H. Copy number variants are a common cause of non-syndromic hearing loss. *Genome Med.* **2014**, *6*, 37. [CrossRef] [PubMed]
27. Nishio, S.-Y.; Usami, S.-I. Frequency of the STRC-CATSPER2 deletion in STRC-associated hearing loss patients. *Sci. Rep.* **2022**, *12*, 1–7. [CrossRef] [PubMed]
28. Yokota, Y.; Moteki, H.; Nishio, S.-Y.; Yamaguchi, T.; Wakui, K.; Kobayashi, Y.; Ohyama, K.; Miyazaki, H.; Matsuoka, R.; Abe, S.; et al. Frequency and clinical features of hearing loss caused by STRC deletions. *Sci. Rep.* **2019**, *9*, 4408. [CrossRef] [PubMed]
29. Riggs, E.R.; Andersen, E.F.; Cherry, A.M.; Kantarci, S.; Kearney, H.; Patel, A.; Raca, G.; Ritter, D.I.; South, S.T.; Thorland, E.C.; et al. Technical standards for the interpretation and reporting of constitutional copy-number variants: A joint consensus recommendation of the American College of Medical Genetics and Genomics (ACMG) and the Clinical Genome Resource (ClinGen). *Genet. Med.* **2020**, *22*, 245–257. [CrossRef]
30. Clift, K.; Macklin, S.; Halverson, C.; McCormick, J.B.; Dabrh, A.M.A.; Hines, S. Patients' views on variants of uncertain significance across indications. *J. Community Genet.* **2020**, *11*, 139–145. [CrossRef]
31. Brown, K.K.; Alkuraya, F.S.; Matos, M.; Robertson, R.L.; Kimonis, V.E.; Morton, C.C. NR2F1 deletion in a patient with a de novo paracentric inversion, inv(5)(q15q33.2), and syndromic deafness. *Am. J. Med. Genet. Part A* **2009**, *149A*, 931–938. [CrossRef]
32. Currall, B.B.; Chen, M.; Sallari, R.C.; Cotter, M.; Wong, K.; Robertson, N.G.; Penney, K.L.; Lunardi, A.; Reschke, M.; E Hickox, A.; et al. Loss of LDAH associated with prostate cancer and hearing loss. *Hum. Mol. Genet.* **2018**, *27*, 4194–4203. [CrossRef]
33. Anger, G.J.; Crocker, S.; McKenzie, K.; Brown, K.K.; Morton, C.C.; Harrison, K.; MacKenzie, J.J. X-Linked Deafness-2 (DFNX2) Phenotype Associated With a Paracentric Inversion Upstream of POU3F4. *Am. J. Audiol.* **2014**, *23*, 1–6. [CrossRef]
34. Brown, K.K.; Reiss, J.A.; Crow, K.; Ferguson, H.L.; Kelly, C.; Fritzsch, B.; Morton, C.C. Deletion of an enhancer near DLX5 and DLX6 in a family with hearing loss, craniofacial defects, and an inv(7)(q21.3q35). *Qual. Life Res.* **2010**, *127*, 19–31. [CrossRef]
35. Doco-Fenzy, M.; Mauran, P.; Marie Lebrun, J.; Bock, S.; Bednarek, N.; Struski, S.; Albuisson, J.; Ardalan, A.; Collot, N.; Schneider, A.; et al. A Child With Marcus Gunn Phenomenon and Multiple Congenital Anomalies. *Am. J. Hum. Genet.* **2006**, *221*, 212–221.
36. Gardner, R.J.M.; Amor, D.J. *Gardner and Sutherland's Chromosome Abnormalities and Genetic Counseling*, 5th ed.; Oxford University Press: Oxford, UK, 2018.
37. Wilch, E.S.; Morton, C.C. Historical and Clinical Perspectives on Chromosomal Translocations. *Chromosome Translocat.* **2018**, *1044*, 1–14.
38. Dong, Z.; Yan, J.; Xu, F.; Yuan, J.; Jiang, H.; Wang, H.; Chen, H.; Zhang, L.; Ye, L.; Xu, J.; et al. Genome Sequencing Explores Complexity of Chromosomal Abnormalities in Recurrent Miscarriage. *Am. J. Hum. Genet.* **2019**, *105*, 1102–1111. [CrossRef] [PubMed]
39. Andermann, A.; Blancquaert, I.; Beauchamp, S.; Déry, V. Revisiting Wilson and Jungner in the genomic age: A review of screening criteria over the past 40 years. *Bull. World Health Organ.* **2008**, *86*, 317–319. [CrossRef]
40. Rotz, S.J.; Kodish, E. Ethical conundrums in pediatric genomics. *Hematology* **2018**, *2018*, 301–306. [CrossRef]

International Journal of
Neonatal Screening

MDPI

Commentary

Newborn Screening Is on a Collision Course with Public Health Ethics

Robert J. Currier

Department of Pediatrics, University of California, San Francisco, CA 94158, USA; robert.currier@ucsf.edu;
Tel.: +1-778-887-9581

Abstract: Newborn screening was established over 50 years ago to identify cases of disorders that were serious, urgent, and treatable, mirroring the criteria of Wilson and Jungner. In the last decade, conditions have been added to newborn screening that do not strictly meet these criteria, and genomic newborn screening is beginning to be discussed. Some of these new and proposed additions to newborn screening entail serious public health ethical issues that need to be explored.

Keywords: newborn screening; ethics; consent; DNA sequencing; genome; genomic newborn screening; Krabbe disease; Pompe disease; adrenoleukodystrophy

1. Introduction

Newborn screening was named by the Centers for Disease Control among the Ten Great Public Health Achievements—United States, 2001–2010 [1]. This decade brought a four-fold increase in the number of screened disorders and the development and adoption of the Recommended Uniform Screening Panel (RUSP) by the Advisory Committee on Heritable Diseases of Newborns and Children (ACHDNC) [2].

Currently newborn screening programs are set up to collect a specimen and send it to the newborn screening laboratory within 48 h of birth, with results returned to the pediatrician, and often a specialist, shortly thereafter. There is no parental consent, although some States allow an "opt out" for religious or personal reasons. On the contrary, the perinatal period is a time when most parents are recovering from birth, consumed by the overwhelming adjustments of parenthood, and excited about the new baby. It is not an opportune time for a detailed discussion of rare events and formal consent.

However, public health newborn screening without formal consent requires justification based on the urgency, severity, and treatability of the diseases targeted [3]. In order for the State to supersede the decision-making authority of parents over the health of their child, the essential argument has been that irreparable harm will be done if the screening does not proceed immediately. This points to both the seriousness and urgency of the screened conditions. Thus, after identification of an affected infant, it is necessary that effective treatment is available that can avert otherwise dire consequences. For this reason, identification of untreatable conditions has never been accepted by newborn screening programs as a goal of newborn screening. The constellation of these factors—seriousness, urgency, and treatability—provides a compelling justification; the vast majority of parents would consent, were they to fully consider the process [4].

Previous studies have considered newborn screening from the perspective of medical ethics or medical economics. Here, we will discuss newborn screening from the perspective of public health ethics within governmental ethics.

2. Discussion

2.1. Public Health Ethics as a Framework for Consideration of Newborn Screening

The State has many roles in conducting a newborn screening program. In addition to providing laboratory testing and interpretation of results or contracting with professionals to do so, the State provides education to medical providers and to parents, coordinates follow-up and provides payment for services in many newborn screening programs, conducts epidemiological monitoring to better understand disease incidence and natural history, regulates the entire newborn screening system, and makes sure that newborn screening is provided for all newborns.

As such, the ethical evaluation of newborn screening can appropriately be located within governmental ethics, and particular, public health ethics. The principles of public health ethics focus primarily on improving population health overall, including health equity, reducing disparities, and removing societal barriers to health. In all of these activities, individual autonomy may be limited, which requires a separate ethical framework for analysis. Cass [5] has organized this framework as a series of six sequential questions that any proposed public health project should be able to answer with supportive data. Responses to these questions with regard to newborn screening for phenylketonuria (PKU, MIM: 261600), the paradigm of newborn screening tests, show how these principles apply.

1. **What are the public health goals of the proposed program?** The goal of newborn screening for PKU is the early detection of PKU to enable treatment (dietary modification) to avoid irremediable damage to the newborn's brain.
2. **How effective is the program in achieving its stated goals?** Newborn screening is applied universally, so its reach is the entire population of newborns. Screening for PKU has been highly effective at identifying cases, to the point that any reported case missed by screening requires an investigation of causes and a plan for remediation.
3. **What are the known or potential burdens of the program?** A universal burden of newborn screening is the loss of parental autonomy with regard to the medical care of their child. Secondary burdens are those relating to positive results caused by other factors than PKU itself. These off-target results require follow-up and a period of uncertainty and anxiety in parents until PKU is ruled out.
4. **Can burdens be minimized? Are there alternative approaches?** Newborn screening without parental involvement is considered unavoidable in order to maintain the universality of the program. Two developments over the course of the decades of screening for PKU have greatly reduced the burdens of off-target results. First, the existence of hyperphenylalaninemia has been recognized, and infants identified with this condition are not required to restrict their diets as severely. Second, the screening test itself has become much more specific, first by the addition of the ratio of phenylalanine to tyrosine, and later by interpretation of a much larger panel of newborn screening markers. These developments have greatly reduced the number of off-target results.
5. **Is the program implemented fairly?** As indicated previously, newborn screening has always been implemented as a universal program. All newborns are tested, without regard to birth location, insurance coverage status, or ability to pay.
6. **How can the benefits and burdens of a program be fairly balanced?** In general, newborn screening for PKU has achieved a very high degree of recognition and satisfaction for the real benefits that it has achieved. The loss of parental autonomy is considered by some to be a reason for eliminating newborn screening entirely, but that is very much a minority opinion.

Some recent additions to newborn screening highlight how problematic some of these principles have become.

2.2. Three Problematic Recent Introductions to Newborn Screening

As newborn screening has evolved and has moved farther from the original principles of Wilson and Jungner [3], disorders have been added to programs that raise issues from the perspective of public health ethics. We look at three specific screened disorders, then apply these public health ethics questions to them. Afterward, we consider the response of some newborn screening programs to these issues.

2.2.1. Krabbe Disease Screening in New York

The Newborn Screening Program of New York State was mandated by the New York legislature to begin screening for Krabbe disease, a lysosomal storage disorder (KD. OMIM:245200) in August, 2006. Orsini et al. reported on the first eight years of screening in 2016 [6]. They found, that of 2,090,910 infants tested, there were 10,199 that required retesting to confirm low enzymatic activity. From these, 620 were reflexed to molecular testing. Within that group, 272 had only benign polymorphisms in the *GALC* gene and 348 were referred for follow-up.

The clinical outcome of these cases identified by screening was reported by Wasserstein et al. [7]. Within the group of 348 infants referred for follow-up, the diagnostic testing found that 203 were at no risk for infantile KD, 92 were at low risk, 37 were at moderate risk, and 14 were at high risk, and 5 of those at high risk had confirmed early infantile Krabbe disease (EIKD). The confirmatory testing included extensive neurological evaluation and measurement of protein in CSF. These 5 families were offered hematopoietic stem cell transplantation (HSCT). One family refused; based on the genetic result for the infant they anticipated that treatment would not be successful. The other four infants were transplanted, between 24 and 41 days of life. Of these infants, two died of transplantation-related complications. The infants who were identified as high-risk but not EIKD were followed for 1 to 9 years, with no symptoms of Krabbe disease.

Ehmann and Lantos [8] considered these data pointed to the positive predictive value of the screening test of only 1.4%, which they characterized as too inefficient. A more recent publication from New York [9] explains the current screening algorithm which involves evaluating a panel of enzyme activities and other newborn screening markers. From a population of roughly 260,000, the number of referrals was reduced from 48 to 10.

An essential tool of this more precise algorithm is the use of the Collaborative Laboratory Integrated Reports (CLIR, Mayo Clinic, Rochester, MN, USA) tools, which use data submitted from multiple programs around the world for affected and unaffected newborns. Combining multiple newborn screening analytes, in this case a panel of enzymes implicated in lysosomal storage diseases, can provide this better separation of high-risk infants warranting referral for diagnosis from other types of results.

Within the group of high-risk infants referred for diagnosis in the New York study, almost two-thirds were ruled out from EIKD. This points to an additional need to refine the screening test to be able to distinguish these subgroups of high-risk infants. Recent work suggests that psychosine is very highly elevated in the EIKD group, and much lower in the rest of the high-risk group. Implementing psychosine testing as a second-tier test within the Krabbe screening algorithm can greatly improve the overall screening performance [10].

Considering the public health ethics framework questions, the question how effective the program is at meeting its goals already points to potential problems. The goal of the screening test is to diagnose and effectively treat EIKD. In the original implementation, there were very many more off-target results than true positive results. Although a more recent publication from New York shows that an alternative algorithm for the screening test reduced the burden of these off-target results substantially, the data on the effectiveness of treatment has been called into question as pointed out by Ehmann and Lantos. Observing these results from New York, several newborn screening programs have declined to implement screening for Krabbe disease. In 2009, the ACHDNC considered screening for Krabbe disease and did not recommend screening based on gaps in evidence. In the intervening years, additional data and improvements in the screening algorithm suggest that reconsideration may be warrented.

2.2.2. X-Linked Adrenoleukodystrophy

Newborn screening for X-linked adrenoleukodystrophy [X-ALD] was added to the RUSP in 2016. X-ALD (MIM:300100) is an X-linked recessive disorder. Like Krabbe disease, X-ALD has a variable phenotypic spectrum, from childhood onset cerebral adrenoleukodystrophy, which is the target of newborn screening, to later onset forms, including isolated adrenal insufficiency without central nervous system involvement.

The evidence review prepared for ACHDNC was definitive:

> It is estimated that about 20% of heterozygote females have VLCFA plasma levels within normal limits. However, because females with X-ALD do not typically experience symptoms until adulthood, if ever, they are not a target of newborn screening. [11] (p. 5)

Nonetheless, screening for X-ALD includes the entire population, males and females. Advocates of screening point to benefits of screening females, including the potential to identify females who might experience symptoms later in life, and the indirect identification of mildly affected older siblings or other male relatives who had been previously undiagnosed.

In newborn screening for X-ALD, the benefits accrue almost entirely to males, and the burdens primarily to females. This suggests that the program as implemented is unfair, and alternative approaches should be considered. In this case, the need for immediate treatment is lower, so it is possible to consider a screening test offered somewhat later by the pediatrician. This would also allow time for discussion and reflection on the part of the parents.

The newborn screening program in the Netherlands decided to go forward with a boys-only newborn screen for X-ALD with a four-tier algorithm. To avoid errors in recording the sex on the heel-prick card, the screening algorithm includes a count of X-chromosomes. Only infants with a single X-chromosome go on to further tiers of screening [12].

2.2.3. Pompe Disease

Pompe disease (MIM:232300) is another lysosomal storage disorder; it was added to the RUSP in 2013. Like the above conditions, Pompe disease has both infantile-onset and late-onset forms, with approximately 28% being infantile-onset. The classical infantile onset form includes cardiomyopathy, a primary cause of neonatal morbidity in this condition.

The screening test as initially implemented had a high false positive rate and consequently a low positive predictive value. More recent research has shown that a larger panel of newborn screening analytes combined with the CLIR tools for lysosomal storage disorders is better able to distinguish between the true positive cases from the false positive/pseudodeficiency cases [13].

Screening for Pompe disease has also highlighted the reality for individuals with late-onset disease identified as newborns [14]. There is no consensus on the clinical care for these patients—what tests to order and how to interpret them, what treatments to consider and when to begin them. Essentially, newborn screening enrolls these patients in an unconsented clinical trial of case management. This cannot be considered a valid goal of newborn screening.

2.3. Genomic Newborn Screening Requires Multiple Ethical Considerations

Over 400 genetic conditions have been identified [15] as meeting the initial screening criteria: pediatric onset, some level of severity, and some ability to intervene. Within this group, there is a smaller subset of disorders with newborn onset that are serious and highly actionable. Some of these, in the absence of any other testing method, could be the targets of a DNA sequencing-based newborn screening test. The goal of this test, like all newborn screening, would be the identification of affected infants and the early treatment of the condition to prevent adverse consequences. It is unlikely that such a screening test could be implemented effectively. The DNA sequence results identify variants in the gene, but the inference of the possible disease state—whether early-onset, late-onset, or not penetrant—is difficult to predict for some conditions. One possibility is to restrict the group of target conditions still further to conditions that have well-developed genotype/phenotype correlations.

In addition, it will be difficult, if not impossible, to implement genomic newborn screening in a way that treats the population equitably. The interpretation of the clinical significance of the variants detected by sequencing relies on genomic databases. However, the existing databases of genetic variants overrepresent the variants found in individuals of European ancestry and underrepresent the variants in individuals of other ancestries. The consequence of this divergence is an increased likelihood of finding a variant of uncertain significance (VUS) in individuals of underrepresented ancestry. Whether VUSs are released to the patient or not, the implication is that the performance of genomic newborn screening will be different for different populations. This issue in particularly important in parts of the United States with large immigrant populations from Mexico, Central and South America. Due to the expense of genetic testing in their home countries, these individuals tend to be underrepresented in genetic databases.

One burden of genomic newborn screening is structural within the public health department. Genomic sequencing is currently more than two orders of magnitude more expensive than any current newborn screening test. Budgets for newborn screening are not limitless, and fees cannot be raised arbitrarily without limit. The introduction of genomic newborn screening has the potential to divert resources from other responsibilities, including follow-up, diagnostic testing, and treatment. The expense of genomic sequencing also has the potential to absorb funds that the larger public health department might need for other priorities. The scale of the funding involved could imply a significantly more convoluted contract management process, with additional levels of State supervision beyond the newborn screening program.

Another population-wide burden arises from sequence data as intensely personal data for the newborn, but which also has implications for the parents. This challenge to trust will require the newborn screening program to practice extreme transparency in how the DNA is used, whether residual DNA is stored, how the sequence data is generated, and how the results will be safeguarded for the future. The possibility of future use of the data or the DNA for the benefit of the individual (by reinterpretation of variants) or for more general public health benefit (from research) must be explicitly communicated. Potential harm to the same person might arise from law enforcement requiring access to DNA or data for future forensic identification purposes of the person or relatives.

The clear alternative is to undertake genomic newborn screening only after detailed discussions with parents about the kinds of results and the implications for diagnosis and treatment. Parental preferences will need to be elicited, recorded, and complied with.

Failure in any of these areas of public health ethics has the potential to dramatically undercut the public's trust that the newborn screening program is acting in the public interest. This increased distrust is one precondition for the crisis to come.

2.4. The Coming Storm

A significant threat to the future of newborn screening is political polarization driven by social media. It is plausible that the social media environment is primed to attack genomic sequencing in newborn screening. Any online discussion of universal DNA sequencing will attract the single-word comment "GATTACA", referring to the dystopian film from 1997 about a eugenic future of genetic determinism. It is easy to imagine that the announcement by a single State of genomic newborn screening without parental involvement will catalyze a group of privacy absolutists who begin with a deep suspicion of governmental activity to mount an online campaign against all newborn screening. With the example of the social media campaign against vaccination for SARS-CoV-2, we can see how a small number of highly influential individuals created dissension that was magnified by millions of followers and amplified by social media algorithms that prioritize controversy and outrage. In addition, there are groups of malign actors who seek not to promote policy, but to foment distrust of government and discord in the population.

The threat of political polarization can already be seen in the controversy over the storage and future use of residual dried blood specimens from newborn screening that are obtained without explicit consent for storage or use, exemplified by the lawsuit Kanuszewski vs. Michigan Department of Health and Human Services, discussed below.

The controversy over dried blood spots points to a second, and potentially more serious, threat to the future of newborn screening: a constitutional challenge to the State's ability to do newborn screening at all. A recent case from Michigan, Kanuszewski vs. Michigan Department of Health and Human Services, was heard by the United States Court of Appeals, Sixth Circuit. This complicated case involves allegations that rights of (a) the newborn and (b) the parents were violated with regard to: (1) the collection of the specimen and (2) the storage and future analysis of the residual dried blood spot. In the Court's ruling, the analysis of standing and the analysis of the claims regarding the newborn and the parents were separated into four combinations. When the Court considered the claim that the newborn's rights had been violated by the specimen collection [ax1], the Court first noted that the State's sovereign immunity precluded the claims. However, the Court further noted that the newborn does not have a right to direct their own medical care, so that there was no constitutional violation. However, when the Court ruled on the parents' claim [bx1], the State's sovereign immunity again precluded the claim, but the Court declined to go further into an analysis of the constitutional issue:

> In contrast with the issue discussed in the previous section [RJC: regarding the rights of the newborn], we cannot easily say, based on the allegations in the Complaint, that the drawing of the children's blood "do[es] not make out a constitutional violation" of the parents' substantive due process right to direct their children's medical care. *Id.* The Supreme Court has suggested that we might decline to exercise our jurisdiction in situations where "it is plain that a constitutional right is not clearly established but far from obvious whether in fact there is such a right". *Pearson*, 555 U.S. at 237, 129 S.Ct. 808. Because this issue presents such a situation, we decline to rule on whether the initial drawing of blood violated the parents' substantive due process rights. [16] (p. 416)

This ruling points to the thinness of the thread that supports newborn screening. Another court, in another jurisdiction, may choose to go further and rule that the collection of the newborn screening specimen is an unconstitutional violation of the Fourth and Fourteenth Amendments. A ruling to that effect would require immediate and radical restructuring of newborn screening, with the possibility of a significant hiatus during the restructuring process resulting in significant irreversible but preventable harm to infants in the short term, and, if the mandate of newborn screening for all were eliminated, in the long term as well.

2.5. Sustaining Newborn Screening Will Require Challenging Adjustments

2.5.1. Establish, Maintain, and Monitor a Very High Standard for the Positive Predictive Values of Newborn Screening Tests

The genetics workforce is under increasing pressure to do more. Furthermore, the number of new genetic counselors, clinical geneticists and medical geneticists being produced is not sufficient to meet the demand. False positive results from newborn screening can produce a larger burden in diagnostic work-up than true positives, because it is a matter of ruling out all possibilities, a process that can require multiple visits to specialists over months to years. As stewards of the human resources of the follow-up programs, newborn screening has the responsibility to avoid excessive false positive results. Each screening test should aim for fewer false positive results than true positive, i.e., for a PPV greater than 50%. The examples of the use of CLIR tools for both Krabbe disease and Pompe disease show that this benchmark can be achieved. It does require a collaborative effort to collect and unify the world-wide data on these rare diseases. Additionally, second-tier genetic testing (either mutation panels or sequencing) applied to a selected group of genes is currently being used in NBS programs to reduce false positive rates. Some of the issues of genetic testing cited above do not apply, principally because the first-tier positive NBS test provides an initial phenotype and indication that further testing is warranted.

2.5.2. Implement Only Screening Tests That Can Single Out Early Onset Forms of a Disorder to Avoid Reporting Late-Onset and Non-Penetrant Forms

Of all results other than true target disorders, late-onset forms create a substantial, and ongoing burden for the follow-up center. The infant will need to be followed periodically to determine if or when clinical indications of disease may appear, and then to plan and monitor an ongoing treatment regimen.

In addition, the parents of infants with a late-onset disorder identified by newborn screening could justifiably feel that their consent should have been obtained before the screening went forward. The larger this cohort becomes, the greater possibility that a group of parents will decide to sue the State to end the practice.

2.5.3. Include in Newborn Screening Only Disorders That Have Serious, Irremediable Consequences within the First Weeks of Life

The only defense that the State can offer to a parental suit alleging a due process violation in the failure to obtain consent for newborn screening is for the State to assert that screening was a matter of preventing death or severe disability for the infant. If the designated follow-up for a disorder identified by newborn screening is watchful waiting and periodic monitoring for the first year of life or more, this defense would not apply, and the suit could prevail.

In the event that the Court rules that screening for a particular disorder without consent is not permitted, the transition to removing that screening test could cause disruptions to the overall screening process. In some LIMS systems, the removal of a screening test would need support from the LIMS vendor. At the same time, parents of infants who were not identified as having the condition could feel that the State did them harm, which might also result in legal liability for the State.

2.5.4. Develop a Life-Course Staged Approach to Public Health Genetic Screening

Disorders that do not meet the urgency criterion above may still be important targets for public health screening. Other medical screening tests, for example colonoscopy, have a schedule of examination tailored to the individual's medical history, including family history, and previous testing. Genetic screening needs to expand the time frame to allow for more complex discussions of what testing will entail, what kinds of results may arise, and what follow-up may ensue. As the child becomes older, they may also have a perspective that needs to be included.

The challenge will be to institute expanded screening beyond the newborn period in a way that makes it available to all, in the same way that newborn screening is. Advocates hoping to include additional disorders in newborn screening underline the importance of identifying all affected infants. A similar assurance that screening will be available to all will need to accompany genetic screening tests carried out later in life, while recognizing that some families may choose not to participate. The Early Check program in North Carolina has begun to explore later newborn screening with consent. This program grew from a desire to implement early screening for Fragile-X syndrome, while recognizing that the testing is unsuitable for the standard newborn screening system [17]. As an additional example, the State of California has made prenatal screening for certain birth defects available to all residents of the State who consent to have it, originally through serum biomarker testing of a maternal blood sample and ultrasound, more recently by analysis of cell-free fetal DNA in maternal blood (noninvasive prenatal testing or screening, referred to as NIPT or NIPS).

2.5.5. Alternatively, Find a Way to Inform Parents about Newborn Screening and Get Genuine Consent

Consent for newborn screening has long been resisted, in the belief that the consent process is too burdensome and poorly comprehended during the period immediately following the birth and that the impact of parental refusal to consent will be primarily borne by disadvantaged populations. There has been substantial research on the effectiveness of prenatal education about newborn screening and about the use of the residual DBS [18]. If the transition from prenatal care to neonatal care were smoother, it might be possible to do much of the education and consent for newborn screening during prenatal care.

3. Conclusions

The issue of consent for newborn screening seems to be fundamental for its future. It seems likely that genomic sequence data will be determined to be Protected Health Information (PHI) as being inherently identifiable. Such a determination is likely to increase pressure on NBS programs that use sequence data to get consent for its generation and storage. New screening tests are likely to take a longer time for development and refinement to meet screening standards. This will imply an extended period of pilot testing, at first with consent; then later, perhaps, without.

Newborn screening has been a tremendously successful public health program. However, the future of newborn screening is not guaranteed. We should not go forward without considering whether what we do today will make its survival more or less likely.

Author Contributions: R.J.C. is responsible for this article. Helpful comments on drafts were received from the individuals named in the acknowledgments and from the anonymous referees. The author have read and agreed to the published version of the manuscript.

Funding: This research received no external funding.

Acknowledgments: I grateful to colleagues on the NBSeq project for extensive discussions about newborn screening, genetics, and ethics. I would particularly like to mention Jennifer Puck, Barbara Koenig, Flavia Chen, and Bob Nussbaum.

Conflicts of Interest: The author declares no conflict of interest.

References

1. MMWR. Ten Great Public Health Achievements—United States, 2001–2010. *MMWR* **2011**, *60*, 619–623. Available online: https://www.cdc.gov/mmwr/preview/mmwrhtml/mm6019a5.htm (accessed on 16 March 2019).
2. Recommended Uniform Screening Panel. Available online: https://www.hrsa.gov/advisory-committees/heritable-disorders/rusp/index.html (accessed on 16 March 2019).
3. Wilson, J.M.G.; Jungner, G. *Principles and Practice of Screening for Disease*; Public Health Paper No. 34; World Health Organisation: Geneva, Switzerland, 1968.
4. Faden, R.R.; Holtzman, N.A.; Chwalow, J. Parental Rights, Child Welfare, and Public Health: The Case of PKU Screening. *Am. J. Public Health* **1982**, *72*, 1396–1400. [CrossRef]
5. Kass, N.E. An ethics framework for public health. *Am. J. Public Health* **2001**, *91*, 1776–1782. [CrossRef] [PubMed]
6. Orsini, J.J.; Kay, D.M.; Saavedra-Matiz, C.A.; Wenger, D.A.; Duffner, P.K.; Erbe, R.W.; Biski, C.; Martin, M.; Krein, L.M.; Nichols, M.; et al. Newborn screening for Krabbe disease in New York State: The first eight years' experience. *Genet. Med.* **2016**, *18*, 239–248. [CrossRef] [PubMed]
7. Wasserstein, M.P.; Andriola, M.; Arnold, G.; Aron, A.; Duffner, P.; Erbe, R.W.; Escolar, M.L.; Estrella, L.; Galvin-Parton, P.; Iglesias, A.; et al. Clinical outcomes of children with abnormal newborn screening results for Krabbe disease in New York State. *Genet. Med.* **2016**, *18*, 1235–1243. [CrossRef] [PubMed]
8. Ehmann, P.; Lantos, J.D. Ethical issues with testing and treatment for Krabbe disease. *Dev. Med. Child Neurol.* **2019**, *61*, 1358–1361. [CrossRef] [PubMed]
9. Martin, M.M.; Wilson, R.; Caggana, M.; Orsini, J.J. The Impact of Post-Analytical Tools on New York Screening for Krabbe Disease and Pompe Disease. *Int. J. Neonatal Screen.* **2020**, *6*, 65. [CrossRef] [PubMed]
10. Kwon, J.M.; Matern, D.; Kurtzberg, J.; Wrabetz, L.; Gelb, M.H.; Wenger, D.A.; Ficicioglu, C.; Waldman, A.T.; Burton, B.K.; Hopkins, P.V.; et al. Consensus guidelines for newborn screening, diagnosis and treatment of infantile Krabbe disease. *Orphanet J. Rare Dis.* **2018**, *13*, 30. [CrossRef] [PubMed]
11. Newborn Screening for X-Linked Adrenoleukodystrophy (X-ALD): A Systematic Review of Evidence. Final Report (v5.01). Available online: https://www.hrsa.gov/sites/default/files/hrsa/advisory-committees/heritable-disorders/rusp/previous-nominations/xald-external-evidence-review-report.pdf (accessed on 16 March 2019).
12. Barendsen, R.W.; Dijkstra, I.M.E.; Visser, W.F.; Alders, M.; Bliek, J.; Boelen, A.; Bouva, M.J.; van der Crabben, S.N.; Elsinghorst, E.; van Gorp, A.G.M.; et al. Adrenoleukodystrophy Newborn Screening in the Netherlands (SCAN Study): The X-Factor. *Front. Cell Dev. Biol.* **2020**, *8*, 499; Erratum in *Front. Cell Dev. Biol.* **2021**, *9*, 631655. [CrossRef] [PubMed]

13. Tortorelli, S.; Eckerman, J.S.; Orsini, J.J.; Stevens, C.; Hart, J.; Hall, P.L.; Alexander, J.J.; Gavrilov, D.; Oglesbee, D.; Raymond, K.; et al. Moonlighting newborn screening markers: The incidental discovery of a second-tier test for Pompe disease. *Genet. Med.* **2018**, *20*, 840–846. [CrossRef] [PubMed]
14. Kwon, J.M.; Steiner, R.D. "I'm fine; I'm just waiting for my disease": The new and growing class of presymptomatic patients. *Neurology* **2011**, *77*, 522–523. [CrossRef] [PubMed]
15. Milko, L.V.; O'Daniel, J.M.; DeCristo, D.M.; Crowley, S.B.; Foreman, A.K.M.; Wallace, K.E.; Mollison, L.F.; Strande, N.T.; Girnary, Z.S.; Boshe, L.J.; et al. An Age-Based Framework for Evaluating Genome-Scale Sequencing Results in Newborn Screening. *J. Pediatr.* **2019**, *209*, 68–76. [CrossRef] [PubMed]
16. Kanuszewski v. MI Dept of Heath & Human Services, 927 F. 3rd 396—Court of Appeals, 6th Circuit. Available online: https://scholar.google.ca/scholar_case?case=335740144033800467&hl=en&as_sdt=6&as_vis=1&oi=scholarr (accessed on 30 November 2021).
17. Okoniewski, K.C.; Wheeler, A.C.; Lee, S.; Boyea, B.; Raspa, M.; Taylor, J.L.; Bailey, D.B., Jr. Early Identification of Fragile X Syndrome through Expanded Newborn Screening. *Brain Sci.* **2019**, *9*, 4. [CrossRef] [PubMed]
18. Botkin, J.R.; Rothwell, E.; Anderson, R.A.; Rose, N.C.; Dolan, S.M.; Kuppermann, M.; Stark, L.A.; Goldenberg, A.; Wong, B. Prenatal Education of Parents About Newborn Screening and Residual Dried Blood Spots: A Randomized Clinical Trial. *JAMA Pediatr.* **2016**, *170*, 543–549. [CrossRef] [PubMed]

International Journal of
Neonatal Screening

MDPI

Opinion

Implications of Genomic Newborn Screening for Infant Mortality

Monica H. Wojcik [1,*] and Nina B. Gold [2]

1 Divisions of Newborn Medicine and Genetics and Genomics, Department of Pediatrics, Boston Children's Hospital and Harvard Medical School, Boston, MA 02115, USA
2 Division of Medical Genetics and Metabolism, Department of Pediatrics, Massachusetts General Hospital, Boston, MA 02114, USA
* Correspondence: monica.wojcik@childrens.harvard.edu; Tel.: +1-617-355-5355

Abstract: Technological advances and decreasing costs of genomic sequencing have paved the way for the increased incorporation of genomics into newborn screening (NBS). Genomic sequencing may complement current NBS laboratory analyses or may be used as a first-tier screening tool to identify disorders not detected by current approaches. As a large proportion of infant deaths occur in children with an underlying genetic disorder, earlier diagnosis of these disorders may improve neonatal and infant mortality rates. This lends an additional layer of ethical consideration regarding genomic newborn screening. We review the current understanding of genomic contributions to infant mortality and explore the potential implications of expanded access to genomic screening for infant mortality rates.

Keywords: mortality; infant; neonate; sequencing; exome; genome; genetic; diagnosis; ethics

1. Introduction

Genetic disorders underlie a substantial proportion of infant deaths, particularly infants with congenital anomalies and those admitted to an intensive care unit. Additionally, genetic diagnoses have also been identified in a large proportion of apparently healthy infants who die unexpectedly, although many genetic conditions likely remain undiscovered due to a lack of testing [1–4]. The early diagnosis of treatable genetic conditions may facilitate access to appropriate therapies. Conversely, the identification of a genetic diagnosis with a poor prognosis may aid families in the decision to withdraw life-sustaining technologies and transition to comfort-focused care [5]. Furthermore, identification of a condition with a high recurrence risk in future pregnancies of the infants' parents may lead to additional options for reproductive planning, thereby avoiding future infant deaths [4]. Current diagnostic genetic workflows are designed to initiate genetic testing after an infant develops disease symptoms, at which time therapies may not be clinically useful [5,6]. There is increasing interest and an international effort to incorporate genome-wide sequencing into newborn screening approaches, though ethical considerations and other implementation concerns remain unresolved. Here, we comment on the implications of this approach for infant mortality reduction.

2. Infant Mortality: The Genomic Landscape

Prior studies have investigated genetic diagnosis in postmortem cohorts [1,3,6–10] and described outcomes that include mortality after diagnostic genetic testing in infants admitted to intensive care units [4,11], as well as mortality outcomes after prenatal diagnosis [12]. These studies have identified varying diagnostic yields that are dependent upon how the cohort was ascertained, with cohorts of sudden, unexpected infant death being identified at a yield of approximately 10% [3,13], while cohorts involving deaths in an intensive care unit setting approach 25–30% [1,4,14].

The spectrum of diagnoses identified also varies by cohort. Genes associated with epilepsy or cardiac arrhythmia are often implicated in cases of sudden, unexpected infant death [3,13] occurring in an apparently healthy infant. Diagnoses identified in cohorts ascertained from intensive care units include multiple malformation syndromes attributed to common aneuploidies or other chromosomal disorders, such as trisomies 13 or 18, or 22q11 deletion syndrome, in addition to monogenic conditions associated with congenital anomalies, severe neurologic conditions, or genetic conditions not typically associated with structural anomalies, such as inborn errors of metabolism [1,15,16].

As these genetic diagnoses are typically identified by a chromosomal microarray or by massively-parallel sequencing technologies, they would be amenable to early detection via genomic sequencing from the dried blood spot obtained for traditional newborn screening, provided appropriate pre-test counseling and consent is obtained [17]. Several genetic conditions, particularly inborn errors of metabolism in addition to spinal muscular atrophy, are already included in newborn screening panels in many programs in the United States that have a selective approach, where conditions are identified for inclusion in newborn screening panels based upon particular criteria—ideally, conditions for which early treatment is available and leads to meaningful improvements [18]. However, many additional conditions leading to death that were once not treatable may now be amenable to precision treatments or other targeted therapy approaches, particularly as anti-sense oligonucleotide and gene therapies are rapidly emerging [19].

3. Current Barriers to Understanding

Our understanding of the depth and breadth of genetic conditions responsible for infant deaths is limited by several factors. First and foremost, the lack of population-based approaches for a comprehensive genomic evaluation of infant deaths limits our abilities to quantify the public health impact of these diagnoses. Conclusions identified from current cohorts are therefore limited by selection bias. In addition, the interpretation of variants identified is limited in the perimortem setting due to a lack of ability for follow-up investigations. Thus, many infants with genetic conditions are never identified, and the experience with genetic diagnosis in pediatric populations suggests that this may disproportionately impact historically underserved populations, though further research is needed into inequities in this realm [20,21]. Thus, this is a public health concern with particular bioethical overtones.

Finally, limited outcome data preclude accurate estimates of mortality rates for conditions that are identified in the perinatal setting. Attempts to quantify these mortality rates have been undertaken for specific diseases, such as genetic leukodystrophy syndromes [22], though accurate estimates are limited by challenges in death reporting, where specific genetic conditions are difficult to identify [23].

4. Impact of Genomic Newborn Screening on Infant Mortality

Genomic newborn screening has the potential to reduce infant mortality by identifying infants with treatable diseases prior to the onset of irreversible symptom progression, leading toward the improved management of neonates and infants with a range of genetic disorders, although the spectrum of possible impacts is not currently well understood. If applied on a population-wide scale, genomic newborn screening techniques may allow for more a comprehensive description of genetic diagnoses associated with infant deaths by eliminating the inherent bias in the access to a clinical diagnostic genetic evaluation, where many infants die before genetic diagnoses can be identified, as our current knowledge of the prognosis for these conditions is biased toward those who survive long enough to have genetic testing. Although prior research suggests that genomic sequencing is a robust method for the detection of treatable conditions [24], issues related to ethical implementation, particularly informed consent, remain to be fully addressed. If newborn screening is not fitting as a system to incorporate this type of genetic screening due to constraints related to costs and timely results, broad genomic sequencing may be introduced as routine outside of newborn screening: e.g., tailored to the newborn population with emerging health issues.

Nonetheless, dedicated efforts must be undertaken to move toward equitable implementation if genomic newborn screening is to be introduced. Additionally, disorders may be identified for which there are current or emerging therapies that lead to improved survival, though, again, ensuring equitable access to such therapies is paramount to upholding the ethical principle of justice in healthcare. Finally, conditions can be identified that have implications for parents' future childbearing, and the identification of a precise genetic diagnosis can aid in pregnancy planning that can further reduce neonatal and infant mortality.

5. Conclusions

Genomic newborn screening presents a unique opportunity not only to identify and manage infants at risk for long-term medical sequelae of a wider range of underlying genetic conditions, but also to understand and potentially reduce rates of infant mortality. Resource availability regarding the broader application of genomic newborn screening remains a valid concern and area of further focus. Still, understanding this approach and its potential as an important public health outcome of infant mortality may provide additional ethical justification. Critical to the success of this approach is the equitable implementation of genomic newborn screening in addition to resources devoted to accurately capturing health outcomes.

Author Contributions: Conceptualization, M.H.W. and N.B.G.; writing—original draft preparation, M.H.W.; writing—review and editing, M.H.W. and N.B.G. All authors have read and agreed to the published version of the manuscript.

Funding: This research was funded by the National Institutes of Health/National Institute of Child Health and Human Development, K23 HD102589 to MHW and K08HG012811 to NBG. The content is solely the responsibility of the authors and does not necessarily represent the official views of the National Institutes of Health.

Institutional Review Board Statement: Not applicable.

Informed Consent Statement: Not applicable.

Data Availability Statement: Not applicable.

Conflicts of Interest: The authors declare no conflict of interest. The funders had no role in the design of the study; in the collection, analyses, or interpretation of data; in the writing of the manuscript; or in the decision to publish the results.

References

1. Wojcik, M.H.; Schwartz, T.S.; Thiele, K.E.; Paterson, H.; Stadelmaier, R.; Mullen, T.E.; VanNoy, G.E.; Genetti, C.A.; Madden, J.A.; Gubbels, C.S.; et al. Infant mortality: The contribution of genetic disorders. *J. Perinatol.* **2019**, *39*, 1611–1619. [CrossRef] [PubMed]
2. Kingsmore, S.F.; Henderson, A.; Owen, M.J.; Clark, M.M.; Hansen, C.; Dimmock, D.; Chambers, C.D.; Jeliffe-Pawlowski, L.L.; Hobbs, C. Measurement of genetic diseases as a cause of mortality in infants receiving whole genome sequencing. *NPJ Genom. Med.* **2020**, *5*, 49. [CrossRef] [PubMed]
3. Koh, H.Y.; Haghighi, A.; Keywan, C.; Alexandrescu, S.; Plews-Ogan, E.; Haas, E.A.; Brownstein, C.A.; Vargas, S.O.; Haynes, R.L.; Berry, G.T.; et al. Genetic Determinants of Sudden Unexpected Death in Pediatrics. *Genet. Med.* **2022**, *24*, 839–850. [CrossRef]
4. Meng, L.; Pammi, M.; Saronwala, A.; Magoulas, P.; Ghazi, A.R.; Vetrini, F.; Zhang, J.; He, W.; Dharmadhikari, A.V.; Qu, C.; et al. Use of Exome Sequencing for Infants in Intensive Care Units: Ascertainment of Severe Single-Gene Disorders and Effect on Medical Management. *JAMA Pediatr.* **2017**, *171*, e173438. [CrossRef]
5. Wojcik, M.H.; Schwartz, T.S.; Yamin, I.; Edward, H.L.; Genetti, C.A.; Towne, M.C.; Agrawal, P.B. Genetic disorders and mortality in infancy and early childhood: Delayed diagnoses and missed opportunities. *Genet. Med.* **2018**, *20*, 1396–1404. [CrossRef]
6. Gubbels, C.S.; VanNoy, G.E.; Madden, J.A.; Copenheaver, D.; Yang, S.; Wojcik, M.H.; Gold, N.B.; Genetti, C.A.; Stoler, J.; Parad, R.B.; et al. Prospective, phenotype-driven selection of critically ill neonates for rapid exome sequencing is associated with high diagnostic yield. *Genet. Med.* **2020**, *22*, 736–744. [CrossRef] [PubMed]
7. Shamseldin, H.E.; Kurdi, W.; Almusafri, F.; Alnemer, M.; Alkaff, A.; Babay, Z.; Alhashem, A.; Tulbah, M.; Alsahan, N.; Khan, R.; et al. Molecular autopsy in maternal-fetal medicine. *Genet. Med.* **2018**, *20*, 420–427. [CrossRef] [PubMed]

8. Quinlan-Jones, E.; Lord, J.; Williams, D.; Hamilton, S.; Marton, T.; Eberhardt, R.Y.; Rinck, G.; Prigmore, E.; Keelagher, R.; McMullan, D.J.; et al. Molecular autopsy by trio exome sequencing (ES) and postmortem examination in fetuses and neonates with prenatally identified structural anomalies. *Genet. Med.* **2019**, *21*, 1065–1073. [CrossRef] [PubMed]
9. Shamseldin, H.E.; AlAbdi, L.; Maddirevula, S.; Alsaif, H.S.; Alzahrani, F.; Ewida, N.; Hashem, M.; Abdulwahab, F.; Abuyousef, O.; Kuwahara, H.; et al. Lethal variants in humans: Lessons learned from a large molecular autopsy cohort. *Genome Med.* **2021**, *13*, 161. [CrossRef]
10. Byrne, A.B.; Arts, P.; Ha, T.T.; Kassahn, K.S.; Pais, L.S.; O'Donnell-Luria, A.; Babic, M.; Frank, M.S.; Feng, J.; Wang, P. Genomic autopsy to identify underlying causes of pregnancy loss and perinatal death. *Nat. Med.* **2023**, *29*, 180–189. [CrossRef]
11. Kingsmore, S.F.; Cakici, J.A.; Clark, M.M.; Gaughran, M.; Feddock, M.; Batalov, S.; Bainbridge, M.N.; Carroll, J.; Caylor, S.A.; Clarke, C.; et al. A Randomized, Controlled Trial of the Analytic and Diagnostic Performance of Singleton and Trio, Rapid Genome and Exome Sequencing in Ill Infants. *Am. J. Hum. Genet.* **2019**, *105*, 719–733. [CrossRef] [PubMed]
12. Tolusso, L.K.; Hazelton, P.; Wong, B.; Swarr, D.T. Beyond diagnostic yield: Prenatal exome sequencing results in maternal, neonatal, and familial clinical management changes. *Genet. Med.* **2021**, *23*, 909–917. [CrossRef] [PubMed]
13. Heathfield, L.J.; Martin, L.J.; Ramesar, R. A Systematic Review of Molecular Autopsy Studies in Sudden Infant Death Cases. *J. Pediatr. Genet.* **2018**, *7*, 143–149. [PubMed]
14. Hudome, S.M.; Kirby, R.S.; Senner, J.W.; Cunniff, C. Contribution of genetic disorders to neonatal mortality in a regional intensive care setting. *Am. J. Perinatol.* **1994**, *11*, 100–103. [CrossRef] [PubMed]
15. Willig, L.K.; Petrikin, J.E.; Smith, L.D.; Saunders, C.J.; Thiffault, I.; Miller, N.A.; Soden, S.E.; Cakici, J.A.; Herd, S.M.; Twist, G.; et al. Whole-genome sequencing for identification of Mendelian disorders in critically ill infants: A retrospective analysis of diagnostic and clinical findings. *Lancet Respir. Med.* **2015**, *3*, 377–387. [CrossRef] [PubMed]
16. Smith, L.D.; Willig, L.K.; Kingsmore, S.F. Whole-Exome Sequencing and Whole-Genome Sequencing in Critically Ill Neonates Suspected to Have Single-Gene Disorders. *Cold Spring Harb. Perspect. Med.* **2015**, *6*, a023168. [CrossRef]
17. Bassaganyas, L.; Freedman, G.; Vaka, D.; Wan, E.; Lao, R.; Chen, F.; Kvale, M.; Currier, R.J.; Puck, J.M.; Kwok, P.Y. Whole exome and whole genome sequencing with dried blood spot DNA without whole genome amplification. *Hum. Mutat.* **2018**, *39*, 167–171. [CrossRef]
18. American College of Medical Genetics Newborn Screening Expert Group. Newborn screening: Toward a uniform screening panel and system—Executive summary. *Pediatrics* **2006**, *117 (5 Pt 2)*, S296–S307. [CrossRef]
19. Vockley, J.; Aartsma-Rus, A.; Cohen, J.L.; Cowsert, L.M.; Howell, R.R.; Yu, T.W.; Wasserstein, M.P.; Defay, T. Whole-genome sequencing holds the key to the success of gene-targeted therapies. *Am. J. Med. Genet. Part C Semin. Med. Genet.* 2022, *online ahead of print*. [CrossRef]
20. Wojcik, M.H.; Bresnahan, M.; del Rosario, M.C.; Ojeda, M.M.; Kritzer, A.; Fraiman, Y.S. Rare diseases, common barriers: Disparities in pediatric clinical genetics outcomes. *Pediatr. Res.* **2022**, *93*, 110–117. [CrossRef]
21. Omorodion, J.; Dowsett, L.; Clark, R.D.; Fraser, J.; Abu-El-Haija, A.; Strong, A.; Wojcik, M.H.; Bryant, A.S.; Gold, N.B. Delayed diagnosis and racial bias in children with genetic conditions. *Am. J. Med. Genet. A* **2022**, *188*, 1118–1123. [CrossRef] [PubMed]
22. Barczykowski, A.L.; Langan, T.J.; Vanderver, A.; Jalal, K.; Carter, R.L. Death rates in the U.S. due to Leukodystrophies with pediatric forms. *Am. J. Med. Genet. A* **2021**, *185*, 2361–2373. [CrossRef] [PubMed]
23. Wojcik, M.H.; Stadelmaier, R.; Heinke, D.; Holm, I.A.; Tan, W.H.; Agrawal, P.B. The Unrecognized Mortality Burden of Genetic Disorders in Infancy. *Am. J. Public Health* **2021**, *111*, S156–S162. [CrossRef] [PubMed]
24. Gold, N.B.; Harrison, S.M.; Rowe, J.H.; Gold, J.; Furutani, E.; Biffi, A.; Duncan, C.N.; Shimamura, A.; Lehmann, L.E.; Green, R.C. Low frequency of treatable pediatric disease alleles in gnomAD: An opportunity for future genomic screening of newborns. *Hum. Genet. Genom. Adv.* **2022**, *3*, 100059. [CrossRef] [PubMed]

International Journal of
Neonatal Screening

MDPI

Opinion

Genomic-Based Newborn Screening for Inborn Errors of Immunity: Practical and Ethical Considerations

Jovanka R. King [1,2,3], Kalle Grill [4] and Lennart Hammarström [5,*]

1 Department of Allergy & Clinical Immunology, Women's and Children's Hospital Network, North Adelaide, SA 5006, Australia; jovanka.king@adelaide.edu.au
2 Immunology Directorate, SA Pathology, Adelaide, SA 5000, Australia
3 Robinson Research Institute and Discipline of Paediatrics, School of Medicine, University of Adelaide, North Adelaide, SA 5006, Australia
4 Department of Historical, Philosophical and Religious Studies, Umeå University, SE-90187 Umeå, Sweden; kalle.grill@umu.se
5 Department of Biosciences and Nutrition, Neo, Karolinska Institutet, SE-14183 Huddinge, Sweden
* Correspondence: lennart.hammarstrom@ki.se

Abstract: Inborn errors of immunity (IEI) are a group of over 450 genetically distinct conditions associated with significant morbidity and mortality, for which early diagnosis and treatment improve outcomes. Newborn screening for severe combined immunodeficiency (SCID) is currently underway in several countries, utilising a DNA-based technique to quantify T cell receptor excision circles (TREC) and kappa-deleting recombination excision circles (KREC). This strategy will only identify those infants with an IEI associated with T and/or B cell lymphopenia. Other severe forms of IEI will not be detected. Up-front, first-tier genomic-based newborn screening has been proposed as a potential approach by which to concurrently screen infants for hundreds of monogenic diseases at birth. Given the clinical, phenotypic and genetic heterogeneity of IEI, a next-generation sequencing-based newborn screening approach would be suitable. There are, however, several ethical, legal and social issues which must be evaluated in detail prior to adopting a genomic-based newborn screening approach, and these are discussed herein in the context of IEI.

Keywords: inborn errors of immunity (IEI); newborn screening; next-generation sequencing (NGS); whole-exome sequencing (WES); whole-genome sequencing (WGS); ethical, legal and social considerations (ELSI)

1. Introduction

The aim of newborn screening programs is to identify infants with a range of significant conditions for which there is a pre-symptomatic phase and effective treatment is available. Since the description of phenylketonuria (PKU) in the 1930s and subsequent establishment of a laboratory assay to identify asymptomatic infants with this condition in the 1950s [1], there have been significant technological advances that have enabled an expansion of the number and range of treatable conditions identified through newborn screening (NBS) programs. Traditionally, newborn screening tests have centred around a tandem mass-spectrometric (MS/MS) approach, which is effective in identifying a range of conditions including inborn errors of metabolism, congenital hypothyroidism and congenital adrenal hyperplasia. Technological advances have driven the expansion of NBS programs to include a wider range of diseases [2], for example, severe inborn errors of immunity (IEI) such as severe combined immunodeficiency (SCID), using DNA-based technologies (measurement of T cell receptor excision circles (TREC) and kappa-deleting recombination excision circles (KREC) by quantitative PCR).

Inborn errors of immunity are a heterogenous group of disorders which manifest as severe, unusual or recurrent infections; immune dysregulation (including autoimmunity);

and other clinical features. There are now over 485 different monogenic IEI which have been described, and this number continues to increase at a rapid rate [3]. Marked diagnostic delay (up to several years) and a long 'diagnostic odyssey' are experienced by many affected individuals. This results in delayed treatment and subsequent increased morbidity, mortality and poorer outcomes. SCID is a particularly severe IEI which presents in infancy and is fatal without definitive treatment with either allogeneic hematopoietic stem cell transplantation (HSCT) or gene therapy (GT). Outcomes are significantly improved if this is undertaken at an early age (preferably prior to 3.5 months of age) to avoid infections and other complications at the time of transplant [4]. This requires a diagnosis to be made in the first few weeks of life. In the absence of a known family history or prenatal diagnosis, this can only be achieved by screening infants in the neonatal period; hence, newborn screening for SCID has commenced in many countries throughout the world [5].

Current screening methodologies for SCID involve assays measuring TREC and/or KREC levels, which are surrogate markers for naïve T and B cell production and enable the identification of a range of IEI where T and/or B cell lymphopenia are a feature [5]. However, IEI are clinically, phenotypically and immunologically heterogeneous; thus, this screening approach will not capture all clinically relevant forms of IEI, including conditions such as neutrophil disorders, complement deficiencies and familial hemophagocytic lymphohistiocytosis (HLH). A range of alternative methodologies, including protein-based assays and copy number variant analyses, have demonstrated a proof of concept that screening for these conditions is possible [6–9]. However, employing a multitude of different methodological strategies for a range of conditions is not practically nor economically feasible. Given that IEI are genetically determined, an alternative approach would be concurrent, parallel screening of hundreds of disease-causing genes using next generation sequencing (NGS), employing either whole-exome sequencing (WES) or whole-genome sequencing (WGS) as an up-front, first-tier testing strategy. This challenges the current paradigm, whereby genetic sequencing is employed as a second- or even third-tier test in newborn screening algorithms. Despite disease heterogeneity, many forms of IEI have one commonality: an identifiable genetic target. This suggests that an NGS-based screening strategy is a rational approach, providing a single platform to screen for hundreds of diseases simultaneously.

An NGS-based screening approach is particularly suitable for the identification of infants with IEI based on disease heterogeneity, lack of a suitable biochemical marker to screen for all conditions simultaneously, and the genetic basis of this group of disorders. At the same time, we believe that there is further scope for its application in newborn screening for other conditions with a monogenic basis, including inborn errors of metabolism and a large range of other conditions. NGS provides a single modality which enables parallel screening for hundreds of different disorders which differ in terms of clinical phenotype and disease-specific biomarkers, making it an attractive option for newborn screening.

The feasibility of a first-tier, rapid WGS-based newborn screening approach has been demonstrated by Kingsmore et al., who identified 388 clinically actionable conditions in 2208 critically unwell neonates in Intensive Care Units with 99.7% specificity and 88.8% sensitivity [10]. Genetic screening of sick newborn infants rarely presents any ethical, legal or social concerns, and is currently regarded a routine medical service. Other studies have also demonstrated the utility of NGS in providing a definitive genetic diagnosis in patients with rare diseases, informing disease prognostication and enabling commencement of effective treatment [11]. This work has demonstrated proof of concept of NGS testing approaches to improve diagnostics and clinical care of acutely unwell infants. In particular, it has provided evidence for the application of this methodology and the provision of rapid results to facilitate time-critical clinical decision making. These findings may be extrapolated to NBS programs, which rely on rapidly available results for early intervention. This approach has been demonstrated to be an effective testing modality to screen for hundreds of different genes simultaneously. There are some differences, however, in that the majority of unselected newborns undergoing screening for disease will be 'healthy'.

Thus, first-tier screening of ALL newborns, as we are advocating, requires careful reflection. This screening approach has already been evaluated in a study of 321 unselected newborns in China, in whom first-tier WGS identified pathogenic or likely pathogenic variants associated with 59 Mendelian disorders in one-third of screened neonates [12]. There is a view to further evaluation in other, larger, prospective newborn screening programs, as is the case with the Genomics England Newborn screening project [13]. Table 1 highlights the findings of NGS-based screening studies to date, including both unwell infants and unselected newborns [10,12,14–19].

There are several considerations which must be made prior to adopting a first-tier NGS-based screening approach for IEI, spanning those of a practical nature (turn-around time, costs, clinical follow-up protocols, etc.) and methodological and technical factors (test characteristics and acceptability, quality assurance, bioinformatic pipelines and analysis, variant calling, etc.) [20]. NGS-based techniques include both WES and WGS, and the choice of methodology is based on a number of factors. The current standard clinical approach to genetic investigation of patients with a suspected IEI involves the evaluation of a 'panel' of IEI-associated genes by WES. This panel-based WES approach has also been used in the majority of NGS-based NBS studies to date. It is anticipated that over time, these panels will expand to include a broader number of genes in alignment with new gene discovery. WGS will further increase the diagnostic yield. Methodological options will, thus, likely evolve and change over time. Importantly, ethical, legal and social issues (ELSI) must also be considered and rigorously evaluated, as this forms an important part of the dialogue around genomic-based screening [20]. These factors will now be discussed in the context of newborn screening for IEI.

1.1. Selection of Disease Candidates for Newborn Screening Programs

Wilson and Jungner published their recommendations for population screening in 1968 [21], outlining criteria to guide disease inclusion in screening programs. There have been recent calls to update these criteria in the context of technological advances and new therapies [22–25]. These updated criteria were recently reviewed in the context of newborn screening for IEI, highlighting the need to both consider alternative approaches and increase the spectrum of screened diseases, particularly in the context of developing new and improved therapies [20]. A more recent set of criteria was subsequently published by the US Advisory Committee on Heritable Diseases in Newborns and Children [26].

Table 1. Outcomes of published studies evaluating rapid, first-tier NGS for both unselected (healthy) and unwell infants.

Author	Methodology	Cohort	Number of Screened Infants	Number of Genes Interrogated	Mendelian Diseases Covered	Key Findings	Reference
Jian et al., 2022	NBS WGS	Unselected neonates	321	251	59	136/321 (33.33%) pathogenic/likely pathogenic/copy number variants identified	[12]
Kingsmore et al., 2022	Simulated NBS rWGS	Critically unwell infants Biobank (healthy) subjects	2208 454,707	317	388 388	Negative predictive value 99.6%, sensitivity 88.8%, sensitivity 99.7%	[10]
Cho et al., 2017	Targeted NGS computational exome analysis, exome analysis	Unwell infants Controls (mutation carriers) (negative controls)	Total: 103 81 22 (10) (12)	307	159	5/25 (20%) known causal mutations in databases 20/25 (80%) rare variants (SNVs, nonsense mutations, short indels, gene duplication or deletion) 7/25 (30%) compound heterozygosity 93% sensitivity for core metabolic conditions	[14]
Bhattacharjee et al., 2015	WES 'NBDx' gene panel, in silico gene filter	Infants with known genetic disorders	36	126	27	75% sensitivity for core metabolic conditions	[15]
Bodian et al., 2016	Research-generated WGS data	Unselected infants	1696	163	28	88.6% true positive and 98.9% true negative rates for state-screened disorders Good genetic coverage of disorders using WGS	[16]
Willig et al., 2015	Rapid trio WGS	Unwell infants, <4 months of age, NICU/PICU	35	5430	20	20/35 (57%) genetic diagnoses achieved	[17]

Table 1. *Cont.*

Author	Methodology	Cohort	Number of Screened Infants	Number of Genes Interrogated	Mendelian Diseases Covered	Key Findings	Reference
Pavey et al., 2017	Trio WGS	Healthy cohort (genotype-first) Re-analysis of cohort with suspected IEI (phenotype-first)	1349 29	329 (IEI-associated genes)		396 (29%) pathogenic/likely pathogenic mutations identified 1/1349 (0.07%) clinically actionable IEI 3 (10%) non-IEI genetic diagnosis	[18]
Ceyhan-Birsoy et al., 2019	Singleton WES (trio re-analysis selected cases) BabySeq Project	Healthy newborns Unwell newborns in NICU	Total: 159 (127) (32)			15/59 (9.4%) risk of childhood-onset disease (10 from healthy cohort, 5 in NICU) 3/85 (3.5%) actionable adult-onset disease 140/159 (88%) carrier status for AR conditions 8/159 (5%) pharmacogenomic variants	[19]

WES: whole-exome sequencing, WGS: whole-genome sequencing, rWGS: rapid WGS, IEI: inborn errors of immunity, NICU/PICU: neonatal/paediatric intensive care unit.

A wealth of information is generated from genetic sequencing; thus, careful consideration must be given to the specific disease candidates and specific disease-associated genes which should be included in NBS programs. In the case of IEI, along with the identification of clear pathogenic mutations in disease-associated genes, there is potential for the discovery of variants of unknown significance (VUS), carrier statuses for diseases which may have relevance for individuals in their later reproductive years and adult-onset conditions. It is anticipated that each individual will be a carrier for one or more conditions. Some clinically heterogenous conditions may be associated with VUS or variants giving rise to sub-clinical disease. In addition, advances in knowledge may lead to the reclassification of variants previously assigned as VUS to pathogenic, with potential implications for the clinical management of individuals. All of these situations, as well as how they will be managed, need careful consideration, including the risk–benefit profile of disclosure (or non-disclosure) of various findings, which poses a challenge both ethically and clinically. It is likely that our approach will change over time as technological and methodological changes and increased knowledge is gained. At the current time, we would advocate that only those genes in which mutations are associated with clinically actionable IEI be included in newborn screening panels [20]. This is also supported by Johnston et al., who recommend screening only for select diseases in NBS programs for which treatment is available, and focusing only on pathogenic mutations [27]. With increased research and experience regarding this approach, and acquisition of knowledge over time, this will be refined. This will include modified disease and gene lists for interrogation, which will be regularly reviewed and updated in accordance with new findings, given that novel monogenic diseases will continue to be described and new therapies will become available. In addition, our ability to better classify and resolve VUS will also improve in the future.

There are now several hundred monogenic IEI which are broadly categorised into ten groups [28], but these are highly variable in terms of disease presentation, severity and available treatment options. These conditions, in the context of future NGS-based NBS programs, were reviewed in detail by King, Notarangelo and Hammarström in 2021 [20]. Although it was highlighted that all forms of IEI have potential interventions which will reduce morbidity and mortality and improve the quality of life of affected individuals, it was advocated that early genomic-based NBS programs should aim to identify infants with well-defined, significant and clinically actionable conditions which have effective treatments [20]. In the first instance, this would include conditions for which potentially curative therapies are available, including SCID, other combined immunodeficiencies and chronic granulomatous disease, which can be cured with successful HSCT or gene therapy. In addition, it was advocated that in the first instance, carefully selected and disease-associated genes be interrogated for known pathogenic mutations giving rise to clinical disease, with a view to expand both gene and variant lists over time in alignment with technological advancements, improved knowledge and increased experience with newly described IEI and IEI-associated variants [20]. There is a significant international effort underway to define, construct, curate and harmonise a comprehensive database of conditions and genes for IEI and a range of other conditions for diagnostic testing [29]. Applications such as PanelApp (https://panelapp.agha.umccr.org/) (accessed on 15 December 2022) are important for facilitating this collaborative process. Such efforts are especially important in the lead-up to NGS-based NBS pilot studies. These lists will no doubt continue to be critically analysed and further developed prior to implementation, and then regularly reviewed and updated once these programs are established.

1.2. Genetic Screening Will Enable Us to Identify a Wider Range of Clinically Actionable Conditions

The ethical, social and legal considerations of first-tier NGS-based screening are closely intertwined with the practical, methodological and technical factors of both the testing itself and the handling of genetic information during and after testing. In addition, our current (and future) medical knowledge determines which conditions can be identified, and with what level of certainty diagnoses can be made relative to the risk of false positives and false negatives. One particularly salient factor is whether NGS-based screening would be used as an exclusive first-tier approach or used in combination with current testing methodologies, based on biochemical and other markers. In the case of IEI, TREC/KREC enumeration is the only current, routinely available screening assay, and would only identify a small proportion of the many forms of IEI. Conversely, some infants returning an abnormal TREC and/or KREC result would not have an identifiable monogenic disease. As such, if used in combination with current techniques, genomic testing will both broaden the range of identified diseases and improve precision. Similarly, there are other conditions in addition to IEI that would not be identified by genetic screening, but would be found by screening based on biochemical or other markers. Given this fact, it remains to be seen whether first-tier NGS-based screening will replace current methodologies, be used where current methodologies do not exist (e.g., for diseases where there is no current MS/MS platform) or be used in tandem, and whether these factors may need to be different for specific diseases in order to increase diagnostic yield. A recent evaluation of MS/MS versus NGS screening approaches for inborn errors of metabolism suggested that the former is superior at the current time in terms of sensitivity and specificity [30], although this suggestion has been challenged [10,12]. This issue requires further evaluation in the future once results of larger, prospective studies evaluating first-tier genomic-based NBS are available. From the perspective of IEI, aside from those conditions identifiable by TREC/KREC screening, as aforementioned, there is no alternative testing strategy currently available. Thus, NGS-based testing would hence be the only option, aside from the few diseases where MS/MS testing may be a possibility (ADA deficiency and purine nucleoside phosphorylase (PNP) deficiency) [31,32].

2. Ethical, Legal and Social Implications (ELSIs) in Screening for IEI

We can distinguish a number of ELSIs that will be relevant to different extents for different screening approaches, including NGS-based NBS for IEI. Many of these are further discussed in detail by Johnston et al. [27]. Herein, we have divided the key ELSIs into two main categories: the relatively direct effects of testing on the individual level, and the more indirect or conditional effects that depend on what solutions are found at the societal level. We will now address these two categories in turn in the context of IEI, while distinguishing within those categories the major, more specific issues, as we see them.

2.1. *Individual: Physical and Psychological Well-Being*

Genomic screening will enable the diagnosis of conditions that would be missed using current testing modalities. As such, this approach will result in both an increase in the breadth of different IEI identified at birth and an increase in the overall number of cases identified. The resulting improvements in health and physical well-being represent the obvious rationale for introducing first-tier genetic screening. More children will be diagnosed with IEI and receive effective treatments earlier. In addition, in the context of pharmacogenomics, the potential for adverse reactions to medications may be identified prior to drug administration, which will enable the prevention of predictable and avoidable adverse outcomes. If the testing method is such that it avoids false negatives, there is also an informational benefit for those who are found not to have any actionable conditions. On the other hand, with a risk of false negatives comes not only the risk of being misinformed about disease susceptibility, but also the risk that a particular condition, such as SCID or XLA, will be under-diagnosed because it is known to be included in a screening program and, thus, physicians may be less aware of it as a differential diagnosis.

Unlike some other screening programs, NBS testing itself involves little medical risk, given that it is currently based on a minimally invasive heel prick. However, health and well-being may be negatively affected by the receipt of an abnormal screening result which may be suggestive of an IEI. Firstly, the result can cause anxiety, particularly for the parents at the time of testing. This risk is greater if parents receive poor pre-test information and post-test counselling, potentially causing misunderstanding or confusion regarding the test results. For example, although the target condition for TREC screening is SCID, an abnormal initial screening result may, in fact, normalise upon re-testing or be of unclear clinical significance for that particular infant. Hence, the weight of this ethical consideration depends, to a very large extent, on the quality and accessibility of both pre-test information and genetic counselling. Secondly, the result can lead parents to request treatment and for physicians to provide it even though it is not warranted. In the words of Lund et al., there is a risk of 'reporting of benign variants or variants for late-onset diseases, leading to unnecessary medicalising of the child, giving unnecessary treatment and creating patients-in-waiting' [33]. Overtreatment can be harmful to the individual and is costly to society.

The balance of both the health benefits and the psychological and social risks will depend on what disease candidates are selected for screening. This selection, therefore, must be a considered process [34]. It is almost universally accepted that target conditions should have an effective treatment option available. It can be argued that all IEI have potential management options, spanning empirical and targeted therapies which may be preventive, supportive or curative [20]. For example, a patient identified to have an IEI affecting JAK-STAT signalling pathways such as *STAT1* or *STAT3* gain-of-function mutations can be offered targeted therapies abrogating abnormal signalling, and those with activated phosphoionositide 3-kinase delta syndrome may be offered specific therapies with mammalian target of rapamycin (mTOR) inhibitors or newly developed targeted small-molecule drugs [20]. The future will see the description of further new genetic mutations and the development of novel, improved targeted therapeutic options, further justifying a broader approach to NBS for IEI.

However, even with current screening programs, non-target conditions without treatment options are being identified, and this should also be considered in the pre-testing information offered to parents. An example of one important, non-target condition identified in SCID screening programs is ataxia–telangiectasia (AT), a condition presenting with progressive neurological decline in early childhood, variable immunodeficiency and reduced life expectancy. There is no curative treatment available at the current time. This has raised the question of whether it is more ethical to inform families of the diagnosis at the outset, as compared to allowing them to experience a typical infancy without disclosure of the diagnosis before the onset of symptoms as toddlers. When Blom et al. interviewed the families of healthy newborns enrolled in the Dutch SCID screening program, eighty-two percent of families indicated that early diagnosis was preferred, based on factors such as options for commencement of early supportive treatment and avoidance of diagnostic uncertainty [35]. These results highlight the importance of not making assumptions about families' preferences, and reinforces the need to carry out further studies evaluating similar questions. Individuals are likely to hold different views, and perhaps information about non-actionable conditions could, to some extent, be individualized based on parents' preferences, which could be registered during pre-delivery visits to the clinic.

Genotype–phenotype correlations in IEI are not uniform, and any selected genetic candidates for screening should be well-defined in terms of clinical features. Other factors such as penetrance must be well-understood [20]. Screening for less well-defined conditions should be avoided, so that only clearly pathogenic variants are reported. Concerns have been raised regarding the management of variants of unknown significance in terms of the risk of potentially causing undue anxiety in families, as well as the wider systemic implications (particularly in terms of workforce burden and cost) of second-tier testing and follow-up. It is anticipated that bioinformatic pipelines and variant-calling will be further refined over time, and reference can be made to population-specific databases to minimise over-calling of non-pathogenic variants. Provision of adequate pre-test information and information regarding the testing strategy may also help to minimise parental anxiety regarding follow-up clinical assessment and further testing.

It is imperative that newborn screening tests are acceptable to families in order to maintain high levels of uptake of these programs. All of the considerations discussed above can potentially impact the overall acceptability of an NGS-based NBS approach, and overall acceptability requires formal evaluation prior to implementation.

2.2. Individual: Autonomy and Informed Consent

The majority of newborn screening programs function on an opt-out basis, where testing will proceed routinely unless families decline it. For some ethicists, the fact that testing is proposed by society presents a threat to the autonomous choice of individuals, or, in the case of newborn screening, their parents [36]. Unlike testing that is actively sought out, screening imposes a pressure to conform because society has deemed testing not just worthwhile to provide, but important enough to initiate. From this perspective, expanding newborn screening for IEI increases the imposition on individual choice. The standard way of mitigating threats to autonomy in medical and many other contexts is, of course, informed consent. If people understand what they are being offered, and that they can opt out of testing without any further adverse consequences, then their voluntary acceptance of the offered testing will go a long way to mitigate any imposition. If one accepts this informed consent approach, then the radical expansion of newborn screening to cover many more conditions, including an increased number of IEI, as well as any increased probability of receiving information about carrier status, may seem problematic. This is because of the much more complex information that becomes relevant to making an informed choice either to accept the testing offered or to opt out [37,38].

However, this concern is arguably misdirected for several reasons. The first factor to note is that NBS is not a standard case of patient consent. The benefactor of newborn screening is primarily the newborn child, who has no capacity to give informed consent. Therefore, there is no basis for requiring outright consent. What might be possible is some sort of hypothetical or proxy consent (typically from parents). However, for individuals who are not and have never been competent to make decisions for themselves, society should arguably adopt a *best interest* approach and aim to further their interests rather than arrange for a substitute decision-making proxy to choose for them, as if they were merely temporarily incompetent [39]. An alternative would be to delay screening until adulthood, when individuals can provide meaningful consent, but at that point it would, of course, be too late to identify and treat many IEI, the majority of which have an early onset. This would be contrary to the overall aims and principles of NBS.

Parents are often considered the legitimate guardians of their children's health in everyday contexts. However, this is arguably a pragmatic solution rather than a principled moral order. There is no general moral right for parents to make medical decisions for their children. This is reflected in the fact that in most jurisdictions, at least those that are somewhat liberal, the government will assume guardianship, to the exclusion of parents, if parents make important decisions that are contrary to the best medical interest of their children. It is, therefore, highly doubtful that any moral or legal right of parents to refuse newborn screening for IEI for their children should be based on respect for *patient* autonomy. Instead, there are arguably two main reasons for such a right: (1) to avoid alienating parents from the health care system, and (2) to respect parents' general right to decide for their children, which prevails in more everyday matters [40,41]. In family ethics, it is a mainstream position that all rights of parents to decide for their children are ultimately based on the child's interest in being parented, rather than in any interest or sui generis moral right of the parents (see Brighouse & Swift [40]). An argument for why parents make informed choices regarding NBS was presented by Nicholls [41]. If parents do not have the moral right to refuse testing of their children for serious immunological conditions, then they need not understand the implications of testing for that reason. However, this argument may not convince everyone. Furthermore, since we do allow parents to opt out, and since we want to preserve the often very high participation in newborn screening for IEI and other conditions, it is important to accommodate any expectations on the part of parents to be informed, or to be treated *as if* they had a moral right to make an informed decision. Doing so will increase acceptance. Hence, it is important to consider whether expanding screening to increase the breadth of detectable IEI will undermine the parental opportunity for informed choice.

In current screening programs, while information about the tests and the conditions tested for is typically available, there are generally modest (if any) attempts to ensure that parents have actively obtained and understood this information (there are variable approaches to pre-screening information provision in different settings [42]). This is not surprising, since the medical details of current screening programs are very difficult to understand and evaluate. In the case of IEI, there are a multitude of different conditions which are highly variable in terms of aetiology, clinical presentation and severity. Typically, in NBS programs, many diverse conditions are tested for, and each condition has a different testing method with varying probabilities for false positives and varying potential for second- and sometimes third-tier testing. In addition, given the complexity of the conditions themselves and the very small probabilities of being affected, to evaluate the overall risks and benefits of such tests is beyond the ability of most parents.

Against this background, it is not clear that an increase in complexity would change the ability of parents to make informed choices. Arguably, the type of information that parents might reasonably expect is not about the details of the testing methods (e.g., biochemical or genetic), nor about which IEI conditions might be identified and their pathogeneses. Rather, information that will be sought includes reassurance that the testing itself is harmless, details regarding the general purpose of screening (to identify very rare, but serious, IEI that can be treated) and perhaps the general possibility of false positive and false negative test results. The provision of this kind of information does not become much more difficult or expensive with expanded screening, nor with a change in methods. We advocate that pre-screening information should be provided to parents as part of an integrated, routine pre-natal care service. The level of information provided could potentially be tailored to the individual family based on their wishes, which could be recorded during their initial clinical encounters.

As highlighted, the approach to obtaining consent for newborn screening raises several ethical and practical issues, with many complexities that warrant consideration, particularly in the context of introducing genomic-based screening methodologies for IEI and other conditions. Importantly, trust in NBS programs is essential [34], and families can be reassured that the programs are well-thought out and established by governments after extensive planning, incorporating the involvement of many stakeholders and advice from experts. There are a multitude of safeguards in place to ensure that only relevant testing is performed.

2.3. Society: Privacy and Protection of Genetic Information

A broad variety of genetically determined IEI can be identified by genetic sequencing, and, as such, are potential candidates for genomic-based screening to identify these conditions in the newborn period. Genetic screening necessitates the processing and, at least for some time, storage of genetic information. This raises ethical, social and legal issues because genetic information is very rich and very personal. A person's genome is a unique identifier, and extensive information can be extracted from DNA. In addition, the familial aspects of genetic data need to be considered, as the information may be relevant for other family members. This is the case for various IEI which may be caused by familial or de novo mutations, with variable modes of inheritance. This portends greater risks involved in the handling of genetic information, with a wider-reaching impact than may be initially anticipated. This also means that genetic information would be, to a large extent, collective, and so it makes sense to seek collective solutions for its handling.

It is crucial to develop testing procedures that protect genetic information. One safety measure would be to destroy all genetic information after analysis, keeping only the list of screened conditions given to the individual and their parents. However, there are potential benefits of long-term storage of the genetic information itself. In the case of IEI, there are ongoing, frequent new gene discoveries, and our understanding of the pathogenicity of genetic variants is always improving. As such, there may be benefits of having stored genomic data available for re-analysis at a later date in light of new information and knowledge. In addition, the evolution of new symptoms suggestive of an IEI in an individual could trigger rapid re-analysis of stored genomic data, reducing diagnostic and treatment delay. It does, however, remain uncertain whether retrospective access to stored genomic data will provide a more efficient, cost-effective process with a higher diagnostic yield compared to prospective indication-based re-sequencing based on clinical need. Firstly, data storage is expensive, and future re-sequencing may potentially be more cost-effective using newer techniques. In addition, technological advances may also result in improved diagnostic capabilities (for example, the ability to identify somatic variants, which underlie some forms of IEI and are not well-captured on current NGS platforms).

It is not medically justified to provide the parents of newborns with all information that may be relevant to the child during their lifetime. On the other hand, some information will be important later in life. As proposed by Biesecker et al., it would be ideal from a health perspective to disclose findings to individuals at a life stage at which interventions are beneficial, in relation to our best scientific knowledge at that time [43]. In the case of IEI, many of which present in infancy and early childhood, the provision of screening and diagnoses is most beneficial if performed early in life. As new conditions are identified and new treatments are developed, existing genetic information could be re-analysed and used to provide new and actionable information to individuals that was not accessible when they were infants, and that may potentially be very important at that later time (Chan and Petros 2019, reviewed by Biesecker et al.) [43]. This may also be applicable to pharmacogenomics, for which an individual's genomic data could be re-visited just prior to the commencement of specific drugs to help predict the risk of adverse events and guide judicious prescription [43]. Although the focus of current genomic-based screening is the identification of monogenic diseases, future advances may also assist in identifying polygenic disorders and help to establish disease risk profiles [43].

On occasion, health systems have given private corporations access to genetic information [44]. On other occasions, law enforcement have been given access to blood samples obtained by population screening [45]. Even if such intentional breaches of confidentiality are avoided in the future, there are also risks of unintentional breaches. Any database that is connected to the internet can be hacked. One relevant example is the hacking of My Heritage, a company that sells genetic testing to individuals for genealogical purposes [46]. People working with genetic databases may make errors or be corrupt. Strict data management strategies are required to safeguard individuals from these risks, and must be maintained in order to minimise them. Proposed models are under evaluation using encryption approaches to safeguard genetic data in order to develop safe, secure data storage and sharing [47].

Another potential concern which has arisen is the impact of genetic screening results on interactions with agencies such as insurance providers, where a known genetic diagnosis of an IEI or other condition might have an impact on access to health insurance. While risks to individuals from insurance complications must be considered, we arguably cannot, as societies, allow the practices of insurance providers to determine how we deal with predictive and preventive medicine. Insurance practices and regulations should adjust to public health policy rather than the other way around. Different jurisdictions have, in practice, taken different approaches to this issue with various degrees of success [48]. Regulations should align with local needs and legal and social norms, as well as with general ethical considerations [49]. Although this may be of concern to some members of the public, in practical terms, this has not proven to be a significant issue, given that many countries have protective legislation in place (such as the Genetic Information Non-Disclosure Act in the US) which precludes the use of genetic information for insurance and other purposes.

When considering the privacy risks of genetic screening, we must also consider the alternatives. If a society does not implement population-wide genomic newborn screening for a range of conditions, including IEI, people may increasingly seek unregulated private or external screening where genetic information may be handled by disparate private actors to a larger extent, and the differences in what information is available for different people will vary depending not only on their own choices, but also on the choices of their relatives. Given the real risks associated with the dissemination of genetic information, it may be preferable that this information be handled by healthcare systems with clear recommendations which uphold regulatory requirements.

2.4. Society: Health and Economic Considerations

Rational and responsible expenditure of the healthcare budget is paramount. It is an ethical and social consideration from the perspective of ensuring that funds are used appropriately and will be of benefit to the community. Formal evaluation of health economic data and cost–benefit analyses for NGS-based NBS for IEI must be undertaken, and should take into account all aspects of NBS program-associated costs, including pre-test information provision, the testing itself, clinical follow-up, further testing and treatment [20]. We are seeing a steady decrease in the costs of genetic sequencing, owing to factors such as widespread uptake and technological improvements which have made NGS more readily available and competitively priced. Similar to the experience with screening for SCID using TREC/KREC analysis, where cost–benefit analyses have been in favour of screening [50–52], we anticipate that early diagnosis of patients with additional forms of IEI will ultimately decrease health-related expenditure. In the case of SCID, these studies have demonstrated that healthcare expenditure was reduced in infants diagnosed and managed early with HSCT, owing to a reduction in the utilisation of resources, including hospital and intensive care unit admissions and costs incurred in the management of serious disease complications. In the case of genomic-based screening for IEI, it is anticipated that the savings will likely outweigh any additional costs from overtreatment due to false positives and variants of unknown significance, especially over time, as healthcare professionals adjust to frequent use of genetic information. Rapid WGS for unwell infants in intensive care units has been shown not only to improve patient outcomes, but also to reduce healthcare expenditure [53]. In addition to cost-effectiveness studies, which directly assess healthcare expenditure at a systemic level, another important health economic consideration relates to Quality of Life Years (QALY) gained through early diagnosis and treatment. These health and economic considerations should be carefully evaluated in the context of NGS-based NBS.

Establishment of any new NBS program or a new approach to NBS, as discussed herein in the context of IEI, is a considerable task that relies not only on robust testing methodologies and pipelines, but personnel and resources to carry out the program effectively. This includes healthcare providers providing pre-test information and post-test counselling to parents, laboratory personnel processing specimens and performing sequencing analysis and clinical input from physicians for follow-up on infants returning abnormal screening results. There are many layers to a successful NBS program, as well as associated costs, which all need to be rigorously evaluated.

2.5. Society: Equity and Access to Newborn Screening

At present, there is wide variability in screening methodologies and screened conditions in different regions, even within the same country. Decisions regarding the addition of new candidate diseases, including IEI, to screening programs are multifactorial and may include considerations such as the population prevalence of specific diseases. In some settings, newborn screening is funded by public health systems and is free of charge to families, whereas in other areas, testing may incur a cost, which may impact upon uptake. These factors all impact the equity of testing and access to NBS, which is another important consideration when considering disease inclusion and the methodologies used in NBS programs.

An additional consideration in the implementation of genomic-based NBS for IEI are reference genome datasets. Current databases are predominantly based upon individuals from Northern European populations, and are, therefore, not representative of other ethnicities [20]. As such, it will be essential to build genomic population databases which are highly representative of different ethnic groups in order to enable robust variant calling and interpretation [20].

As noted above, healthcare screening should be compared to the alternative. If testing is a market good provided by commercial companies, access will depend on ability to pay as well as on education, access to information and other social factors. Commercial testing will also more likely lack robust clinical processes and genetic counselling capabilities, potentially resulting in less judicious testing with lower clinical utility [38]. This is particularly the case for IEI, as there is significant complexity owing to disease heterogeneity, requiring specialist clinical oversight of test interpretation and reporting. This, once again, reinforces the need for careful regulation of NBS and for NBS services to be linked with the appropriate clinical services to provide follow-up and treatment for any abnormal results received.

3. Conclusions

Up-front, first-tier genomic-based newborn screening shows promise for the identification of infants with IEI, a group of conditions for which there is significant clinical and phenotypic heterogeneity, through enabling the concurrent analysis of hundreds of genes. There are many factors which must be taken into account prior to adopting this approach to screening for IEI relating to practical, methodological and technical aspects, and, importantly, a range of ethical, legal and social considerations which must be fully evaluated. In particular, assessing the acceptability of the testing strategy is imperative to avoid undermining existing successful systems with very high uptakes, and we have discussed some of the issues in this context. Ethical, legal and social issues sometimes interact in non-obvious ways. While informed consent from parents may not be needed to safeguard autonomy, since newborns are not autonomous and so should rather have their best interest protected, it is important to provide parents with both information and the ability to opt-out so as to preserve the very high uptake. As technology advances, we are likely to see ongoing evolution in the approach to genomic newborn screening for IEI, starting with an initial, limited WES gene panel which will expand over time to include more genes. progresses to This is expected to then be replaced by WGS in order to improve diagnostic yield and expand screening capabilities for this broad group of disorders. Ongoing evaluation of all of these factors is essential in the planning for and implementation of genomic-based approaches to newborn screening for inborn errors of immunity and other clinically significant conditions.

Author Contributions: Writing—original draft preparation, review and editing: J.R.K., K.G. and L.H. All authors have read and agreed to the published version of the manuscript.

Funding: This research received no external funding.

Institutional Review Board Statement: Not applicable.

Informed Consent Statement: Not applicable.

Data Availability Statement: Not applicable.

Conflicts of Interest: The authors declare no conflict of interest.

References

1. Centerwall, S.A.; Centerwall, W.R. The discovery of phenylketonuria: The story of a young couple, two retarded children, and a scientist. *Pediatrics* **2000**, *105*, 89–103. [CrossRef] [PubMed]
2. Cornel, M.C.; Rigter, T.; Jansen, M.E.; Henneman, L. Neonatal and carrier screening for rare diseases: How innovation challenges screening criteria worldwide. *J. Community Genet.* **2021**, *12*, 257–265. [CrossRef]

3. Tangye, S.G.; Al-Herz, W.; Bousfiha, A.; Chatila, T.; Cunningham-Rundles, C.; Etzioni, A.; Franco, J.L.; Holland, S.M.; Klein, C.; Morio, T.; et al. Human Inborn Errors of Immunity: 2022 Update on the Classification from the International Union of Immunological Societies Expert Committee. *J. Clin. Immunol.* **2022**, *42*, 1473–1507. [CrossRef] [PubMed]
4. Brown, L.; Xu-Bayford, J.; Allwood, Z.; Slatter, M.; Cant, A.; Davies, E.G.; Veys, P.; Gennery, A.R.; Gaspar, H.B. Neonatal diagnosis of severe combined immunodeficiency leads to significantly improved survival outcome: The case for newborn screening. *Blood* **2011**, *117*, 3243–3246. [CrossRef] [PubMed]
5. King, J.R.; Hammarström, L. Newborn Screening for Primary Immunodeficiency Diseases: History, Current and Future Practice. *J. Clin. Immunol.* **2017**, *38*, 56–66. [CrossRef] [PubMed]
6. Dezfouli, M.; Bergström, S.; Skattum, L.; Abolhassani, H.; Neiman, M.; Torabi-Rahvar, M.; Jarava, C.F.; Martin-Nalda, A.; Balaguer, J.M.F.; Slade, C.A.; et al. Newborn Screening for Presymptomatic Diagnosis of Complement and Phagocyte Deficiencies. *Front. Immunol.* **2020**, *11*, 455. [CrossRef] [PubMed]
7. Hamsten, C.; Skattum, L.; Truedsson, L.; von Döbeln, U.; Uhlén, M.; Schwenk, J.M.; Hammarström, L.; Nilsson, P.; Neiman, M. Heat differentiated complement factor profiling. *J. Proteom.* **2015**, *126*, 155–162. [CrossRef]
8. Borte, S.; Meeths, M.; Liebscher, I.; Krist, K.; Nordenskjöld, M.; Hammarström, L.; von Döbeln, U.; Henter, J.-I.; Bryceson, Y.T. Combined newborn screening for familial hemophagocytic lymphohistiocytosis and severe T- and B-cell immunodeficiencies. *J. Allergy Clin. Immunol.* **2014**, *134*, 226–228. [CrossRef]
9. Janzi, M.; Sjöberg, R.; Wan, J.; Fischler, B.; von Döbeln, U.; Isaac, L.; Nilsson, P.; Hammarström, L. Screening for C3 deficiency in newborns using microarrays. *PLoS ONE* **2009**, *4*, e5321. [CrossRef]
10. Kingsmore, S.F.; Smith, L.D.; Kunard, C.M.; Bainbridge, M.; Batalov, S.; Benson, W.; Blincow, E.; Caylor, S.; Chambers, C.; Del Angel, G.; et al. A genome sequencing system for universal newborn screening, diagnosis, and precision medicine for severe genetic diseases. *Am. J. Hum. Genet.* **2022**, *109*, 1605–1619. [CrossRef]
11. Smedley, D.; Smith, K.R.; Martin, A.; Thomas, E.A.; McDonagh, E.M.; Cipriani, V.; Ellingford, J.M.; Arno, G.; Tucci, A.; Vandrovcova, J.; et al. 100,000 Genomes Pilot on Rare-Disease Diagnosis in Health Care-Preliminary Report. *N. Engl. J. Med.* **2021**, *385*, 1868–1880.
12. Jian, M.; Wang, X.; Sui, Y.; Fang, M.; Feng, C.; Huang, Y.; Liu, C.; Guo, R.; Guan, Y.; Gao, Y.; et al. A pilot study of assessing whole genome sequencing in newborn screening in unselected children in China. *Clin. Transl. Med.* **2022**, e843. [CrossRef] [PubMed]
13. Pichini, A.; Ahmed, A.; Patch, C.; Bick, D.; Leblond, M.; Kasperaviciute, D.; Deen, D.; Wilde, S.; Noriega, S.G.; Matoko, C.; et al. Developing a National Newborn Genomes Program: An Approach Driven by Ethics, Engagement and Co-design. *Front. Genet.* **2022**, *13*, 866168. [CrossRef]
14. Cho, Y.; Lee, C.-H.; Jeong, E.-G.; Kim, M.-H.; Hong, J.H.; Ko, Y.; Lee, B.; Yun, G.; Kim, B.J.; Jung, J.; et al. Prevalence of Rare Genetic Variations and Their Implications in NGS-data Interpretation. *Sci. Rep.* **2017**, *7*, 9810. [CrossRef]
15. Bhattacharjee, A.; Sokolsky, T.; Wyman, S.K.; Reese, M.G.; Puffenberger, E.; Strauss, K.; Morton, H.; Parad, R.B.; Naylor, E.W. Development of DNA Confirmatory and High-Risk Diagnostic Testing for Newborns Using Targeted Next-Generation DNA Sequencing. *Genet. Med.* **2015**, *17*, 337–347. [CrossRef] [PubMed]
16. Bodian, D.L.; Klein, E.; Iyer, R.K.; Wong, W.S.W.; Kothiyal, P.; Stauffer, D.; Huddleston, K.C.; Gaither, A.D.; Remsburg, I.; Khromykh, A.; et al. Utility of whole-genome sequencing for detection of newborn screening disorders in a population cohort of 1696 neonates. *Genet. Med.* **2016**, *18*, 221–230. [CrossRef] [PubMed]
17. Willig, L.K.; Petrikin, J.E.; Smith, L.D.; Saunders, C.J.; Thiffault, I.; Miller, N.A.; Soden, S.E.; Cakici, J.A.; Herd, S.M.; Twist, G.; et al. Whole-genome sequencing for identification of Mendelian disorders in critically ill infants: A retrospective analysis of diagnostic and clinical findings. *Lancet Respir. Med.* **2015**, *3*, 377–387. [CrossRef] [PubMed]
18. Pavey, A.R.; Bodian, D.L.; Vilboux, T.; Khromykh, A.; Hauser, N.S.; Huddleston, K.; Klein, E.; Black, A.; Kane, M.S.; Iyer, R.K.; et al. Utilization of genomic sequencing for population screening of immunodeficiencies in the newborn. *Genet. Med.* **2017**, *19*, 1367–1375. [CrossRef]
19. Ceyhan-Birsoy, O.; Murry, J.B.; Machini, K.; Lebo, M.S.; Yu, T.W.; Fayer, S.; Genetti, C.A.; Schwartz, T.S.; Agrawal, P.B.; Parad, R.B.; et al. Interpretation of Genomic Sequencing Results in Healthy and Ill Newborns: Results from the BabySeq Project. *Am. J. Hum. Genet.* **2019**, *104*, 76–93. [CrossRef]
20. King, J.R.; Notarangelo, L.D.; Hammarström, L. An appraisal of the Wilson & Jungner criteria in the context of genomic-based newborn screening for inborn errors of immunity. *J. Allergy Clin. Immunol.* **2021**, *147*, 428–438.
21. Wilson, J.; Jungner, G. *The Principles and Practice of Screening for Disease*; World Health Organization: Geneva, Switzerland, 1968.
22. Dobrow, M.J.; Hagens, V.; Chafe, R.; Sullivan, T.; Rabeneck, L. Consolidated principles for screening based on a systematic review and consensus process. *CMAJ* **2018**, *190*, E422–E429. [CrossRef]
23. Petros, M. Revisiting the Wilson-Jungner criteria: How can supplemental criteria guide public health in the era of genetic screening? *Genet. Med.* **2012**, *14*, 129–134. [CrossRef]
24. Andermann, A.; Blancquaert, I.; Beauchamp, S.; Déry, V. Revisiting Wilson and Jungner in the genomic age: A review of screening criteria over the past 40 years. *Bull. World Health Organ.* **2008**, *86*, 317–319. [CrossRef] [PubMed]
25. Bick, D.; Ahmed, A.; Deen, D.; Ferlini, A.; Garnier, N.; Kasperaviciute, D.; Leblond, M.; Pichini, A.; Rendon, A.; Satija, A.; et al. Newborn Screening by Genomic Sequencing: Opportunities and Challenges. *Int. J. Neonatal. Screen* **2022**, *8*, 40. [CrossRef] [PubMed]

26. Children UACoHDiNa; Administration HRaS. Committee Approach to Evaluating the Condition Review Report (Decision Matrix). 2022. Available online: https://www.hrsa.gov/advisory-committees/heritable-disorders/decision-matrix (accessed on 15 December 2022).
27. Johnston, J.; Lantos, J.D.; Goldenberg, A.; Chen, F.; Parens, E.; Koenig, B.A. Sequencing Newborns: A Call for Nuanced Use of Genomic Technologies. *Hastings Cent. Rep.* **2018**, *48* (Suppl. 2), S2–S6. [CrossRef]
28. Tangye, S.G.; Al-Herz, W.; Bousfiha, A.; Skogstrand, K.; Bækvad-Hansen, M. Human Inborn Errors of Immunity: 2019 Update on the Classification from the International Union of Immunological Societies Expert Committee. *J. Clin. Immunol.* **2020**.
29. DiStefano, M.T.; Goehringer, S.; Babb, L.; Alkuraya, F.S.; Amberger, J.; Amin, M.; Austin-Tse, C.; Balzotti, M.; Berg, J.S.; Birney, E.; et al. The Gene Curation Coalition: A global effort to harmonize gene–disease evidence resources. *Genet. Med.* **2022**, *24*, 1732–1742. [CrossRef]
30. Adhikari, A.N.; Gallagher, R.C.; Wang, Y.; Currier, R.J.; Amatuni, G.; Bassaganyas, L.; Chen, F.; Kundu, K.; Kvale, M.; Mooney, S.D.; et al. The role of exome sequencing in newborn screening for inborn errors of metabolism. *Nat. Med.* **2020**, *26*, 1392–1397. [CrossRef] [PubMed]
31. la Marca, G.; Canessa, C.; Giocaliere, E.; Romano, F.; Duse, M.; Malvagia, S.; Lippi, F.; Funghini, S.; Bianchi, L.; Della Bona, M.L.; et al. Tandem mass spectrometry, but not T-cell receptor excision circle analysis, identifies newborns with late-onset adenosine deaminase deficiency. *J. Allergy Clin. Immunol.* **2013**, *131*, 1604–1610. [CrossRef] [PubMed]
32. la Marca, G.; Canessa, C.; Giocaliere, E.; Romano, F.; Malvagia, S.; Funghini, S.; Moriondo, M.; Valleriani, C.; Lippi, F.; Ombrone, D.; et al. Diagnosis of immunodeficiency caused by a purine nucleoside phosphorylase defect by using tandem mass spectrometry on dried blood spots. *J. Allergy Clin. Immunol.* **2014**, *134*, 155–159. [CrossRef]
33. Lund, A.M.; Wibrand, F.; Skogstrand, K.; Bækvad-Hansen, M.; Gregersen, N.; Andresen, B.S.; Hougaard, D.M.; Dunø, M.; Olsen, R.K.J. Use of Molecular Genetic Analyses in Danish Routine Newborn Screening. *Int. J. Neonatal Screen* **2021**, *7*, 50. [CrossRef]
34. Goldenberg, A.J.; Lloyd-Puryear, M.; Brosco, J.P.; Therrell, B.; Bush, L.; Berry, S.; Brower, A.; Bonhomme, N.; Bowdish, B.; Chrysler, D.; et al. Including ELSI research questions in newborn screening pilot studies. *Genet. Med.* **2019**, *21*, 525–533. [CrossRef] [PubMed]
35. Blom, M.; Schoenaker, M.H.D.; Hulst, M.; de Vries, M.C.; Weemaes, C.M.R.; Willemsen, M.A.A.P.; Henneman, L.; van der Burg, M. Dilemma of Reporting Incidental Findings in Newborn Screening Programs for SCID: Parents' Perspective on Ataxia Telangiectasia. *Front. Immunol.* **2019**, *10*, 2438. [CrossRef]
36. Juth, N.; Munthe, C. *The Ethics of Screening in Health Care and Medicine: Serving Society or Serving the Patient?* Springer: Berlin/Heidelberg, Germany, 2012.
37. Nijsingh, N.; Juth, N.; Munthe, C. *International Encyclopedia of Public Health*, 2nd ed.; Academic Press (Elsevier): Amsterdam, The Netherlands, 2017.
38. Esquerda, M.; Palau, F.; Lorenzo, D.; Cambra, F.J.; Bofarull, M.; Cusi, V.; Bioetica, G.I.E. Ethical questions concerning newborn genetic screening. *Clin. Genet.* **2021**, *99*, 93–98. [CrossRef] [PubMed]
39. Dawson, A. The determination of the best interests in relation to childhood immunisation. *Bioethics* **2005**, *19*, 72–89. [CrossRef]
40. Brighouse, H.; Swift, A. *Family Values: The Ethics of Parent-Child Relationships*; Princeton University Press: Princeton, NJ, USA, 2014.
41. Nicholls, S.G. Knowledge or Understanding? Informed Choice in the Context of Newborn Bloodspot Screening. *Public Health Ethics* **2010**, *3*, 128–136. [CrossRef]
42. Franková, V.; Driscoll, R.O.; Jansen, M.E.; Loeber, J.G.; Kožich, V.; Bonham, J.; Borde, P.; Brincat, I.; Cheillan, D.; Dekkers, E.; et al. Regulatory landscape of providing information on newborn screening to parents across Europe. *Eur. J. Hum. Genet.* **2021**, *29*, 67–78. [CrossRef]
43. Biesecker, L.G.; Green, E.D.; Manolio, T.; Solomon, B.D.; Curtis, D. Should all babies have their genome sequenced at birth? *BMJ* **2021**, *375*, n2679. [CrossRef] [PubMed]
44. Powles, J.; Hodson, H. Google DeepMind and healthcare in an age of algorithms. *Health Technol.* **2017**, *7*, 351–367. [CrossRef]
45. Hårstrån kan Fälla Gärningsmannen. 2004. Available online: https://www.dn.se/arkiv/inrikes/harstran-kan-falla-garningsmannen/ (accessed on 15 December 2022).
46. 2018. Available online: https://blog.myheritage.com/2018/06/myheritage-statement-about-a-cybersecurity-incident/ (accessed on 15 December 2022).
47. Hasan, M.Z.; Mahdi, M.S.R.; Sadat, M.N.; Mohammed, N. Secure count query on encrypted genomic data. *J. Biomed. Inform.* **2018**, *81*, 41–52. [CrossRef]
48. Prince, A.E.R. Comparative perspectives: Regulating insurer use of genetic information. *Eur. J. Hum. Genet.* **2019**, *27*, 340–348. [CrossRef] [PubMed]
49. Pugh, J. Genetic information, insurance and a pluralistic approach to justice. *J. Med. Ethics* **2021**, *47*, 473. [CrossRef]
50. Gardulf, A.; Winiarski, J.; Thorin, M.; Heibert Arnlind, M.; von Dobeln, U.; Hammarstrom, L. Costs associated with treatment of severe combined immunodeficiency-rationale for newborn screening in Sweden. *J. Allergy Clin. Immunol.* **2016**, *139*, 1713–1716.e6. [CrossRef]
51. Chan, K.; Davis, J.; Pai, S.Y.; Bonilla, F.A.; Puck, J.M.; Apkon, M. A Markov model to analyze cost-effectiveness of screening for severe combined immunodeficiency (SCID). *Mol. Genet. Metab.* **2011**, *104*, 383–389. [CrossRef] [PubMed]

52. Ding, Y.; Thompson, J.D.; Kobrynski, L.; Ojodu, J.; Zarbalian, G.; Grosse, S.D. Cost-Effectiveness/Cost-Benefit Analysis of Newborn Screening for Severe Combined Immune Deficiency in Washington State. *J. Pediatr.* **2016**, *172*, 127–135. [CrossRef]
53. Farnaes, L.; Hildreth, A.; Sweeney, N.M.; Clark, M.M.; Chowdhury, S.; Nahas, S.; Cakici, J.A.; Benson, W.; Kaplan, R.H.; Kronick, R.; et al. Rapid whole-genome sequencing decreases infant morbidity and cost of hospitalization. *NPJ Genom. Med.* **2018**, *3*, 10. [CrossRef] [PubMed]

International Journal of
Neonatal Screening

Opinion

Age-Based Genomic Screening during Childhood: Ethical and Practical Considerations in Public Health Genomics Implementation

Laura V. Milko * and Jonathan S. Berg

Department of Genetics, University of North Carolina at Chapel Hill, 120 Mason Farm Rd., Chapel Hill, NC 27599-7264, USA; jonathan_berg@med.unc.edu
* Correspondence: laura_milko@med.unc.edu; Tel.: +1-919-829-5747

Abstract: Genomic sequencing offers an unprecedented opportunity to detect inherited variants that are implicated in rare Mendelian disorders, yet there are many challenges to overcome before this technology can routinely be applied in the healthy population. The age-based genomic screening (ABGS) approach is a novel alternative to genome-scale sequencing at birth that aims to provide highly actionable genetic information to parents over the course of their child's routine health care. ABGS utilizes an established metric to identify conditions with high clinical actionability and incorporates information about the age of onset and age of intervention to determine the optimal time to screen for any given condition. Ongoing partnerships with parents and providers are instrumental to the co-creation of educational resources and strategies to address potential implementation barriers. Implementation science frameworks and informative empirical data are used to evaluate strategies to establish this unique clinical application of targeted genomic sequencing. Ultimately, a pilot project conducted in primary care pediatrics clinics will assess patient and implementation outcomes, parent and provider perspectives, and the feasibility of ABGS. A validated, stakeholder-informed, and practical ABGS program will include hundreds of conditions that are actionable during infancy and childhood, setting the stage for a longitudinal implementation that can assess clinical and health economic outcomes.

Keywords: genetics; newborn screening (NBS); stakeholder engagement; dissemination; implementation science; health equity

1. Introduction

Public health newborn screening (NBS) epitomizes the early detection of individuals with rare genetic conditions to allow the initiation of effective treatments before symptoms develop. Currently, the number of detectable conditions is limited by the technology employed. Exome and genome sequencing (collectively referred to here as "genome-scale sequencing") has profoundly advanced the ability to diagnose and manage patients affected with rare Mendelian conditions [1–3] and could vastly expand the range of conditions detected in the general population through predictive screening [4]. Furthermore, the promise of many cutting-edge gene and cell therapies for early onset genetic conditions is contingent on their timely ascertainment in the healthy pediatric population [5].

Proponents of expanding public health NBS to include genome-scale sequencing advocate for the predictive—and, potentially, future diagnostic—utility of providing all newborns with a sequenced genome [6]. However, despite some interest among a subset of the population, there are well-founded doubts about whether and how genome-scale sequencing should be implemented [7–10]. It is clear that the addition of genome-scale sequencing to routine NBS would raise substantial ethical, societal, and practical concerns related to parental consent and in determining the kind of information that should be sought and disclosed [11–13], making its implementation in NBS programs untenable at present. However, if costs are low enough and the value is high enough, predictive genomic analysis could become accessible in a way that reduces barriers to obtaining highly actionable information with the greatest chance of societal benefit.

We suggest that focusing on genome-scale sequencing at birth overlooks a crucial opportunity to deliver actionable information closer to the point of care across the lifespan. Beyond newborn screening, routine pediatric preventive care interventions continue throughout childhood, such as growth charting, vaccinations, and hearing/vision screening, all of which have individual utility and are also widely accepted because of their public health impact. The periodicity schedule for these interventions is reviewed in an evidence-based manner [14] and establishes policies for insurance coverage under the Affordable Care Act. Practitioners are accustomed to standard workflows, and parents expect to receive anticipatory guidance and screens for potential health concerns for their child over time. Given the rapid development of next-generation sequencing capabilities, could population-based genomic screening for monogenic conditions that are actionable in childhood be incorporated into the existing practice of well-child care?

An age-based genomic screening (ABGS) approach seeks to deliver discrete, predictive genomic information at intervention-oriented time-points during well-child care, including neonatally, and provide clinically useful results in easily digestible portions for both parents and providers. Thus, ABGS addresses many, but not all, of the ethical concerns about genomic sequencing in children, while retaining most of the benefits. By interrogating panels of highly actionable conditions at relevant time points during infancy and childhood [15], the focused approach of ABGS simplifies parental decision-making around the types of genetic information that should be sought and disclosed in a healthy child by screening only for conditions with the highest degree of clinical actionability at the most clinically relevant intervals. As an alternative to screening newborns for every detectable condition at birth, including those that will likely not manifest until later in childhood, ABGS ameliorates loss to the follow-up of individuals for whom there is a protracted latency between the discovery of the genetic diagnosis and the actionability of that information. Periodic engagement about genomic screening between providers and parents (and gradual exposure of the child over time) has the added benefit of building knowledge about genetics and confidence in the ability to make recommendations or decisions, thus improving genomic literacy. If implemented throughout the lifespan, ABGS could represent a cost-effective and tractable way to capitalize on advances in genomic medicine that would seamlessly connect with genomic screening programs designed for adults [16,17].

The implementation of ABGS as a public health care service, offered in diverse populations with varying geographic, sociodemographic, and cultural backgrounds will require ongoing partnerships in clinics and communities to ensure broad accessibility to parents across all segments of society. Frameworks, theories, and models from implementation science can be used to identify potential barriers and strategies to overcome them, as well as harmonized measures developed by genomic medicine consortia [18–21], which can be used to standardize data collection, knowledge integration, and inform best practices for future implementation trials [22].

The lag in the clinical adoption of genomic interventions, including population screening, into routine clinical practice has been attributed to various factors related to the impending shift from genetic specialty providers to primary care providers, including contextual factors (e.g., a perceived lack of knowledge, expertise, and supporting resources) and process factors (e.g., an engagement of organizational leadership and provider buy-in) [22–24]. The development of educational and clinical decision support tools for non-genetics clinicians is growing; however, research to develop and evaluate strategies to effectively integrate genomic screening into diverse clinical settings is largely unexplored, particularly in settings with limited resources and other structural barriers to implementing public health innovations [25,26]. Engagement with clinical providers and staff will be needed to develop and provide resources to support the integration of ABGS into the clinical workflow. Key stakeholders from pediatric clinics in diverse communities will need to be involved, including the perspectives of providers and parents to develop strategies and resources to facilitate the equitable uptake of genomic screening [27].

2. Identifying Appropriate Conditions for Screening during Childhood

Current NBS focuses on a small number of conditions with unambiguous health benefits (for the most part) and bypasses explicit parental informed consent due to its public health importance. Genetic sequencing would introduce a much wider range of possible findings for NBS, including conditions with less clinical actionability and later ages of onset that would likely invoke a paradigm shift to a new "opt-in" model of screening. Decisions about which conditions to include as part of a public health genomic screening program must take into account the value to society and various interested parties.

Partitioning the genome into interpretable groupings based on the clinical actionability and natural history characteristics of genetic conditions can facilitate informed decision-making and preference setting by individuals and parents [28]. ABGS will rely on a semi-quantitative metric (SQM) for scoring clinical actionability based on five key parameters (the severity and likelihood of disease manifestations, the efficacy and acceptability of interventions, and a knowledge base about the condition) [29] that was previously developed by our research group and subsequently adopted with minor modifications by the ClinGen Actionability and Pediatric Actionability Working Groups [30,31]. We utilized this approach to define a subset of conditions that qualified for disclosure to research participants as a "next-generation sequencing newborn screen" [32] and further analyzed SQM scores for a comparison of commercial panels that are being offered to parents as expanded newborn screening options [33].

Although clinical actionability is an important criterion for determining eligibility for screening purposes, it is not the only factor involved. The latency between information and action (the time that elapses between learning information about a newborn's future health condition and the time at which actions can be taken to ameliorate adverse outcomes) will influence the efficacy of the genomic screening intervention. For example, a long delay could induce unnecessary stress on the family and/or child, or even impact the effectiveness of the intervention (for example, if the molecular diagnosis is not followed up on effectively, or forgotten, over the course of many years). The economic implications of genomic screening are also likely to be influenced by the duration and nature of interventions that are prompted by a positive finding, with greater downstream costs associated with prolonged periods of surveillance by medical specialists before symptoms manifest and/or definitive prophylactic or therapeutic interventions are deployed.

An ABGS approach will therefore categorize groups of conditions based on high clinical actionability, natural history pattern (age of symptom onset), and current recommendations for age of intervention. Clustering conditions in panels that can be offered at specific time points will optimally balance early detection with proximity to a recommended course of action to prevent or ameliorate symptoms. Sequencing panels will ideally be informed by and synchronized with existing pediatric preventive care visits to maximize efficiency for clinical workflows. There are clear trade-offs in terms of gene content, number of panels, and timing of testing, requiring multidisciplinary and multisource input and consensus.

3. Sequencing Healthy Newborns and Children: Start Small, Grow with Time

The generation of genome-scale data at birth is viewed by some as an efficient and cost-effective way to incorporate public health screening for a much broader range of conditions. Once sampled, sequenced, and stored, whole genome sequence data theoretically offers the ability to repeatedly interrogate the data if undiagnosed conditions with a suspected genetic etiology arise, and for additional screening once a child reaches the age of consent. However, the wide range of possible results from genome-scale sequencing, including conditions with differing levels of clinical actionability and ages of onset, immediately raises questions about what information should be sought and disclosed in healthy newborns.

Parental reactions might include anxiety regarding: the range of possible choices about what information they wish to have disclosed to them; perceptions that elective genome sequencing is less important due to other factors in their lives that take precedence; concerns about out-of-pocket expense; worries about data privacy and legal implications for their child in the future, such as insurability; or uncertainty about whether to learn about health conditions that are out of their control. If genome-scale sequencing were adopted as part of routine public health NBS, these concerns would need to be addressed through comprehensive educational programs and detailed parental decision-making processes, which would require substantial changes to the current procedures. The neonatal period, which is clearly challenging for most parents, may not be an ideal time to make such complex decisions, and could result in parents opting out of NBS entirely [34]. Therefore, we suggest that initial public health genomic screening in newborns should focus narrowly on conditions that would be highly actionable in the neonatal period, with additional layers of screening throughout childhood—with parental informed consent—gradually expanding the number and range of conditions that are screened for across the lifespan.

Generation of genome-wide data also introduces many passionately argued ethical concerns that could impede the widespread adoption of genomic screening in infants and children. It is unlikely that extensive pre-test genetic counseling will be feasible for a population-level genomic screening program, whereas highly focused sequencing panels provide a streamlined opt-in choice for parents and providers. While it is possible to sequence the genome or exome and then limit the informatic analysis to subsets of genes, this approach requires justification as to why certain information is not being disclosed and may result in challenges with parental requests for the full set of raw data. The ABGS approach is to start by interrogating the small fraction of genes that do meet that standard, determine how best to implement genomic screening in diverse populations, and then scale it to the general population to obtain the greatest impact, for the most people, at the least expense.

A targeted sequencing approach would reduce technical issues and privacy concerns related to accessing, interpreting, and securely maintaining the enormous volume of data generated by genome-scale sequencing, including potential ethical questions about data interpretation and ownership that could hinder widespread acceptance. Finally, economic arguments about various sequencing methods can be fraught with assumptions, given the highly subsidized nature of large-scale sequencing in both the research and commercial settings, differences in economies of scale at different steps of the sequencing process, and the rapid and unpredictable advances in technology. Sequencing costs will invariably continue to reduce over time, making serial resequencing progressively less expensive, while taking advantage of newer technology and avoiding data storage and reanalysis costs (which could be substantial but are often ignored). A persistent desire to utilize better sequencing technologies as a person grows is to be expected, rather than relying on old sequence data generated at birth. Studying a population-level implementation of targeted screening (either through specific biochemical enrichment strategies or via informatics approaches to selectively analyze virtual panels) is a cost-effective and ethically feasible way to identify rare individuals with highly actionable conditions. However, at an individual level, this approach can also lay the groundwork for additional tiers of optional conditions that could be analyzed over time based on parental decision-making in consultation with a primary care provider or genetic specialist.

4. Using Implementation Science to Advance Innovations in Genomic Screening

We argue that ABGS of healthy children for monogenic conditions is initially and inherently an implementation challenge that must be researched and conducted in a rigorous, transparent, and relatively cautious manner in order to build public health buy-in and avoid "putting the cart before the horse" by overextending the reach of expanded genomic NBS and causing iatrogenic harm to parents and families. An early implementation of ABGS will require ongoing engagement with primary care providers and parents in order to develop an evidence-based and contextually appropriate program and responsive implementation strategies for the clinical adoption and inclusion of representative populations. Implementation science provides frameworks and models to guide the planning and conduct of implementation, as well as the evaluation of multilevel outcomes in serial implementation phases [35,36]. These frameworks and models are increasingly used to inform the design and evaluation of health interventions with a diverse reach to improve adoption and increase health equity in underserved and marginalized communities [37,38].

Implementation science approaches developed and evaluated by genomic medicine consortia will be used to standardize data collection, integrate knowledge, and inform best practices for future pragmatic clinical trials. The genomic medicine integrative research (GMIR) framework [39] developed by the National Human Genome Research Institute (NHGRI)-funded Implementing Genomics in Practice (IGNITE) network [40] and the Clinical Sequencing Evidence-Generating Research (CSER) consortium [21] has a strong theoretical basis in the consolidated framework for implementation research (CFIR) [41] and provides an organizational structure for key domains of the greatest relevance to genomic medicine researchers [42]. The GMIR framework provided an effective model to modify for ABGS study activities and will enable us to link our constructs and outcomes with those of other genomic medicine research studies and consortia [43,44] (Figure 1).

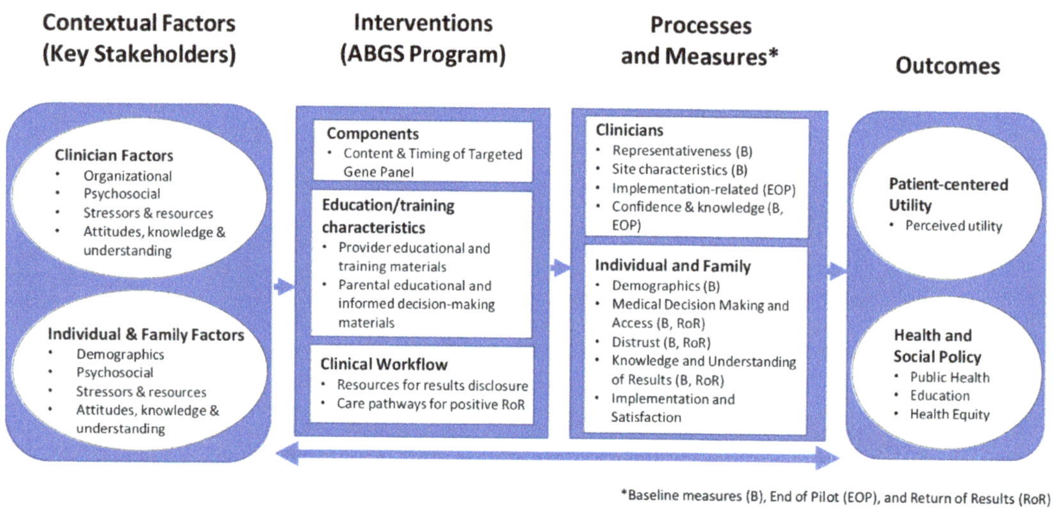

Figure 1. The Genomic Medicine Integrative Research (GMIR) framework developed by the National Human Genome Research Institute (NHGRI)-funded Implementing Genomics in Practice (IGNITE) network and the Clinical Sequencing Evidence-Generating Research (CSER) consortium provides an organizational structure for the key domains of the greatest relevance to genomic medicine researchers. The ABGS-adapted GMIR framework shown here will facilitate linking our constructs and outcomes with those of other genomic medicine research studies and consortia.

5. Multilevel Partnerships with Parents and Providers

The involvement of primary care providers and parents will be critical to identify and address barriers that could impair the successful clinical implementation of ABGS [45–47]. The understanding of negative/normal results [48] by parents and providers, and their perspectives about the future health of the child, need to be studied. Even true positive findings can have highly varying clinical utility depending on the condition, the age at which sequencing is performed, and the age at which actions need to be taken to prevent adverse health outcomes [49,50]. There are important ethical concerns that presymptomatic genomic sequencing could impair parental bonding, create "patients in waiting", or impinge on the future autonomy of the child [51–54]. Extensive multi-level engagement and collaboration with parent and provider partners throughout the process will be crucial for developing the ABGS program and exploring key contextual factors for individuals and families, as well as providers and clinics, the psychosocial aspects of participation, and the broader outcomes for health and social policy.

Collaboration with primary care specialties (family medicine, internal medicine, and pediatrics) and a strong representation of minority populations will facilitate a broad perspective about the needs for ABGS implementation and foster an organizational culture that is receptive to this new clinical innovation. Partnerships with community clinics and health providers in diverse settings will help elucidate organizational readiness and identify local barriers and facilitators for the implementation of ABGS. Ongoing and iterative feedback from clinical staff and providers will be needed to guide the development of strategies and supports that are responsive to the needs of health providers and parent partners.

The effective and equitable integration of genomic screening into health care for infants and children will require building trust with community partners in diverse settings to understand the kinds of information that should be sought after and how best to communicate that information. One method to forge such a relationship is through community advisory boards that have an iterative role in the development of research objectives and resources and providing guidance and recommendations as research advances [27]. Bidirectional and ongoing relationships between researchers, providers, and communities can promote trust and genetic literacy, develop resources to facilitate informed decision-making by families, and work toward an equitable uptake of genomic screening [55].

6. Conclusions

ABGS transforms the thought process from "what information should be returned?" (if genome-scale sequencing is performed) to "what information should we seek out, and when?" (for the greatest benefit in the general population). Although divergent from the currently prevailing notion that genome-scale sequencing will be imminently adopted as part of routine clinical care, ABGS could establish a new clinical practice paradigm and ultimately form a stable foundation for a more widespread adoption of evidence-based and genome-driven health care. It is also entirely compatible with a future in which genome-scale sequencing is in fact routine, providing a framework for supporting decision-making, analysis, and result disclosure that would allow parents to obtain periodic analyses of actionable conditions that are highly relevant to their child's developmental stage, and prepare individuals to receive sequencing results for carrier screening and actionable adult-onset conditions when they are able to assent or consent. Ultimately, our overarching goal should be to make the advances of genome sciences broadly available to the general population, maximizing the benefits and minimizing the harms.

Author Contributions: All authors have read and agreed to the published version of the manuscript.

Funding: This study was funded by NHGRI R01HG012271.

Conflicts of Interest: The authors declare no conflict of interest. The funders had no role in the design of the study; in the collection, analyses, or interpretation of data; in the writing of the manuscript, or in the decision to publish the results.

References

1. Biesecker, L.G.; Green, R.C. Diagnostic clinical genome and exome sequencing. *N. Engl. J. Med.* **2014**, *370*, 2418–2425. [CrossRef] [PubMed]
2. Strande, N.T.; Berg, J.S. Defining the Clinical Value of a Genomic Diagnosis in the Era of Next-Generation Sequencing. *Annu. Rev. Genomics Hum. Genet.* **2016**, *17*, 303–332. [CrossRef] [PubMed]
3. Willig, L.K.; Petrikin, J.E.; Smith, L.D.; Saunders, C.J.; Thiffault, I.; Miller, N.A.; Soden, S.E.; Cakici, J.A.; Herd, S.M.; Twist, G.; et al. Whole-genome sequencing for identification of Mendelian disorders in critically ill infants: A retrospective analysis of diagnostic and clinical findings. *Lancet Respir. Med.* **2015**, *3*, 377–387. [CrossRef]
4. Berg, J.S.; Powell, C.M. Potential Uses and Inherent Challenges of Using Genome-Scale Sequencing to Augment Current Newborn Screening. *Cold Spring Harb. Perspect. Med.* **2015**, *5*. [CrossRef] [PubMed]
5. Bailey, D.B. A window of opportunity for newborn screening. *Mol. Diagn. Ther.* **2022**, *26*, 253–261. [CrossRef] [PubMed]

6. Kingsmore, S.F.; Smith, L.D.; Kunard, C.M.; Bainbridge, M.; Batalov, S.; Benson, W.; Blincow, E.; Caylor, S.; Chambers, C.; Del Angel, G.; et al. A genome sequencing system for universal newborn screening, diagnosis, and precision medicine for severe genetic diseases. *Am. J. Hum. Genet.* **2022**, *109*, 1605–1619. [CrossRef]
7. Brothers, K.B.; Vassy, J.L.; Green, R.C. Reconciling opportunistic and population screening in clinical genomics. *Mayo Clin. Proc.* **2019**, *94*, 103–109. [CrossRef]
8. Joshi, E.; Mighton, C.; Clausen, M.; Casalino, S.; Kim, T.H.M.; Kowal, C.; Birken, C.; Maguire, J.L.; Bombard, Y. Primary care provider perspectives on using genomic sequencing in the care of healthy children. *Eur. J. Hum. Genet.* **2020**, *28*, 551–557. [CrossRef]
9. Kerruish, N. Parents' experiences 12 years after newborn screening for genetic susceptibility to type 1 diabetes and their attitudes to whole-genome sequencing in newborns. *Genet. Med.* **2016**, *18*, 249–258. [CrossRef]
10. Moultrie, R.R.; Paquin, R.; Rini, C.; Roche, M.I.; Berg, J.S.; Powell, C.M.; Lewis, M.A. Parental views on newborn next generation sequencing: Implications for decision support. *Matern. Child Health J.* **2020**, *24*, 856–864. [CrossRef]
11. Botkin, J.R.; Belmont, J.W.; Berg, J.S.; Berkman, B.E.; Bombard, Y.; Holm, I.A.; Levy, H.P.; Ormond, K.E.; Saal, H.M.; Spinner, N.B.; et al. Points to consider: Ethical, legal, and psychosocial implications of genetic testing in children and adolescents. *Am. J. Hum. Genet.* **2015**, *97*, 6–21. [CrossRef] [PubMed]
12. Ross, L.F.; Saal, H.M.; David, K.L.; Anderson, R.R. American Academy of Pediatrics; American College of Medical Genetics and Genomics Technical report: Ethical and policy issues in genetic testing and screening of children. *Genet. Med.* **2013**, *15*, 234–245. [CrossRef] [PubMed]
13. Johnston, J.; Lantos, J.D.; Goldenberg, A.; Chen, F.; Parens, E.; Koenig, B.A. Members of the NSIGHT Ethics and Policy Advisory Board Sequencing newborns: A call for nuanced use of genomic technologies. *Hastings Cent. Rep.* **2018**, *48 Suppl 2*, S2–S6. [CrossRef]
14. The American Academy of Pediatrics and Bright Futures 2017 recommendations for preventive pediatric health care. *Pediatrics* **2017**, *139*, e20170254. [CrossRef]
15. Mollison, L.; Berg, J.S. Genetic screening: Birthright or earned with age? *Expert Rev. Mol. Diagn.* **2017**, *17*, 735–738. [CrossRef] [PubMed]
16. Evans, J.P.; Berg, J.S.; Olshan, A.F.; Magnuson, T.; Rimer, B.K. We screen newborns, don't we?: Realizing the promise of public health genomics. *Genet. Med.* **2013**, *15*, 332–334. [CrossRef] [PubMed]
17. Murray, M.F.; Evans, J.P.; Khoury, M.J. DNA-Based Population Screening: Potential Suitability and Important Knowledge Gaps. *JAMA* **2020**, *323*, 307–308. [CrossRef]
18. Orlando, L.A.; Sperber, N.R.; Voils, C.; Nichols, M.; Myers, R.A.; Wu, R.R.; Rakhra-Burris, T.; Levy, K.D.; Levy, M.; Pollin, T.I.; et al. Developing a common framework for evaluating the implementation of genomic medicine interventions in clinical care: The IGNITE Network's Common Measures Working Group. *Genet. Med.* **2018**, *20*, 655–663. [CrossRef]
19. Weitzel, K.W.; Alexander, M.; Bernhardt, B.A.; Calman, N.; Carey, D.J.; Cavallari, L.H.; Field, J.R.; Hauser, D.; Junkins, H.A.; Levin, P.A.; et al. IGNITE Network The IGNITE network: A model for genomic medicine implementation and research. *BMC Med. Genomics* **2016**, *9*, 1. [CrossRef]
20. Zebrowski, A.M.; Ellis, D.E.; Barg, F.K.; Sperber, N.R.; Bernhardt, B.A.; Denny, J.C.; Dexter, P.R.; Ginsburg, G.S.; Horowitz, C.R.; Johnson, J.A.; et al. Qualitative study of system-level factors related to genomic implementation. *Genet. Med.* **2019**, *21*, 1534–1540. [CrossRef]
21. Amendola, L.M.; Berg, J.S.; Horowitz, C.R.; Angelo, F.; Bensen, J.T.; Biesecker, B.B.; Biesecker, L.G.; Cooper, G.M.; East, K.; Filipski, K.; et al. The Clinical Sequencing Evidence-Generating Research Consortium: Integrating Genomic Sequencing in Diverse and Medically Underserved Populations. *Am. J. Hum. Genet.* **2018**, *103*, 319–327. [CrossRef] [PubMed]
22. Khoury, M.J.; Feero, W.G.; Chambers, D.A.; Brody, L.C.; Aziz, N.; Green, R.C.; Janssens, A.C.J.W.; Murray, M.F.; Rodriguez, L.L.; Rutter, J.L.; et al. A collaborative translational research framework for evaluating and implementing the appropriate use of human genome sequencing to improve health. *PLoS Med.* **2018**, *15*, e1002631. [CrossRef]
23. Murray, M.F.; Evans, J.P.; Angrist, M.; Uhlmann, W.R.; Lochner Doyle, D.; Fullerton, S.M.; Ganiats, T.G.; Hagenkord, J.; Imhof, S.; Rim, S.H.; et al. A Proposed Approach for Implementing Genomics-Based Screening Programs for Healthy Adults. *NAM Perspectives* **2018**. [CrossRef]
24. Shen, E.C.; Srinivasan, S.; Passero, L.E.; Allen, C.G.; Dixon, M.; Foss, K.; Halliburton, B.; Milko, L.V.; Smit, A.K.; Carlson, R.; et al. Barriers and facilitators for population genetic screening in healthy populations: A systematic review. *Front. Genet.* **2022**, *13*, 865384. [CrossRef] [PubMed]
25. Sharma, Y.; Cox, L.; Kruger, L.; Channamsetty, V.; Haga, S.B. Evaluating primary care providers' readiness for delivering genetic and genomic services to underserved populations. *Public Health Genomics* **2021**, *25*, 1–10. [CrossRef]
26. Kaphingst, K.A.; Bather, J.R.; Daly, B.M.; Chavez-Yenter, D.; Vega, A.; Kohlmann, W.K. Interest in cancer predisposition testing and carrier screening offered as part of routine healthcare among an ethnically diverse sample of young women. *Front. Genet.* **2022**, *13*, 866062. [CrossRef] [PubMed]
27. Griesemer, I.; Staley, B.S.; Lightfoot, A.F.; Bain, L.; Byrd, D.; Conway, C.; Grant, T.L.; Leach, B.; Milko, L.; Mollison, L.; et al. Engaging community stakeholders in research on best practices for clinical genomic sequencing. *Per. Med.* **2020**, *17*, 435–444. [CrossRef]

28. Berg, J.S.; Khoury, M.J.; Evans, J.P. Deploying whole genome sequencing in clinical practice and public health: Meeting the challenge one bin at a time. *Genet. Med.* **2011**, *13*, 499–504. [CrossRef]
29. Berg, J.S.; Foreman, A.K.M.; O'Daniel, J.M.; Booker, J.K.; Boshe, L.; Carey, T.; Crooks, K.R.; Jensen, B.C.; Juengst, E.T.; Lee, K.; et al. A semiquantitative metric for evaluating clinical actionability of incidental or secondary findings from genome-scale sequencing. *Genet. Med.* **2016**, *18*, 467–475. [CrossRef]
30. Hunter, J.E.; Irving, S.A.; Biesecker, L.G.; Buchanan, A.; Jensen, B.; Lee, K.; Martin, C.L.; Milko, L.; Muessig, K.; Niehaus, A.D.; et al. A standardized, evidence-based protocol to assess clinical actionability of genetic disorders associated with genomic variation. *Genet. Med.* **2016**, *18*, 1258–1268. [CrossRef]
31. Hunter, J.E.; Jenkins, C.L.; Bulkley, J.E.; Gilmore, M.J.; Lee, K.; Pak, C.M.; Wallace, K.E.; Buchanan, A.H.; Foreman, A.K.M.; Freed, A.S.; et al. ClinGen ClinGen's Pediatric Actionability Working Group: Clinical actionability of secondary findings from genome-scale sequencing in children and adolescents. *Genet. Med.* **2022**, *24*, 1328–1335. [CrossRef] [PubMed]
32. Milko, L.V.; O'Daniel, J.M.; DeCristo, D.M.; Crowley, S.B.; Foreman, A.K.M.; Wallace, K.E.; Mollison, L.F.; Strande, N.T.; Girnary, Z.S.; Boshe, L.J.; et al. An Age-Based Framework for Evaluating Genome-Scale Sequencing Results in Newborn Screening. *J. Pediatr.* **2019**, *209*, 68–76. [CrossRef] [PubMed]
33. DeCristo, D.M.; Milko, L.V.; O'Daniel, J.M.; Foreman, A.K.M.; Mollison, L.F.; Powell, B.C.; Powell, C.M.; Berg, J.S. Actionability of commercial laboratory sequencing panels for newborn screening and the importance of transparency for parental decision-making. *Genome Med.* **2021**, *13*, 50. [CrossRef] [PubMed]
34. van der Pal, S.M.; Wins, S.; Klapwijk, J.E.; van Dijk, T.; Kater-Kuipers, A.; van der Ploeg, C.P.B.; Jans, S.M.P.J.; Kemp, S.; Verschoof-Puite, R.K.; van den Bosch, L.J.M.; et al. Parents' views on accepting, declining, and expanding newborn bloodspot screening. *PLoS ONE* **2022**, *17*, e0272585. [CrossRef]
35. Brownson, R.C.; Shelton, R.C.; Geng, E.H.; Glasgow, R.E. Revisiting concepts of evidence in implementation science. *Implement. Sci.* **2022**, *17*, 26. [CrossRef]
36. Milko, L.V.; Khoury, M.J. Editorial: DNA-based population screening for precision public health. *Front. Genet.* **2022**, *13*, 1061329. [CrossRef]
37. Kwan, B.M.; Brownson, R.C.; Glasgow, R.E.; Morrato, E.H.; Luke, D.A. Designing for dissemination and sustainability to promote equitable impacts on health. *Annu. Rev. Public Health* **2022**, *43*, 331–353. [CrossRef]
38. Shelton, R.C.; Adsul, P.; Oh, A.; Moise, N.; Griffith, D.M. Application of an antiracism lens in the field of implementation science (IS): Recommendations for reframing implementation research with a focus on justice and racial equity. *Implement. Res. Pract.* **2021**, *2*, 263348952110494. [CrossRef]
39. Horowitz, C.R.; Orlando, L.A.; Slavotinek, A.M.; Peterson, J.; Angelo, F.; Biesecker, B.; Bonham, V.L.; Cameron, L.D.; Fullerton, S.M.; Gelb, B.D.; et al. The genomic medicine integrative research framework: A conceptual framework for conducting genomic medicine research. *Am. J. Hum. Genet.* **2019**, *104*, 1088–1096. [CrossRef]
40. Ginsburg, G.S.; Horowitz, C.R.; Orlando, L.A. What will it take to implement genomics in practice? Lessons from the IGNITE Network. *Per. Med.* **2019**, *16*, 259–261. [CrossRef]
41. Damschroder, L.J.; Aron, D.C.; Keith, R.E.; Kirsh, S.R.; Alexander, J.A.; Lowery, J.C. Fostering implementation of health services research findings into practice: A consolidated framework for advancing implementation science. *Implement. Sci.* **2009**, *4*, 50. [CrossRef] [PubMed]
42. Kirk, M.A.; Kelley, C.; Yankey, N.; Birken, S.A.; Abadie, B.; Damschroder, L. A systematic review of the use of the Consolidated Framework for Implementation Research. *Implement. Sci.* **2016**, *11*, 72. [CrossRef] [PubMed]
43. IGNITE Toolbox. Available online: https://gmkb.org/ignite-toolbox-overview/ (accessed on 3 March 2020).
44. Clinical Sequencing Evidence-Generating Research CSER Research Materials. Available online: https://cser-consortium.org/cser-research-materials (accessed on 12 August 2020).
45. Halley, M.C.; Young, J.L.; Fernandez, L.; Kohler, J.N.; Undiagnosed Diseases Network; Bernstein, J.A.; Wheeler, M.T.; Tabor, H.K. Perceived utility and disutility of genomic sequencing for pediatric patients: Perspectives from parents with diverse sociodemographic characteristics. *Am. J. Med. Genet. A* **2022**, *188*, 1088–1101. [CrossRef] [PubMed]
46. Downie, L.; Halliday, J.; Lewis, S.; Amor, D.J. Principles of genomic newborn screening programs: A systematic review. *JAMA Netw. Open* **2021**, *4*, e2114336. [CrossRef] [PubMed]
47. Goldenberg, A.J. Considering equity in assessing familial benefit from the return of genomic research results. *Pediatrics* **2019**, *144*, e20193111. [CrossRef]
48. Henderson, G.E.; Ewing, M.; Kuczynski, K.J.; Cadigan, R.J.; Waltz, M.; Butterfield, R.M.; Rini, C.; Weck, K.; Berg, J.S.; Edwards, T.P. Development and validation of a measure of comprehension of genomic screening-negative results (CoG-NR). *Eur. J. Hum. Genet.* **2020**, *28*, 1394–1402. [CrossRef]
49. Hendricks-Sturrup, R.M.; Linsky, A.; Lu, C.Y.; Vassy, J.L. Genomic testing is best integrated into clinical practice when it is actionable. *Per. Med.* **2020**, *17*, 5–8. [CrossRef]
50. Waltz, M.; Meagher, K.M.; Henderson, G.E.; Goddard, K.A.; Muessig, K.; Berg, J.S.; Weck, K.E.; Cadigan, R.J. Assessing the implications of positive genomic screening results. *Per. Med.* **2020**, *17*, 101–109. [CrossRef]
51. Borry, P.; Goffin, T.; Nys, H.; Dierickx, K. Attitudes regarding predictive genetic testing in minors: A survey of European clinical geneticists. *Am. J. Med. Genet. C Semin. Med. Genet.* **2008**, *148C*, 78–83. [CrossRef]

52. Borry, P.; Evers-Kiebooms, G.; Cornel, M.C.; Clarke, A.; Dierickx, K. Public and Professional Policy Committee (PPPC) of the European Society of Human Genetics (ESHG) Genetic testing in asymptomatic minors: Background considerations towards ESHG Recommendations. *Eur. J. Hum. Genet.* **2009**, *17*, 711–719. [CrossRef]
53. Knoppers, B.M.; Sénécal, K.; Borry, P.; Avard, D. Whole-genome sequencing in newborn screening programs. *Sci. Transl. Med.* **2014**, *6*, 229cm2. [CrossRef] [PubMed]
54. Shkedi-Rafid, S.; Fenwick, A.; Dheensa, S.; Lucassen, A.M. Genetic testing of children for adult-onset conditions: Opinions of the British adult population and implications for clinical practice. *Eur. J. Hum. Genet.* **2015**, *23*, 1281–1285. [CrossRef] [PubMed]
55. Powell, S.N.; Byfield, G.; Bennetone, A.; Frantz, A.M.; Harrison, L.K.; James-Crook, E.R.; Osborne, H.; Owens, T.H.; Shaw, J.L.; O'Daniel, J.; et al. Parental guidance suggested: Engaging parents as partners in research studies of genomic screening for a pediatric population. *Front. Genet.* **2022**, *13*, 867030. [CrossRef] [PubMed]

International Journal of
Neonatal Screening

MDPI

Review

Select Ethical Aspects of Next-Generation Sequencing Tests for Newborn Screening and Diagnostic Evaluation of Critically Ill Newborns

Kuntal Sen [1], Jennifer Harmon [2] and Andrea L. Gropman [1,*]

1 Division of Neurogenetics and Developmental Pediatrics, Center for Neuroscience and Behavioral Medicine, Children's National Hospital, Washington, DC 20010, USA; ksen2@childrensnational.org
2 Rare Disease Institute, Children's National Hospital, Washington, DC 20010, USA; jharmon2@childrensnational.org
* Correspondence: agropman@childrensnational.org; Tel.: +1-202-476-3511; Fax: +1-202-476-4336

Abstract: In this review, we analyze medical and select ethical aspects of the increasing use of next-generation sequencing (NGS) based tests in newborn medicine. In the last five years, there have been several studies exploring the role of rapid exome sequencing (ES) and genome sequencing (GS) in critically ill newborns. While the advantages include a high diagnostic yield with potential changes in interventions, there have been ethical dilemmas surrounding consent, information about adult-onset diseases and resolution of variants of uncertain significance. Another active area of research includes a cohort of studies funded under Newborn Sequencing in Genomic Medicine and Public Health pertaining to the use of ES and GS in newborn screening (NBS). While these techniques may allow for screening for several genetic disorders that do not have a detectable biochemical marker, the high costs and long turnaround times of these tests are barriers in their utilization as public health screening tests. Discordant results between conventional NBS and ES-based NBS, as well as challenges with consent, are other potential pitfalls of this approach. Please see the Bush, Al-Hertani and Bodamer article in this Special Issue for the broader scope and further discussion.

Keywords: critically ill newborns; ethics; genomic sequencing; newborn screening; policy; rapid whole exome sequencing; rapid whole genome sequencing

1. Introduction

With the rapid evolution of molecular genetics, next-generation sequencing (NGS) testing methods such as exome sequencing (ES) and genome sequencing (GS) are being increasingly used for diagnostic evaluation of critically ill infants as well as for newborn screening (NBS) [1–3]. They have been applauded for the promise they hold for the prompt and precise diagnosis of pre-symptomatic as well as sick infants. However, there are several psychosocial and ethical dilemmas surrounding the use of these tests under these circumstances that require discussion. Many of these issues have been historically associated with ES and GS, in general; however, other challenges are unique regarding their use in neonatal medicine.

2. Next-Generation Sequencing for Newborn Screening

In the past few years, there have been several studies by various groups to explore the use of NGS-based tests such as ES and GS for NBS. While these techniques may enable clinicians to screen for rare diseases that do not have any reliable biochemical markers, there are several moral caveats to be considered. [1,2,4].

NBS was designed as a universal cost-effective screening test aimed at early detection of treatable hereditary (and a few non-hereditary) conditions to prevent long-term mortality and morbidity [5]. The test utilizes dried blood spots from heel prick samples obtained typically on day one of life. The test screens for an array of monogenic inborn errors of metabolism (IEM), in addition to endocrine disorders, hemoglobinopathies and immunodeficiency syndromes [6]. The Advisory Committee on Hereditary Disorders in Newborns and Children (ACHDNC) makes recommendations to the individual states I the USA regarding potential new disorders to be added to the NBS. Currently, there are 35 core and 26 secondary conditions on the recommended uniform screening panel (RUSP). The American College of Medical Genetics publishes action sheets (or ACT sheets) for positive screens, to provide uniform practice guidelines for pediatricians, neonatologists and biochemical geneticists [7]. Some conditions which may present with metabolic crisis (e.g., organic acidemia) and warrant prompt evaluation in an inpatient setting, whereas others with insidious onset (e.g., phenylketonuria) are followed up in an outpatient setting.

Robert Guthrie devoted several years to developing the first screening test utilizing the bacterial inhibition assay for phenylketonuria [8]. The NBS is often referred to as 'the PKU test,' which remains a testimony to his career. The introduction of tandem mass spectrometry (MS/MS) revolutionized the landscape of NBS as the technique allowed screening for many disorders due to its ability to measure several analytes (plasma amino acids and the acylcarnitine profile) simultaneously [9]. The testing laboratories utilize national databases to determine the cut-off values for analytes and sometimes may involve second-tier tests. In the last decade, with the discovery of novel therapies, other disorders including storage diseases, X-linked adrenoleukodystrophy (X-ALD) and spinal muscular atrophy have been included in the RUSP for several states, which use different technologies for the screening test [10–14]. The literature suggests that screening for X-ALD poses a plethora of dilemmas, and there have been ongoing modifications to the follow-up protocol. The challenges include establishing contact with other family members across different generations who may be affected based on an X-linked inheritance pattern, and care co-ordination with sequential neuroimaging to identify those who will develop the cerebral form of the disease [15]. Massively parallel sequencing such as ES and GS has been used abundantly for diagnostic evaluation of pediatric genetic diseases, and clinical researchers finally decided to interrogate its potential for NBS [14]. The National Human Genome Research Institute funded a cohort of studies to evaluate the medical, economic and psychosocial effects of integrating exome sequencing (ES) for NBS, which led to the formation of Newborn Sequencing in Genomic Medicine and Public Health.

North Carolina Newborn Exome Sequencing for Universal Screening (NC NEXUS) enrolled 106 newborns and children with previously diagnosed metabolic diseases and hearing loss, and ES results confirmed an underlying diagnosis in 88% and 18% of the patients, respectively. The results included pathogenic variants in hereditary cancer syndromes in two children, and 1.8 variants per patient showing a carrier status for recessive conditions [1]. The BabySeq Project is another noteworthy study from this cohort. The group enrolled and randomized half of the families of newborns from Brigham Women's Hospital and Boston Children's Hospital to receive ES-based NBS. Out of 159 newborns enrolled, 15 were found to be at risk of childhood-onset conditions. Risk of adult-onset diseases, a carrier status and pharmacogenomic variants were detected in 3.5%, 88% and 5% of subjects, respectively. Testing parental samples resulted in interpretation of variants in 8% of cases [2,4].

Utilization of ES-based NBS is advantageous as it allows for screening of several monogenic conditions that do not have a consistent analyte that can be measured using MS/MS. For instance, mitochondrial disorders and proximal urea cycle disorders have historically been impossible to screen, despite the availability of therapies and interventions [16,17]. ES-based NBS could also shorten the diagnostic odysseys for those genetic diseases where there is no precise treatment, but where early diagnosis can have a significant impact on the medical care and parental perspectives. However, this rationale defies the very ethos of the Wilson and Jungner criteria, which emphasize the actionability of the disorder and cost-effectiveness of the test as the core principles of NBS [18]. The high costs and long turnaround times of NGS are obvious barriers in the current scenario, which hinder its integration as a widespread public health screening test [6]. There are also studies that suggest that the results of conventional NBS and ES-based NBS may be discordant, and the latter alone may not very specific in screening for IEM [19,20].

While shortening the diagnostic journey for infants who are sick can substantially change family's viewpoints, diagnosis of childhood-onset conditions and carrier status can cause untold and unwarranted anxiety [1,3,4]. The BabySeq project did include an option to disclose the results of adult-onset conditions and applied a post-consent survey to better delineate parental perspectives [2]. NBS has always been an 'opt out' rather than an 'opt in' test, where families are required to actively decline it if they do not wish for their newborn to receive it. This is based on the dramatic success of the program, which has led to the slogan "newborn screening saves lives." Parents often do not understand the purpose and process of NBS. If ES or GS were ever to become a standardized screening tool, the consenting process would need to be robust and standardized, as was proposed in the pilot studies. Reporting and resolution of variants of uncertain significance may pose several challenges for the molecular genetics laboratories as well as the clinical teams following up with these families [21]. The follow-up testing and clinic visits secondary to unclear results have been known to cause substantial financial and psychological strain for families even with the conventional NBS, and this can only be accentuated with the incorporation of ES-based NBS, unless meticulous consent and education can be ensured [2,6,22,23]. As per recommendations from the Pediatric Task Force of the Global Alliance for Genomics and Health, each jurisdiction needs to resolve ethical and policy issues regarding the disclosure of incidental or secondary findings to families, as well as the ownership, appropriate storage and sharing of genomic data. Ultimately, the best interests of children should form the basis of all decisions [21]. Since medical geneticists, genetic counsellors and metabolic dietitians are still a small group, such a drastic upgrade in NBS may also cause disruption to the access to and uniformity of care [24].

3. Next-Generation Sequencing for Diagnostic Evaluation of Critically Ill Newborns

While the newborn screening programs and the BabySeq project have focused on predicting and preventing future disease in pre-symptomatic infants with genetic disorders, another active area of investigation has focused on the use of rapid genomic sequencing techniques in the evaluation of critically ill infants.

Studies have estimated that genetic diseases are present in approximately 16% of neonates in regional ICUs; furthermore, there is high mortality in infants with genetic diseases, which accounts for an estimated 20% of deaths in this age group, and in one center, accounted for an estimated 45% of neonatal intensive care unit (NICU) deaths over a ten-year period [25,26]. It is proposed that the primary benefits of early genetic diagnosis in these patients include both the rapid implementation of targeted interventions that may decrease morbidity, as well as the rapid identification of likely futile intensive care in the course of what may otherwise be a protracted diagnostic approach during, which parents may experience "inappropriate hope" or "needless guilt." Meanwhile, secondary benefits may include guiding parents regarding the risk of recurrence in future children as well as possible overall healthcare cost reductions [1,27].

Since 2015, several studies have sought to investigate the clinical utility of genomic sequencing in the NICU setting (Table 1). In these studies, the percentage of patients receiving a genetic diagnosis as a result of NGS has ranged from 21 to 57%, with results returned in a range of 2.3 to 95 days and the majority of studies utilizing rapid exome or genome sequencing and returning the results in fewer than 21 days (Table 2) [28–34]. Comparatively, a retrospective study comparing the diagnostic yield of genomic testing showed similar diagnostic sensitivity of rapid whole genome sequencing (rWGS), with 43% of infants receiving a genetic diagnosis compared to only 10% diagnostic sensitivity in infants who underwent a standard genetic testing protocol; similarly, another research group obtained a genetic diagnosis for 8/20 critically ill newborns using a targeted gene panel approach based on phenotypic presentation, and was able to obtain a genetic diagnosis for an additional five patients when whole exome sequencing (WES) was offered to those patients with a negative gene panel [35,36]. Interestingly, one study showed that the phenotype of neonates was a poor predictor of the underlying genotype in 90% of patients evaluated in the ICU setting with WGS, suggesting that standard genetic evaluation would likely delay the diagnosis for the majority of these critically ill patients [31]. These conclusions were supported by the results of the NSIGHT2 trial, in which a subset of patients was selected to receive ultrarapid whole genome sequencing (urWGS) as a first-tier diagnostic; in general, these patients were more unstable and had differential diagnoses that included rare disorders requiring specific targeted therapies to prevent morbidity and mortality [34]. While urWGS was more costly than the other testing modalities (rWES and rWGS) evaluated in this study, the percentage of patients that received a genetic diagnosis was significantly greater in the urWGS cohort, with a similarly greater proportion of infants in that group receiving a diagnosis for which immediate intervention was available [33].

Table 1. Summary of studies investigating clinical feasibility and utility of NGS in critically ill neonates.

Authors	Year Published	Study Design	Patient Location	Type of Test	Medium Turnaround Time
Willig et al.	2015	Retrospective	NICU/PICU	Trio rWGS	23 days
Van Diemen et al.	2017	Prospective	NICU/PICU (Age < 1 year)	rWGS	12 days
Meng et al.	2017	Retrospective	NICU/PICU/CICU	WES (proband only/trio/rapid trio)	Proband WES: 95 days Trio WES: 51 days rWES: 13 days
French et al.	2019	Prospective	NICU/PICU	Trio rWGS	27 days
Elliott et al.	2019	Prospect	NICU	Trio rWES	7.2 days *
Kingsmore et al.	2019	RCT	NICU/PICU/CICU	urWGS/rWGS/rWES	urWGS: 2–3 days rWGS/rWES: 11.8 days
Freed et al.	2020	Prospective	NICU/PICU/CICU	Trio rWES	9 days

NICU, neonatal intensive care unit; PICU, pediatric intensive care unit; CICU, cardiac intensive care unit; WES, whole exome sequencing; WGS, whole genome sequencing; rWES, rapid whole exome sequencing; rWGS, rapid whole genome sequencing; urWGS, ultra-rapid whole genome sequencing, RCT, randomized clinical trial. * Time to preliminary results.

Table 2. Results of studies investigating clinical feasibility and utility of NGS in critically ill neonates.

Authors	Number of Participants	Number of Diagnoses	Number with Changes in Management	Number with Escalation of Care	Number with Limitation of Care
Willig et al.	35	rWGS 20/35 (57%)	13	6	6
Van Diemen et al.	23	7/23 (30%)	Not reported	Not reported	Not reported
Meng et al.	278	102 (36.7%) Subset: rWES 32/63 (50.8%)	53 Subset rWES: 23/32	12	19
French et al.	195	40 (21%)	12	5	7
Elliott et al.	25	18 (72%)	15	4	3
Kingsmore et al.	213	49 (24%) urWGS 11/24 (46%) rWGS 18/94 (19%) rWES 19/95 (20%)	Not reported	Not reported	Not reported
Freed et al.	46	20 (43%)	24	5	5

rWES, rapid whole exome sequencing; rWGS, rapid whole genome sequencing; urWGS, ultra-rapid whole genome sequencing.

The majority of these studies have quantified changes in management as a secondary measure and have shown repeatedly that these NGS results and subsequent genetic diagnoses have a direct impact on the decisions made by clinicians and families. These changes have encompassed both escalation in patient care (e.g., placement of a gastrotomy tube in a patient determined to have chronic feeding difficulties), as well as limitations in care (e.g., deferral of heart transplant in a patient expected to have a poor neurological prognosis) [28,30–32,34]. In addition to exploring the impact of rWES on acute ICU management, the most recent study reported by Freed et al. demonstrated the feasibility of implementing a rapid genomic sequencing protocol using a commercial send-out lab rather than an internal research-based testing platform, and included a full informed consent process with the option to receive secondary results [34]. As these studies have continued to consistently show a high yield of diagnoses contributing to alterations in management, and as commercial platforms have made these diagnostic modalities more accessible, a question has emerged: should rapid genomic sequencing be considered the standard of care for initial genetic diagnostic evaluation in critically ill infants? At the same time, a second question has also moved more clearly into focus: what are the ethical implications and challenges of utilizing genomic sequencing in the intensive care setting?

While the feasibility of rapid genomic sequencing for the timely diagnosis of suspected monogenic disorders in critically ill newborns has emerged only over the last decade, much accompanying literature over the same time period explores the potential technical and ethical concerns that may limit the widespread adoption of this testing approach. These include the current payer system that typically reimburses only outpatient genomic studies, the challenge of timely resolution of variants of unknown significance (VUS) and the possible impacts of rapid transition to genetic testing on parental anxiety and subsequent parent-infant bonding [27,37]. One of the most often and extensively discussed ethical concerns is the question of secondary findings, including the reporting of childhood-onset diseases not related to the patient's clinical presentation at the time of testing, and even more fraught, the reporting of adult-onset diseases. One case report in the literature from the BabySeq project highlights the moral distress felt by study researchers upon finding a *BRCA2* mutation in a male infant whose parents had not consented to receive information regarding adult-onset disease [38]. As a result of this moral distress, the research team approached the IRB for permission to re-consent the family to receive information regarding adult-onset disease. In this case, the study protocol was changed so as to enroll only families who would consent to receiving information about adult-onset diseases, so as to avoid further ethical dilemmas and subsequent moral distress for laboratory personnel who could ostensibly know information regarding an actionable disease with no recourse to provide that information to the person it most directly affected [38]. While some researchers have argued that testing for genetic susceptibilities to adult-onset diseases is a potential violation of the future autonomy of the infant who has undergone genomic testing, others have developed ethical models that consider the interests of the family as a unit, in which the wellbeing of the infant undergoing testing is dependent on the wellbeing of the family unit as a whole [39,40]. With the specific example of this child found to have a *BRCA2* mutation, the potential impact of this autosomal, dominant adult-onset condition on the health and mortality of the child's affected parent was considered a threat to the wellbeing of the family unit, which posed a credible downstream threat to the patient's health as well [40,41].

Another ethical consideration is access to these technologies, which is limited by several factors, including availability of in-house testing and the associated costs of genomic testing in the setting of uncertainty regarding the likelihood of insurance reimbursement for these testing strategies. Several studies have suggested that panel-based testing could prove a reasonable alternative strategy to accomplish rapid diagnosis in the ICU setting, with the proposed benefits of ensuring that a greater number of patients in need of these rapid diagnoses receive them, while also decreasing costs. In one study, a panel of 4503 genes was utilized for rapid evaluation of critically ill neonates; in the study, this panel-based approach yielded a diagnosis in 10/20 (50%) cases and a partial diagnosis in an additional 1/20 (5%) cases, similar to those results reported in the genomic sequencing studies referenced in Table 2 [42]. Furthermore, the panel-based approach cost $6000 in this study compared to the ~$16,000–$17,500 cost reported for rWGS in other studies [42]. Despite these encouraging results suggesting possible non-inferiority of the panel-based approach, issues may arise from inconsistencies in variant detection between two modalities; for example, the GEMINI study, which directly compared the results of a sequencing panel containing 1722 genes to rWGS, demonstrated discordance between the two platforms in 27% of diagnoses [43]. While many of these were due to technical differences between the platforms, generally stemming from the known inability of the sequencing panel to detect copy number variants, a number resulted from discordance in variant analysis both with respect to the algorithms used to detect and filter variants as well as the methods used to analyze the pathogenicity of detected variants [43]. These findings demonstrate that technical factors add an additional layer of complexity into this process, necessitating an even more nuanced consideration when balancing all the factors that may influence the utility of one diagnostic strategy over another, especially regarding the potentially extensive amount of data analysis required for interpretation of genomic sequencing compared to the inherently more focused datasets resulting from panel-based approaches.

As sequencing platforms and informatic systems designed to quickly analyze large amounts of genomic data become increasingly agile, and as these testing modalities become increasingly available through commercial means, the likelihood that institutions will transition toward genomic sequencing as a first-line genetic testing strategy continues to increase. As such, our resolve to tackle and mitigate the ethical concerns that accompany these testing modalities must continue to strengthen as well.

4. Conclusions

This paper reviewed select ethical aspects regarding the use of ES and GS in NBS and in the diagnostic evaluation of critically ill newborns (please see the Bush, Al-Hertani and Bodamer article in this Special Issue for the broader scope and further discussion). The clinical utility and cost-effectiveness of NGS-based NBS are yet to be established. Dr. Francis Collins, NIH Director, has remarked: " … *whether you like it or not, a complete sequencing of newborns is not far away*" [44]. Genomic sequencing has caused a paradigm shift in the diagnosis of orphan diseases and will inevitably become a part of newborn screening in the near future. Yet, communities of medical geneticists, neonatologists, molecular geneticists and policymakers need to come together as a team to carefully analyze the findings of the pilot studies and improve on the shortcomings of the technique before this can become a reality. In the critically ill population, despite the potential pitfalls, multiple studies have demonstrated that both clinicians and parents have overwhelmingly positive impressions of the impact of rapid genomic sequencing in the ICU setting, regardless of whether the result returned was diagnostic [45–47].

Author Contributions: Conceptualization, A.L.G. and J.H.; methodology, K.S. and J.H.; software, N/A; validation, N/A formal analysis, K.S. and J.H.; investigation, K.S. and J.H.; resources, K.S. and J.H.; data curation, K.S. and J.H.; writing—original draft preparation, K.S. and J.H.; writing—review and editing, K.S., A.L.G. and J.H.; visualization, K.S. and J.H.; supervision, A.L.G.; project administration, A.L.G.; funding acquisition, A.L.G. All authors have read and agreed to the published version of the manuscript.

Funding: This research received no external funding.

Conflicts of Interest: The authors declare no conflict of interest.

References

1. Roman, T.S.; Crowley, S.B.; Roche, M.I.; Foreman, A.K.M.; O'Daniel, J.M.; Seifert, B.A.; Lee, K.; Brandt, A.; Gustafson, C.; DeCristo, D.M.; et al. Genomic Sequencing for Newborn Screening: Results of the NC NEXUS Project. *Am. J. Hum. Genet.* **2020**, *107*, 596–611. [CrossRef]
2. Holm, I.A.; Agrawal, P.B.; Ceyhan-Birsoy, O.; Christensen, K.D.; Fayer, S.; Frankel, L.A.; Genetti, C.A.; Krier, J.B.; LaMay, R.C.; Levy, H.L.; et al. The BabySeq project: Implementing genomic sequencing in newborns. *BMC Pediatr.* **2018**, *18*, 225. [CrossRef] [PubMed]

3. Saunders, C.J.; Miller, N.A.; Soden, S.E.; Dinwiddie, D.L.; Noll, A.; Alnadi, N.A.; Andraws, N.; Patterson, M.L.; Krivohlavek, L.A.; Fellis, J.; et al. Rapid whole-genome sequencing for genetic disease diagnosis in neonatal intensive care units. *Sci. Transl. Med.* **2012**, *4*, 154ra135. [CrossRef]
4. Ceyhan-Birsoy, O.; Murry, J.B.; Machini, K.; Lebo, M.S.; Yu, T.W.; Fayer, S.; Genetti, C.A.; Schwartz, T.S.; Agrawal, P.B.; Parad, R.B.; et al. Interpretation of Genomic Sequencing Results in Healthy and Ill Newborns: Results from the BabySeq Project. *Am. J. Hum. Genet.* **2019**, *104*, 76–93. [CrossRef]
5. El-Hattab, A.W.; Almannai, M.; Sutton, V.R. Newborn Screening: History, Current Status, and Future Directions. *Pediatr. Clin. N. Am.* **2017**, *65*, 389–405. [CrossRef] [PubMed]
6. Fabie, N.A.V.; Pappas, K.B.; Feldman, G.L. The Current State of Newborn Screening in the United States. *Pediatr. Clin. N. Am.* **2019**, *66*, 369–386. [CrossRef] [PubMed]
7. American College of Medical Genetics Newborn Screening Expert Group. Newborn screening: Toward a uniform screening panel and system–executive summary. *Pediatrics* **2006**, *117*, S296–S307. [CrossRef]
8. Guthrie, R.; Susi, A. A simple phenylalanine method for detecting phenylketonuria in large populations of newborn infants. *Pediatrics* **1963**, *32*, 338–343. [PubMed]
9. Millington, D.S.; Kodo, N.; Norwood, D.L.; Roe, C.R. Tandem mass spectrometry: A new method for acylcarnitine profiling with potential for neonatal screening for inborn errors of metabolism. *J. Inherit. Metab. Dis.* **1990**, *13*, 321–324. [CrossRef]
10. Matern, D.; Gavrilov, D.; Oglesbee, D.; Raymond, K.; Rinaldo, P.; Tortorelli, S. Newborn screening for lysosomal storage disorders. *Semin. Perinatol.* **2015**, *39*, 206–216. [CrossRef]
11. Wasserstein, M.P.; Andriola, M.; Arnold, G.; Aron, A.; Duffner, P.; Erbe, R.W.; Escolar, M.L.; Estrella, L.; Galvin-Parton, P.; Iglesias, A.; et al. Clinical outcomes of children with abnormal newborn screening results for Krabbe disease in New York State. *Genet. Med.* **2016**, *18*, 1235–1243. [CrossRef]
12. Kemper, A.R.; Brosco, J.; Comeau, A.M.; Green, N.; Grosse, S.D.; Jones, E.; Kwon, J.M.; Lam, W.K.; Ojodu, J.; Prosser, L.A.; et al. Newborn screening for X-linked adrenoleukodystrophy: Evidence summary and advisory committee recommendation. *Genet. Med.* **2016**, *19*, 121–126. [CrossRef]
13. Boardman, F.K.; Young, P.J.; Griffiths, F.E. Newborn screening for spinal muscular atrophy: The views of affected families and adults. *Am. J. Med. Genet. A* **2017**, *173*, 1546–1561. [CrossRef]
14. Botkin, J.R.; Rothwell, E. Whole Genome Sequencing and Newborn Screening. *Curr. Genet. Med. Rep.* **2016**, *4*, 1–6. [CrossRef]
15. Hall, P.L.; Li, H.; Hagar, A.F.; Jerris, S.C.; Wittenauer, A.; Wilcox, W. Newborn Screening for X-Linked Adrenoleukodystrophy in Georgia: Experiences from a Pilot Study Screening of 51,081 Newborns. *Int. J. Neonatal. Screen.* **2020**, *6*, 81. [CrossRef] [PubMed]
16. Vasquez-Loarte, T.; Thompson, J.D.; Merritt, J.L., 2nd. Considering Proximal Urea Cycle Disorders in Expanded Newborn Screening. *Int. J. Neonatal. Screen.* **2020**, *6*, 77. [CrossRef]
17. Peretz, R.H.; Mew, N.A.; Vernon, H.J.; Ganetzky, R.D. Prospective diagnosis of MT-ATP6-related mitochondrial disease by newborn screening. *Mol. Genet. Metab.* **2021**, *134*, 37–42. [CrossRef]
18. Wilson, J.; Jungner, J. *Principles and Practices of Screening for Disease*; Public Health Papers; World Health Organization: Geneva, Switzerland, 1968; p. 34.
19. Adhikari, A.N.; Gallagher, R.C.; Wang, Y.; Currier, R.J.; Amatuni, G.; Bassaganyas, L.; Chen, F.; Kundu, K.; Kvale, M.; Mooney, S.D.; et al. The role of exome sequencing in newborn screening for inborn errors of metabolism. *Nat. Med.* **2020**, *26*, 1392–1397. [CrossRef] [PubMed]
20. Wojcik, M.H.; Zhang, T.; Ceyhan-Birsoy, O.; Genetti, C.A.; Lebo, M.S.; Yu, T.W.; Parad, R.B.; Holm, I.A.; Rehm, H.L.; Beggs, A.H.; et al. Discordant results between conventional newborn screening and genomic sequencing in the BabySeq Project. *Genet. Med.* **2021**, *23*, 1372–1375. [CrossRef]
21. Friedman, J.M.; Cornel, M.C.; Goldenberg, A.J.; Lister, K.J.; Sénécal, K.; Vears, D.F.; Global Alliance for Genomics and Health Regulatory and Ethics Working Group Paediatric Task Team. Genomic newborn screening: Public health policy considerations and recommendations. *BMC Med. Genom.* **2017**, *10*, 9. [CrossRef] [PubMed]
22. Tarini, B.A.; Goldenberg, A.J. Ethical issues with newborn screening in the genomics era. *Annu. Rev. Genom. Hum. Genet.* **2012**, *13*, 381–393. [CrossRef] [PubMed]
23. Ross, L.F.; Saal, H.M.; David, K.L.; Anderson, R.R.; American Academy of Pediatrics; American College of Medical Genetics and Genomics. Technical report: Ethical and policy issues in genetic testing and screening of children. *Genet. Med.* **2013**, *15*, 234–245. [CrossRef]
24. Reinstein, E. Challenges of using next generation sequencing in newborn screening. *Genet. Res.* **2015**, *97*, e21. [CrossRef] [PubMed]
25. Kingsmore, S.F.; Henderson, A.; Owen, M.J.; Clark, M.M.; Hansen, C.; Dimmock, D.; Chambers, C.D.; Jeliffe-Pawlowski, L.L.; Hobbs, C. Measurement of genetic diseases as a cause of mortality in infants receiving whole genome sequencing. *NPJ Genom. Med.* **2020**, *5*, 49. [CrossRef] [PubMed]
26. Weiner, J.; Sharma, J.; Lantos, J.; Kilbride, H. How infants die in the neonatal intensive care unit: Trends from 1999 through 2008. *Arch. Pediatr. Adolesc. Med.* **2011**, *165*, 630–634. [CrossRef] [PubMed]
27. Berg, J.S.; Agrawal, P.B.; Bailey, D.B.; Beggs, A.H.; Brenner, S.E.; Brower, A.M.; Cakici, J.A.; Ceyhan-Birsoy, O.; Chan, K.; Chen, F.; et al. Newborn Sequencing in Genomic Medicine and Public Health. *Pediatrics* **2017**, *139*, e20162252. [CrossRef]

28. Willig, L.K.; Petrikin, J.E.; Smith, L.D.; Saunders, C.J.; Thiffault, I.; Miller, N.A.; Soden, S.E.; Cakici, J.A.; Herd, S.M.; Twist, G.; et al. Whole-genome sequencing for identification of Mendelian disorders in critically ill infants: A retrospective analysis of diagnostic and clinical findings. *Lancet Respir. Med.* **2015**, *3*, 377–387. [CrossRef]
29. Van Diemen, C.C.; Kerstjens-Frederikse, W.S.; Bergman, K.A.; De Koning, T.J.; Sikkema-Raddatz, B.; Van Der Velde, J.K.; Abbott, K.M.; Herkert, J.C.; Löhner, K.; Rump, P.; et al. Rapid Targeted Genomics in Critically Ill Newborns. *Pediatrics* **2017**, *140*, e20162854. [CrossRef]
30. Meng, L.; Pammi, M.; Saronwala, A.; Magoulas, P.; Ghazi, A.R.; Vetrini, F.; Zhang, J.; He, W.; Dharmadhikari, A.V.; Qu, C.; et al. Use of Exome Sequencing for Infants in Intensive Care Units: Ascertainment of Severe Single-Gene Disorders and Effect on Medical Management. *JAMA Pediatr.* **2017**, *171*, e173438. [CrossRef]
31. French, C.E.; Delon, I.; Dolling, H.; Sanchis-Juan, A.; Shamardina, O.; Mégy, K.; Abbs, S.; Austin, T.; Bowdin, S.; Branco, R.G.; et al. Whole genome sequencing reveals that genetic conditions are frequent in intensively ill children. *Intensive Care Med.* **2019**, *45*, 627–636. [CrossRef]
32. Elliott, A.M.; du Souich, C.; Lehman, A.; Guella, I.; Evans, D.M.; Candido, T.; Tooman, L.; Armstrong, L.; Clarke, L.; Gibson, W.; et al. RAPIDOMICS: Rapid genome-wide sequencing in a neonatal intensive care unit—Successes and challenges. *Eur. J. Pediatr.* **2019**, *178*, 1207–1218. [CrossRef] [PubMed]
33. Kingsmore, S.F.; Cakici, J.A.; Clark, M.M.; Gaughran, M.; Feddock, M.; Batalov, S.; Bainbridge, M.N.; Carroll, J.; Caylor, S.A.; Clarke, C.; et al. A Randomized, Controlled Trial of the Analytic and Diagnostic Performance of Singleton and Trio, Rapid Genome and Exome Sequencing in Ill Infants. *Am. J. Hum. Genet.* **2019**, *105*, 719–733. [CrossRef] [PubMed]
34. Freed, A.S.; Clowes Candadai, S.V.; Sikes, M.C.; Thies, J.; Byers, H.M.; Dines, J.N.; Ndugga-Kabuye, M.K.; Smith, M.B.; Fogus, K.; Mefford, H.C.; et al. The Impact of Rapid Exome Sequencing on Medical Management of Critically Ill Children. *J. Pediatr.* **2020**, *226*, 202–212.e1. [CrossRef] [PubMed]
35. Farnaes, L.; Hildreth, A.; Sweeney, N.M.; Clark, M.M.; Chowdhury, S.; Nahas, S.; Cakici, J.A.; Benson, W.; Kaplan, R.H.; Kronick, R.; et al. Rapid whole-genome sequencing decreases infant morbidity and cost of hospitalization. *NPJ Genom. Med.* **2018**, *3*, 10. [CrossRef]
36. Kernohan, K.D.; Hartley, T.; Naumenko, S.; Armour, C.M.; Graham, G.E.; Nikkel, S.M.; Lines, M.; Geraghty, M.T.; Richer, J.; Mears, W.; et al. Diagnostic clarity of exome sequencing following negative comprehensive panel testing in the neonatal intensive care unit. *Am. J. Med. Genet. A* **2018**, *176*, 1688–1691. [CrossRef] [PubMed]
37. Kingsmore, S.F. Is Rapid Exome Sequencing Standard of Care in the Neonatal and Pediatric Intensive Care Units? *J. Pediatr.* **2020**, *226*, 14–15. [CrossRef] [PubMed]
38. Ross, L.F.; Clayton, E.W. Ethical Issues in Newborn Sequencing Research: The Case Study of BabySeq. *Pediatrics* **2019**, *144*, e20191031. [CrossRef]
39. Bunnik, E.M.; de Jong, A.; Nijsingh, N.; de Wert, G.M.W.R. The New Genetics and Informed Consent: Differentiating Choice to Preserve Autonomy: The New Genetics and Informed Consent: Differentiating Choice to Preserve Autonomy. *Bioethics* **2013**, *27*, 348–355. [CrossRef]
40. Holm, I.A.; McGuire, A.; Pereira, S.; Rehm, H.; Green, R.C.; Beggs, A.H.; BabySeq Project Team. Returning a Genomic Result for an Adult-Onset Condition to the Parents of a Newborn: Insights from the BabySeq Project. *Pediatrics* **2019**, *143*, S37–S43. [CrossRef]
41. Van der Meer, L.; van Duijn, E.; Wolterbeek, R.; Tibben, A. Adverse childhood experiences of persons at risk for Huntington's disease or BRCA1/2 hereditary breast/ovarian cancer. *Clin. Genet.* **2012**, *81*, 18–23. [CrossRef]
42. Brunelli, L.; Jenkins, S.M.; Gudgeon, J.M.; Bleyl, S.B.; Miller, C.E.; Tvrdik, T.; Dames, S.A.; Ostrander, B.; Daboub, J.A.F.; Zielinski, B.A.; et al. Targeted gene panel sequencing for the rapid diagnosis of acutely ill infants. *Mol. Genet. Genom. Med.* **2019**, *7*, e00796. [CrossRef] [PubMed]
43. Maron, J.L.; Kingsmore, S.F.; Wigby, K.; Chowdhury, S.; Dimmock, D.; Poindexter, B.; Suhrie, K.; Vockley, J.; Diacovo, T.; Gelb, B.D.; et al. Novel Variant Findings and Challenges Associated with the Clinical Integration of Genomic Testing: An Interim Report of the Genomic Medicine for Ill Neonates and Infants (GEMINI) Study. *JAMA Pediatr.* **2021**, *175*, e205906. [CrossRef]
44. Elroy, M. *Researchers and Policymakers Point to Successes and Challenges in Personalized Medicine*; American Association for the Advancement of Science (AAAS): Washington, DC, USA, 2009.
45. Dimmock, D.P.; Clark, M.M.; Gaughran, M.; Cakici, J.A.; Caylor, S.A.; Clarke, C.; Feddock, M.; Chowdhury, S.; Salz, L.; Cheung, C.; et al. An RCT of Rapid Genomic Sequencing among Seriously Ill Infants Results in High Clinical Utility, Changes in Management, and Low Perceived Harm. *Am. J. Hum. Genet.* **2020**, *107*, 942–952. [CrossRef] [PubMed]
46. Cakici, J.A.; Dimmock, D.P.; Caylor, S.A.; Gaughran, M.; Clarke, C.; Triplett, C.; Clark, M.M.; Kingsmore, S.F.; Bloss, C.S. A Prospective Study of Parental Perceptions of Rapid Whole-Genome and -Exome Sequencing among Seriously Ill Infants. *Am. J. Hum. Genet.* **2020**, *107*, 953–962. [CrossRef] [PubMed]
47. Australian Genomics Health Alliance Acute Care Flagship; Lunke, S.; Eggers, S.; Wilson, M.; Patel, C.; Barnett, C.P.; Pinner, J.; Sandaradura, S.A.; Buckley, M.F.; Krzesinski, E.I.; et al. Feasibility of Ultra-Rapid Exome Sequencing in Critically Ill Infants and Children with Suspected Monogenic Conditions in the Australian Public Health Care System. *JAMA* **2020**, *323*, 2503–2511.

International Journal of
Neonatal Screening

Article

Genomics and Newborn Screening: Perspectives of Public Health Programs

Aaron J. Goldenberg [1,*], Roselle Ponsaran [1], Amy Gaviglio [2], Dalton Simancek [3] and Beth A. Tarini [4]

1 Department of Bioethics, Case Western Reserve University School of Medicine, Cleveland, OH 44106, USA; rsp10@case.edu
2 G2S Corporation/CDC Newborn Screening and Molecular Biology Branch, Atlanta, GA 30341, USA; pxd9@cdc.gov
3 Child Health Evaluation & Research (CHEAR) Unit, Division of General Pediatrics, University of Michigan, Ann Arbor, MI 48109, USA; dsimancek@gmail.com
4 Children's Research Institute, Children's National Health System, Washington, DC 20012, USA; btarini@childrensnational.org
* Correspondence: aaron.goldenberg@case.edu; Tel.: +1-216-368-8729; Fax: +1-216-368-8713

Abstract: This study assesses the benefits and challenges of using genomics in Newborn Screening Programs (NBS) from the perspectives of State program officials. This project aims to help programs develop policies that will aid in the integration of genomic technology. Discussion groups were conducted with the NBS Program and Laboratory Directors in the seven HRSA Regional Genomics Collaboratives (August 2014–March 2016). The discussion groups addressed expected uses of genomics, potential benefits, and challenges of integrating genomic technology, and educational needs for parents and other NBS stakeholders: Twelve focus groups were conducted, which included participants from over 40 state programs. Benefits of incorporating genomics included improving screening modalities, supporting diagnostic procedures, and screening for a wider spectrum of disorders. Challenges included the costs of genomics, the ability to educate parents and health care providers about results, and the potential negative psychosocial impact of genomic information. Attempts to address the challenges of integrating genomics must focus on preserving the child welfare goals of NBS programs. Health departments will need to explore how genomics could be used to enhance programs while maintaining universal access to screening.

Keywords: newborn screening; genomic testing; next generation genomic sequencing

1. Introduction

Over its 50-year history, the expansion of newborn screening (NBS) has been fueled by the development of new testing technologies. In accordance with this history, there is now a growing interest in utilizing next generation genomic sequencing (NGGS) for a variety of NBS purposes from sequencing of a single gene, to creating sequencing panels of a state's entire set of screened conditions, to sequencing a whole exome or a whole genome [1]. There are a number of potential benefits to integrating NGGS into NBS programs. As an adjunct to current screening tests, NGGS may help NBS programs identify specific genotyps, or pathogenic variants, that could shorten a family's "diagnostic odyssey" after a positive screen [2]. While its benefits are currently limited to a few conditions, a recent paper by a group of NBS experts highlighted that more genomic information may increasingly help providers to refine potential treatment plans by giving them "more accurate genotype-phenotype information" to inform prognoses, such as "severity of disease or age of onset" [2]. The implementation of NGGS would also allow programs to screen newborns for a much wider range of conditions, including risks for later-onset or chronic conditions.

Alternatively, the use of NGGS in NBS will present a number of programmatic and policy challenges for NBS programs [3–5]. For example, genomic sequencing platforms in NBS could represent a dramatic shift in the kinds of information generated through this public health program. The uses of NGGS in clinical settings have already highlighted the difficulties involved in managing, interpreting, and communicating to patients the large amounts of data generated through these sequencing platforms [6]. From a programmatic and policy perspective, NBS programs will have to address the long-term management of and access to the vast amounts of genetic data generated from NGGS. NBS programs must balance suppression of certain results, moral obligations to disclose potentially valuable health information to families, and parents' rights regarding their children's genomic information [4]. NBS programs also need to consider the potential harms of disclosing findings with uncertain or ambiguous implications for newborns that parents and their health care providers would find exceedingly difficult to interpret [7–9]. When a positive NBS result is discovered, parents and PCPs are typically informed of the results and work together to communicate with medical genetics professionals and/or other specialists to coordinate diagnostic steps and future care. In dealing with potentially complex genomic information, NBS programs may need to develop new approaches to these communication processes in order to adequately educate and counsel parents. However, attempts to address these programmatic and policy challenges must be addressed within the existing NBS mission, which is to safeguard child welfare and improve outcomes for newborns and their families.

There have been a number of recent empirical research projects and expert workgroups, that have examined the risks and benefits of using genomic technologies in a newborn population, compared the effectiveness of NGGS to traditional screening modalities, and described the various ethical, social, and practical challenges of genomic NBS [2,10–15]. However, none of these projects have explicitly done so from a public health program perspective. This perspective is crucial given that the challenges associated with the integration of NGGS technology into NBS programs may interfere with the successful functioning of the existing system and impair its ability to deliver care to children and their families. We aim to fill this gap by presenting results from a study that assesses key benefits and challenges of integrating NGGS into NBS programs from the perspectives of the State NBS program officials themselves. Identifying these challenges early will enable NBS programs to proactively develop policies and practices to aid the integration of NGGS technology into NBS programs in ways and, in doing so, preserve the effectiveness of the NBS system and, in turn, improve health outcomes for newborns and their families.

2. Methods

2.1. Participants

Investigators partnered with the seven Regional Genetics Collaboratives (RCs), whose mission is to promote the translation of genetic medicine into public health and healthcare services with the ultimate goal of improving the health of children and their families [16]. Each RC has about 7–8 state NBS program members. These collaboratives represent a diversity of expertise related to genetics and newborn screening from each of the states within that region. These RCs allowed investigators to host focus groups during events such as their regional meetings and conference calls, which are attended by state NBS program officials and other program stakeholders. Leaders of the RCs helped investigators recruit representatives from each of the three stakeholder categories for the focus groups, (1) NBS Program Directors or Coordinators; (2) NBS Laboratory Directors; (3) Newborn Screening Follow-Up Coordinators. This study was reviewed and approved by the Institutional Review Board (IRB).

2.2. Discussion Groups

Discussion groups were facilitated by either Dr. Goldenberg or Dr. Tarini and one of the project's Research Assistants. Research assistants or the non-moderating PI served as notetakers. Consent forms were signed at the beginning of the session if done in person; for focus groups done over the phone, consent was taken verbally. Focus groups were digitally audiotaped and transcribed for analysis. Each focus group lasted approximately one hour. The discussion group guide was developed through a combination of literature reviews on NGGS in NBS and iterative team conversations with our team which includes clinicians, social science and health services researchers, and representatives from state NBS programs. The focus group guide (Table 1) addressed the following major thematic areas: (1) Current or expected uses of NGGS in NBS programs; (2) Potential Benefits and Challenges of Using NGGS in NBS; (3) Educational or communications needs for parents and other NBS stakeholders; and (4) Policy needs for states regarding NGGS in NBS.

Table 1. List of primary focus group guide questions.

Thematic Area	Specific Questions
Current or expected uses	• How have new technologies been integrated into your programs in the past? What is the process? Were any policy changes necessary when these changes were made? • Do your programs utilize genomic sequencing technologies now? • Have any of your programs had any conversations or made any plans to prepare for genomic technologies and their implications? Have you discussed this as a adjunct technologies to current screening modalities or as a new replacement technology for current MS/MS screening?
Potential Benefits and Challenges	• What would you see as the benefits of integrating genomic sequencing into your NBS program? • What would you see as the major challenges/barriers of integrating genomic sequencing into your NBS program? • Do you think there would be any ethical/social implications of utilizing these kinds of screening tests? • What would be the programmatic implications of genomics as an adjunct test? As a replacement test? • How do you think genomic information should be communicated to parents? How should they be educated about screening? • Do you think that the integration of genomic sequencing should impact the mandatory nature of your programs? Should consent be utilized? How might you implement this kind of authorization?
Educational or communications needs	• What kinds of training/education do you think your programs would need to integrate genomics into NBS? • What kinds of parental or public education do you think your programs would need to integrate genomics into NBS?
Policy needs	• Do you believe your current policies would allow for the integration of genomics into your programs? If not, then what types of policies do you think would be necessary to allow for this kind of integration? • What kinds of protections do you think would need to be built into your policies regarding how to collect, store, and manage genomic data?

2.3. Data Analysis

Standard procedures for analyzing qualitative data were employed, based on successive coding passes by two independent coders, beginning with open coding of content at the level closest to the content of the text, and through broader and more analytic codes [16]. All identifying information was removed from the audio and transcripts, and transcripts were imported into Dedoose, a computer program for managing text data [17]. Thematic domains were identified through a process of intense review of transcript data. Every transcript was coded by at least two team members, and a process of iterative group discussions were used to review and settle any discrepancies between coders.

3. Results

3.1. Participant Characteristics

In total, twelve focus groups were conducted—four in person and the remainder were conducted during over the phone conference calls. The number of participants in each group ranged from 5–25. Over 100 participants were included in all the focus groups, including NBS officials from over 40 state programs. All seven of the RCs were represented by at least one focus group. The following sections detail the primary themes discussed across our discussion groups, and Supplemental Table S1 contains additional representative quoted associated with each thematic area.

3.2. Benefits of Using NGGS in NBS

Participants were asked to describe the advantages or benefits of incorporating genomics into NBS. These perceived benefits were mostly related to the possibility of using NGGS technology to improve the current quality or effectiveness of current screening modalities for conditions already screened within state programs.

Reducing Burden of False Positives: For example, many participants discussed the potential for reducing the number of false positives within NBS results. Participants noted that, following up on out of range initial NBS results, many of which turn out to be false positives, can take a great deal of time, and that reducing that delay by using additional technologies would be helpful. One noted their own experience incorporating genomics as a primary technology into testing for a single condition.

> *"... we just had so many false-positives and that created so much work both in the lab and for the short-and the long-term follow-up that we had to find ways to you know reduce the false-positive rate, and that kind of helped us do that, but that's just one condition."*

Participants also discussed how the use of genomic technologies could also help ease the burden of false-positives for families by reducing the need for additional samples and long waiting times for additional results.

> *"And that's kind of what we started, because I found that having to call families about probably false-positives and having them go get blood drawn, it just creates a lot of burden and then you have all this excess worry. Whereas if we're able to do the gene study and find no mutations and have a repeat on some of these disorders, then we can feel pretty comfortable that that's not it."*

Provision of Detailed Risk Information: Yet another potential benefit a few participants noted was the ability for genomic results to provide more detailed risk information to the family. Some described families that had received sequencing results from private companies. One participant noted: "... *there's this need from the community also to say 'We want everything you know about us"*.

Assist with Future Reproductive Decisions: For other participants, genomics in NBS could provide that additional genetic information that may not only help the affected child directly, but also assist the families in making future reproductive decisions.

> *"Yeah, and at this point, you know the resources that parents have can be different. So if a child qualifies for Medicaid and some things can be done, they can be done for the child. They reflect back on the parents, but the parents themselves may not have coverage to get their own sequencing done or even you know identification of some kind of abnormal something, and so especially the fathers. It's like 'That's out of the question. We can't test dad. You will have to pay for it completely.' At least if you have a more definitive something in the baby, you can you know reflect back at least that amount of knowledge securely to the parents, even if they themselves can't get the same or afford the same kind of diagnosis-seeking."*

Screen for Disorders Not Otherwise Possible: While it was not seen as a primary benefit, some participants did discuss the possibility that genomics could allow NBS programs to include a wider spectrum of disorders into the panel via genomics, especially for conditions that would be difficult or impossible to screen with current MS/MS testing modalities.

> *"another benefit would be you know maybe the ability to screen for more disorders where right now there's you know no biochemical assay, for instance, (and) that lends itself to screening on a population basis."*

Equitable Access to Genomic Services: Finally, a number of participants noted that one benefit of integrating NGGS into state NBS programs would be the potential to support access to genomic services to all newborns in the US. These participants felt that, because one of the foundational goals of NBS was universal access regardless of socioeconomic states, state programs might be in a position to provide more equitable access to genomic services.

> *"it's one of the only places in life where there's not healthcare [disparities] ... that's our mantra, right, is universal health? The only time in your life you really could get it [genomics], and so where can we fit in there to benefit our population"?*

3.3. Challenges of Using NGGS in NBS

Even as they acknowledged the potential benefits, participants were much more inclined to raise concerns about the technical and ethical challenges of incorporating genomic testing into NBS. The challenges and concerns they raised fell along a number of areas.

Impact of Workforce and Budgets: A primary concern for the stakeholders was the impact of genomics on their workforce and on their budgets. While the lab directors described the cost of upgrading equipment and space, and the ability to justify and acquire the larger budgets that would be needed, as a significant barrier, an even greater overall concern was the ability of staff to handle the follow-up and counseling needed to address the information provided by genomic sequencing. One program official noted that "we just don't have the manpower to provide information to providers and counsel the families."

3.4. Low Genetic Literacy among Public and Providers

In addition to workforce concerns, many participants also felt that their ability to educate both parents and health care providers would pose a significant challenge to increasing the medical utility of genomic information for families. They worried that, given a lack of genetic literacy among the public and health providers, there would be a steep learning curve for being able to effectively understand complex genomic data—especially in the case of whole exome or genome sequencing. One participant stated that "the doctor has to understand the results, and then the patient has to be taught how to understand the results ... The general pediatrician may not know what to do or how to describe it, and then once they give the wrong message, it gets perpetuated incorrectly in the patient population".

Participants anticipated that, for parents and families, the learning curve could be even greater. Additionally, clarity and transparency about the newborn screening process, and what purposes genetic information may be used for, would be even more important to parents making decisions about NBS screening.

> *"They are scared of just even the word "DNA" being used, let alone sequencing a whole genome ... There are many parents that don't even know newborn screening happens, or they just remember, 'Oh yeah, they took some blood, put it on a card.' The public would have to be very, very educated that this was happening."*

Lessons of Past Technology Integration: Many participants referenced earlier experiences of technology change–specifically, the introduction of tandem mass spectrometry (MS/MS) into newborn screening. These program officials warned that their experience with integrating MS/MS should serve as a cautionary tale for integrating genomic technology into NBS.

> *"I think we should not repeat the mistakes of the past, because I remember when we expanded newborn screening with tandem mass spectrometry, everybody jumped the gun. So, I think we need to be smart in the way that we should gather some information on those conditions, get an idea of when to start treatment, how to follow these patients before we start the [genomic] screening."*

Participants were asked to consider using genomics as an adjunct rather than replacement technology. Most participants felt that, in most cases, using genomics as a secondary or adjunct test would allow a more gradual introduction which would lend itself to a controlled and specific use of the technology.

> *"I think using it as an adjunct technology would kind of ease us into it, so to speak, and you know and help us to gradually adopt it in small doses and build our knowledge and understanding and the capacity to deal with the information ... As replacement technology, I feel it's like really diving into the deep end and just feel very unprepared for that."*

NGGS as Replacement Technology: Participants were asked to specifically consider the prospect of potentially moving towards whole genome or whole exome sequencing as a replacement technology. Generally, this was especially worrisome for participants who were concerned about number and types of results that would need to be returned to parents—especially in the context of a mandatory screening test.

> *"you really can't put that burden on parents that we have a mandatory test with a bunch of things that we can't figure out what's happening with their kids ' ... I mean it's hard enough making sure that kids are in nurturing families to suddenly throw on them that 'We've mandatorily tested your child for x, y, z. We have no idea what this mean, but good luck with that,' right ... I don't want to tell a family that 'Your child has this late onset disorder. There's nothing we can do for it, and shouldn't show any symptoms 'til maybe later on, some muscle weakness or whatever. Have fun. Good luck with your newborn ... I'm not going to do that to a parent."*

Furthermore, participants also worried about how programs would need to decide what kinds of results to return to parents. For programs, this was complicated by unclear guidelines about how to determine which results may be actionable and whether it was appropriate for public health institutions to be making the decisions about which results to return.

> *"We need to be very clear about like the definition of an actionable result ... we would need some guidelines about 'What are actionable results ... So to understand that just because we can do the test, doesn't mean we're prepared to deal with the results, and maybe we shouldn't, as public health systems."*

Finally, participants expressed concerns that too broad use of genomics would in fact hurt the original intention of state newborn screening.

> *"Clearly, we need to keep screening for things that have safe, effective treatment, that that's what newborn screening is based on, and that's finding out about all these other things that are untreatable or unknowable at this point. So, I think that that clearly goes against the ethics of newborn screening."*

4. Discussions and Conclusions

This study found that key NBS program stakeholders perceived a number of structural, technical, and ethical challenges to the integration of NGGS technology into state NBS programs. While participants understood that there may be some compelling benefits to incorporating genomics in their programs, they had significant concerns, particularly around costs and data management, interpretation and communication of results, psychosocial harms associated with uncertain or ambiguous genomic data, and deviation from the core goals of NBS programs. Most notably, participants raised concerns that failure to address programmatic and policy challenges from the integration of NGGS technology into NBS programs could disrupt the functioning and reduce the benefits of these programs for newborns and their families. For example, management of the genomic data could overwhelm the current capacity of NBS programs and lead to an interruption in key functions. Program officials further raised a number of issues related to the impact this information may have on families. First, the public could raise significant concerns about the potential for misuse or unintended harm from genetic data, such as genetic discrimination or possession of genetic information by a government agency. Second, there may be added concerns about giving families information that either would inform parents about their own genetic risk or reveal carrier status or adult onset information about newborns, which may further move beyond the current ethical justifications for population based screening and violate a newborns right not to know certain genetic results that will not be relevant until they reach adulthood. Finally, and most possibly most concerning, the complexity of information or increased uncertainty about results could also prompt parents to opt out of NBS screening altogether, thus negating the potential benefits of screening for their newborns. Addressing these and other as yet unidentified issues requires systematic research about the kinds of genomic information that should be returned to parents and how best to communicate it, as well as how to address public policy concerns about the use of genomic data by a public health program. The international NBS community will need to clarify the important distinctions between adding genomic sequencing into current NBS approaches and a larger paradigm shift to "genomic screening" of newborns which could include whole genome or exome sequencing of all newborns. This shift may further move programs away from their core goals and disrupt the benefits of NBS, especially if the addition of genomics adds significant increases in uncertain results being returned to families. Furthermore, many international NBS stakeholders, including the EUNENBS network of newborn screening experts, have noted the important differences between screening and diagnostic approaches [18], and thus a shift to more diagnostic genomic sequencing may again further move programs away from their primary goals of population based screening.

Another related overarching message from NBS program stakeholders focused on the history of challenges associated with using new testing modalities in NBS programs. Advances in testing technology have always been both the greatest benefit and the greatest challenge to NBS programs' ability to improve health outcomes for newborns and their families [19]. For example, tandem mass spectrometry (MS/MS) technology allowed programs to screen for more disorders without significantly increasing screening costs. However, the increased number of tests was accompanied by an increase in the number of false positive results [20], inadequate education of primary care physicians about newly-screened disorders [21], and indeterminate results [8]. Many of our participant stakeholders felt that the integration of NGGS technology into NBS programs would pose similar challenges. They noted the need for programs to work together to avoid some of the mistakes of the past, while finding effective ways to utilize new technologies and improve programs [22–24].

It seems that, moving forward, it is critical that NBS programs share strategies and lessons as they work to incorporate NGGS into NBS. Such a widespread collaborative approach to complex problems in NBS is not new. In fact, the Collaborative Improvement and Innovation Network (COINN) for Timeliness in Newborn Screening is an example of such an approach to addressing the challenges of ensuring timely collection and processing of NBS specimens. This initiative provides a potentially valuable and useful model for NBS programs as they contend with the challenges of integrating NGGS.

As with all studies, there are limitations that should be noted. This was a qualitative study whose goal was to identify and address the programmatic and policy challenges raised by the integration of NGGS technology into NBS programs. It was not designed to examine the scope and severity of these challenges, but to identify consistent emerging issues for additional investigations. Our participants were leaders and officials within state

NBS programs. While beyond the scope of this study, we acknowledge that gathering additional stakeholder viewpoints will also prove critical as NBS programs grapple with the integration of NGGS technology. We chose to focus on the state NBS programs because theirs is often an underrepresented voice in discussions about NBS technology. We believe their perspective is critical to the goal of maintaining the current benefits of NBS, while exploring how genomic screening technologies may be used to enhance or expand those benefits in the genomic era. Given their experiences with the introduction of tandem mass spectrometry, it is understandable that many of the NBS stakeholders would approach NGGS with caution. These experiences also provide a chance to apply the lessons of the past as the programs to the opportunities of the future [25].

As NBS programs continue to evolve, attempts to address challenges must keep child welfare and patient-centered outcomes front and center. This includes ensuring adequate communication between the state programs and primary care providers, ensuring that patients and providers have access to appropriate education and counseling regarding genomic findings, and providing coordination of care with the medical home for follow-up and treatment [26]. The actual impact of NGGS technology will depend in large part on the ability of health departments to address these concerns in comprehensive ways that maintain the current benefits of programs and ensure universal access to screening, while exploring how these screening technologies may also be used to enhance or expand the benefits of newborn screening services [27,28]. If the programmatic and policy challenges from the integration of NGGS technology into NBS programs are not addressed, they could ultimately disrupt the functioning and reduce the benefits of these programs for newborns. Addressing the challenges identified through this project will require further systematic research about the what kinds of genomic information parents may want to know about their newborns, how to effectively communicate those findings, and assess any potential harms associated with receiving genomic screening results. It will also be crucial to address any public policy concerns about the use of genomic data by a public health program.

Supplementary Materials: Supplementary materials can be found at https://www.mdpi.com/article/10.3390/ijns8010011/s1.

Author Contributions: All authors contributed to the design and implementation of the research and to the analysis of the results. A.J.G., R.P. and B.A.T. wrote the paper with input and edits from A.G. and D.S. All authors have read and agreed to the published version of the manuscript.

Funding: Research reported in this publication was supported by the Health Resources and Services Administration (HRSA), U.S. Department of Health and Human Services under award number R40MC26805.

Institutional Review Board Statement: The subjects have given their written or verbal informed consent and the study protocol was approved by the Case Western Reserve University Institutional Review Board. IRB-2014-793 5/8/2014.

Informed Consent Statement: The subjects have given their written or verbal informed consent and the study protocol. Informed consent was obtained from all subjects involved in the study.

Conflicts of Interest: The authors declare no conflict of interest.

References

1. National Institutes of Health. *Genomic Sequencing and Newborn Screening Disorders (U19 Cooperative Agreement)*; National Institutes of Health: Bethesda MD, USA, 2013.
2. Johnston, J.; Lantos, J.D.; Goldenberg, A.; Chen, F.; Parens, E.; Koenig, B.A.; Board, A.K. Sequencing newborns: A call for nuanced use of genomic technologies. *Hastings Cent. Rep.* **2018**, *48*, S2–S6. [CrossRef] [PubMed]
3. Tarini, B.A.; Goldenberg, A.J. Ethical issues with newborn screening in the genomics era. *Annu. Rev. Genom. Hum. Genet.* **2012**, *13*, 81–93. [CrossRef]
4. Goldenberg, A.J.; Sharp, R.R. The ethical hazards and programmatic challenges of genomic newborn screening. *JAMA* **2011**, *307*, 461–462. [CrossRef] [PubMed]
5. Clayton, E.W. Currents in contemporary ethics. State run newborn screening in the genomic era, or how to avoid drowning when drinking from a fire hose. *J. Law Med. Ethics* **2010**, *38*, 697–700. [CrossRef] [PubMed]

6. Sharp, R.R. Downsizing genomic medicine: Approaching the ethical complexity of whole-genome sequencing by starting small. *Genet. Med.* **2011**, *13*, 191–194. [CrossRef]
7. Kwon, J.M.; Steiner, R.D. "I'm fine; I'm just waiting for my disease": The new and growing class of presymptomatic patients. *Neurology* **2011**, *77*, 522–523. [CrossRef]
8. Timmermans, S.; Buchbinder, M. Patients-in-waiting: Living between sickness and health in the genomics era. *J. Health Soc. Behav.* **2010**, *51*, 408–423. [CrossRef]
9. Comeau, A.M.; Parad, R.B.; Dorkin, H.L.; Dovey, M.; Gerstle, R.; Haver, K.; Lapey, A.; O'Sullivan, B.P.; Waltz, D.A.; Zwerdling, R.G.; et al. Population-based newborn screening for genetic disorders when multiple mutation DNA testing is incorporated: A cystic fibrosis newborn screening model demonstrating increased sensitivity but more carrier detections. *Pediatrics* **2004**, *113*, 1573–1581. [CrossRef]
10. Goldenberg, A.J.; Dodson, D.S.; Davis, M.M.; Tarini, B.A. Parents' interest in whole-genome sequencing of newborns. *Genet. Med.* **2014**, *16*, 78–84. [CrossRef]
11. Ceyhan-Birsoy, O.; Murry, J.B.; Machini, K.; Lebo, M.; Yu, T.; Fayer, S.; Genetti, C.A.; Schwartz, T.S.; Agrawal, P.B.; Parad, R.B.; et al. Interpretation of Genomic Sequencing Results in Healthy and Ill Newborns: Results from the BabySeq Project. *Am. J. Hum. Genet.* **2019**, *104*, 76–93. [CrossRef]
12. Knoppers, B.M.; Sénécal, K.; Borry, P.; Avard, D. Whole-genome sequencing in newborn screening programs. *Sci. Transl. Med.* **2014**, *6*, 229cm2. [CrossRef] [PubMed]
13. Bodian, D.L.; Klein, E.; Iyer, R.K.; Wong, W.S.W.; Kothiyal, P.; Stauffer, D.; Huddleston, K.C.; Gaither, A.D.; Remsburg, I.; Khromykh, A.; et al. Utility of whole-genome sequencing for detection of newborn screening disorders in a population cohort of 1696 neonates. *Genet. Med.* **2016**, *18*, 221. [CrossRef] [PubMed]
14. Bombard, Y.; Miller, F.A.; Hayeems, R.Z.; Barg, C.; Cressman, C.; Carroll, J.C.; Wilson, B.J.; Little, J.; Avard, D.; Painter-Main, M.; et al. Public views on participating in newborn screening using genome sequencing. *Eur. J. Hum. Genet.* **2014**, *22*, 1248. [CrossRef] [PubMed]
15. National Coordinating Center for the Regional Genetic and Newborn Screening Service Collaboratives. About Us. 2013. Available online: http://www.nccrcg.org/AM/Template.cfm?Section=About3 (accessed on 15 July 2021).
16. Denzin, N.; Lincoln, Y. *Handbook of Qualitative Research*, 2nd ed.; Sage Publications: Thousand Oaks, CA, USA, 2000.
17. Dedoose. Available online: http://www.dedoose.com (accessed on 12 October 2021).
18. Cornel, M.C.; Rigter, T.; Weinreich, S.S.; Burgard, P.; Hoffmann, G.F.; Lindner, M.; Loeber, J.G.; Rupp, K.; Taruscio, D.; Vittozzi, L. A framework to start the debate on neonatal screening policies in the EU: An Expert Opinion Document. *Eur. J. Hum. Genet.* **2014**, *22*, 12–17. [CrossRef]
19. Tarini, B.A. The current revolution in newborn screening: New technology, old controversies. *Arch. Pediatr. Adolesc. Med.* **2007**, *161*, 767–772. [CrossRef]
20. Tarini, B.A.; Christakis, D.A.; Welch, H.G. State newborn screening in the tandem mass spectrometry era: More tests, more false-positive results. *Pediatrics* **2006**, *118*, 448–456. [CrossRef]
21. Kemper, A.R.; Uren, R.L.; Moseley, K.L.; Clark, S.J. Primary care physicians' attitudes regarding follow-up care for children with positive newborn screening results. *Pediatrics* **2006**, *118*, 1836–1841. [CrossRef]
22. McCandless, S.E.; Chandrasekar, R.; Linard, S.; Kikano, S.; Rice, L. Sequencing from dried blood spots in infants with "false positive" newborn screen for MCAD deficiency. *Mol. Genet. Metab.* **2013**, *108*, 51–55. [CrossRef]
23. Genetic Alliance. Beyond Bloodspot: How Will Emerging Technologies Shape Detection & Clinical Care? 2013. Available online: http://beyondbloodspot.eventbrite.com/?utm_source=Genetic+Alliance+Announcements+and+Newsletters&utm_campaign=84c008278e-Beyond_the_Bloodspot_Summit7_29_2013&utm_medium=email&utm_term=0_182db72825-84c008278e-67666581 (accessed on 15 July 2021).
24. Eunice Kennedy Shriver National Institute of Child Health and Human Development (NICHD). Newborn Screening in the Genomic Era: Setting a Research Agenda. 2010. Available online: http://www.nichd.nih.gov/sites/default/files/about/meetings/2010-retired/Documents/Newborn_Research_Agenda.pdf (accessed on 12 October 2021).
25. Botkin, J.R.; Clayton, E.W.; Fost, N.C.; Burke, W.; Murray, T.H.; Baily, M.A.; Wilfond, B.; Berg, A.; Ross, L.F. Newborn screening technology: Proceed with caution. *Pediatrics* **2006**, *117*, 1793–1799. [CrossRef]
26. American Academy of Pediatrics Newborn Screening Authoring Committee. Newborn screening expands: Recommendations for pediatricians and medical homes—implications for the system. *Pediatrics* **2008**, *121*, 192–217. [CrossRef]
27. Stoddard, J.J.; Farrell, P.M. State-to-state variations in newborn screening polices. *Arch. Pediatr. Adolesc. Med.* **1997**, *151*, 561–564. [CrossRef] [PubMed]
28. McCann, P.J. Agency discretion and public health service delivery. *Health Serv. Res.* **2009**, *44*, 1897–1908. [CrossRef] [PubMed]

International Journal of
Neonatal Screening

MDPI

Article

A Public Dialogue to Inform the Use of Wider Genomic Testing When Used as Part of Newborn Screening to Identify Cystic Fibrosis

Suzannah Kinsella [1], Henrietta Hopkins [1], Lauren Cooper [2] and James R. Bonham [3,*]

[1] Hopkins Van Mill, 6 Deans Yard, London SW1P 3NP, UK; suzannah@hopkinsvamil.co.uk (S.K.); henrietta@hopkinsvanmil.co.uk (H.H.)
[2] NHS England & NHS Improvement, Wellington House, 133-155 Waterloo Road, London SE1 8UG, UK; lauren.cooper0@nhs.net
[3] Sheffield Childrens (NHS) FT, Western Bank, Sheffield S10 2TH, UK
* Correspondence: j.bonham@nhs.net

Abstract: Cystic fibrosis (CF) has been included within the UK national newborn screening programme since 2007. The approach uses measures of immunoreactive trypsin (IRT) in dried blood spot samples obtained at day 5 of life. Samples which reveal IRT results >99.5th centile go on to be tested for a limited panel of CF mutations. While the programme works well and achieves a high level of sensitivity and specificity, it relies upon repeat testing in some cases and identifies probable carriers, both potentially provoking parental anxiety. In addition, the limited CF mutation panel may not fully reflect the ethnic diversity within the UK population. The use of wider genomic screening, made possible by next-generation sequencing to replace more limited panels, can be used to avoid these shortcomings. However, the way in which this approach is employed can either be designed to maximise specificity by limiting reporting to combinations of known pathogenic mutations or can maximise sensitivity by also reporting combinations of pathogenic mutations together with variants of uncertain significance. The latter approach also increases the number of Cystic Fibrosis Screen-Positive Inconclusive Diagnosis (CFSPID) designations reported, resulting in uncertainty for parents. To help consider the design of the programme, a dialogue was commissioned by the UK National Screening Committee (UKNSC) to elicit the views of members of the public without direct experience of CF, to determine if there was a preference for maximising the sensitivity or the specificity of CF screening. The participants initially expressed a clear preference to maximise sensitivity and avoid missing CF cases, but after time to reflect and consider the implications of their choice, a number changed their views so as to tolerate some missed cases if this resulted in greater certainty of outcome; this became the majority view. It is proposed that it may be a generalisable finding that the public, when facing whole-population screening programmes, may require significant time and information to inform and make their choices and may attach great importance to clarity and certainty of outcome in the screening process.

Keywords: cystic fibrosis; next-generation sequencing; newborn screening

1. Introduction

Newborn screening for cystic fibrosis (CF) aims to identify babies with classical CF before symptoms develop; the detection of these babies shortly after birth enables the early initiation of high-quality care and an optimum long-term health outcome. Screening for CF has formed part of the Newborn Blood Spot Screening (NBS) programme [1] in the UK since 2007. Since that time, there has been a notable expansion in newborn screening for CF across Europe. In 2007, there were only two national NBS programmes, while in the present day there are more than 20 national programs for CF in Europe, each with their own protocols and algorithms [2].

The current approach to newborn screening for CF in the UK relies upon an initial test to quantitate immunoreactive trypsin (IRT) in dried blood spot samples collected five days after birth. When this is elevated above a cut-off designed to reflect the 99.5th centile in the population, the sample is tested for a limited panel of four common mutations. If two disease-causing mutations can be identified, the baby is referred for clinical investigation [3].

If only one mutation is identified, a wider panel is then used that is capable of identifying 50 mutations. If this identifies a further disease-causing mutation, the baby is referred; if it does not, IRT measurement is repeated at 21 days of life. When this is elevated, the baby is referred; if the result is normal, the baby is reported to be a probable CF carrier.

As a safeguard and to help avoid missed cases, if the initial IRT is very elevated, defined in England as greater than >120 μg/mL, a repeat IRT test is performed at 21 days, even if genetic testing is uninformative. When this repeat IRT test is elevated, the baby is referred for clinical investigation.

This combination of IRT measurement followed by limited genetic testing and repeat IRT measurement, if needed, is applied in varying forms by many national screening programmes. The UK approach to newborn screening for CF aims to improve the specificity of testing by the inclusion of genetic testing while seeking to maintain sensitivity by repeating IRT measurement where genetic testing may not be fully informative. This approach, sometimes referred to as IRT/DNA/IRT, has been proven to be robust over many years; nevertheless, it has some significant disadvantages and some limitations.

In particular, the initial and extended mutation panels used may not accurately reflect the wide array of disease-causing mutations encountered in an increasingly ethnically diverse population; the algorithm requires repeat testing at day 21 of life in a significant number of babies, resulting in stress for the family and an organisational cost for the service; a proportion of babies are reported as 'probable carriers', with resultant ambiguity for parents in a screening programme whose primary aim is not carrier detection. In addition, a normal second IRT result is associated with false negative cases in some children [4].

With the advent of relatively inexpensive and technically reliable 'next-generation sequencing' (NGS) able to identify a greater range of CF disease-causing mutations, it is possible to consider an approach that is less reliant on repeat IRT testing and which would more closely reflect the ethnic diversity in the population while avoiding reporting 'probable carrier' results. This approach has begun to be adopted by some CF newborn programmes in the US and elsewhere. An early US study explored the technical feasibility of screening for cystic fibrosis using next-generation sequencing technology [5]. The NGS assay proved concordant with mutations identified by alternate methods and the authors suggested that an IRT/extended NGS algorithm could improve both the sensitivity and specificity of screening. Denmark adopted NGS as part of their newborn CF screening program and their findings identified close to the expected numbers of infants when screening for CF using an IRT algorithm [6].

One of the challenges faced by those wishing to use NGS and related technologies is to decide whether to restrict reporting to combinations of known disease-causing mutations and therefore maximise 'specificity' or to include 'variants of unknown significance' and maximise the 'sensitivity' of CF detection. These choices will, in turn, also influence the number of Cystic Fibrosis Screen-Positive Inconclusive Diagnosis (CFSPID) designations reported to parents. Terlizzi et al. [7] recently performed a review of data of CFSPID cases and concluded that while genetic analysis can improve the positive predictive value of screening, it also increased the number of CFSPID cases reported.

In order to help inform these difficult decisions, a dialogue involving members of the public without direct personal experience of cystic fibrosis was organised to explore their views about the use of wider genomic testing in screening and, in particular, the relative importance placed upon the uncertainty of receiving a CFSPID designation when compared with the potential to miss a true case of CF. It is intended that the current study will be complemented by similar research to determine the views of both patients and families living with CF together with those of the health professionals charged with their treatment and care. The results of these three distinct projects will be used to inform the decision-making of the UK National Screening Committee in relation to the potential incorporation of NGS when screening for CF as part of the national newborn screening programme.

It is worth noting that in either scenario, whether to restrict reporting to combinations of known disease-causing mutations or to include 'variants of unknown significance', the proposed use of NGS would no longer report carriers but only combinations of mutations of varying types and significance. As the purpose of the newborn screening programme is the identification of CF, the bioinformatics pipeline would be designed so that carriers would no longer be identified.

2. Participants and Methods

This dialogue reengaged with a subset of participants who had already taken part in another recently organised dialogue to explore the implications of whole-genome sequencing (WGS) for newborn screening. This group was used to ensure that participants had some familiarity with newborn screening, genetic testing, and cystic fibrosis.

Nineteen people took part in this smaller and more targeted dialogue, their age and geographic distribution is shown in Table 1; the number invited reflected the budgetary constraints of the project while providing access to a reasonable cross-section of the public. In terms of bias, we asked the prospective participants, who had already participated in the WGS study, to indicate on a scale of 1–5 how positive they felt about the use of genomic sequencing in newborn screening. We used these responses to help inform the selection of the 19 for this mini-dialogue, including both those with positive and less positive views. The participants included a range of ages, locations, and socioeconomic backgrounds. Given the life stage associated with a decision to accept newborn screening and so that the new screening approaches will better reflect the ethnic mix in the UK population, the number of participants from ethnic minorities and those of a younger adult age were enriched.

Table 1. Dialogue participant demographics.

Male	8	England	11
Female	10	Scotland [1]	3
Other	1	Wales [1]	1
Age: 18–30	5	Northern Ireland	4
Age: 31–45	7	Ethnic minority	4
Age: 46–65	7	Disability	4

[1] Participant dropouts were from Scotland and Wales.

Frontline NHS staff and people with CF or family members of people with CF were excluded as they would have had greater knowledge and potential for strong influence on the other participants.

Previous experience within the research group indicates that groups of 6–7 are optimal to support active participation in online discussion and this enabled three parallel small group discussions comprising a range of ages, genders, ethnicities, and socioeconomic backgrounds during the sessions.

A public dialogue approach was seen as helpful as it provided sufficient time to learn about the issues by engaging with specialists and reviewing stimulus materials, consider diverse points of view, discover key tensions and values, and generate new ideas and understanding.

The dialogue process involved:

- A pre-task;

- A two-hour online (Zoom) workshop with a mix of plenary and small group discussions to understand what the wider genomic approaches are, their impacts, and how CF and CFSPID are diagnosed and treated;
- A homework task between workshops 1 and 2;
- A final two-hour online workshop to discuss final considerations.

Participants were given a two-week period between the first and final workshop, to provide sufficient time to complete the homework task and consider the potential impact of the two approaches before the final deliberations. The process is set out in Figure 1.

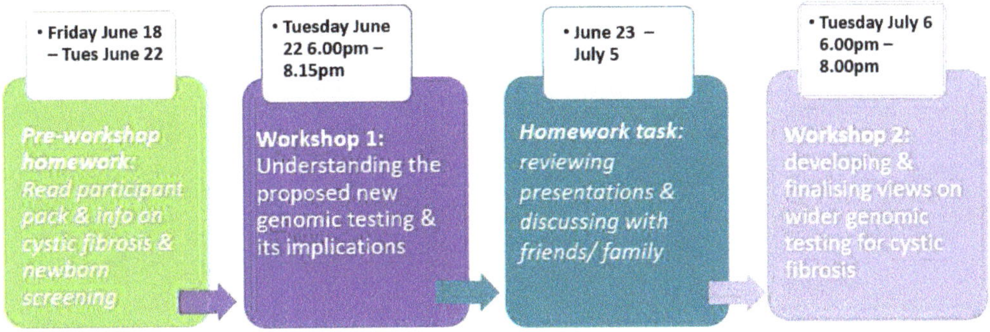
• Friday June 18 – Tues June 22
Pre-workshop homework: Read participant pack & info on cystic fibrosis & newborn screening
• Tuesday June 22 6.00pm – 8.15pm
Workshop 1: Understanding the proposed new genomic testing & its implications
• June 23 – July 5
Homework task: reviewing presentations & discussing with friends/ family
• Tuesday July 6 6.00pm – 8.00pm
Workshop 2: developing & finalising views on wider genomic testing for cystic fibrosis

Figure 1. The mini-dialogue process: June–July 2021.

The pre-task asked participants to review the welcome pack and remind themselves of information shared in the previous public dialogue about newborn screening, cystic fibrosis, and genomic sequencing. The first online workshop of two hours involved hearing from and questioning three specialists in newborn screening and cystic fibrosis: a laboratory scientist involved in the current newborn screening programme for CF; a respiratory paediatrician with extensive experience in receiving referrals from newborn screening when CF is suspected; and a researcher in medical ethics with experience of families and children with CF and CFSPID.

During the homework task, participants discussed the different wider genomic sequencing approaches with friends and family members to gather their views. The second online workshop focused on discussing and finalising considerations on the merits of the two approaches. During both online workshops, three small groups were formed for discussion and each comprised no more than seven participants working with one facilitator throughout the dialogue. Facilitators followed workshop process plans designed in discussion with the UKNSC Project Team.

The questions posed to the dialogue participants were: How should wider genomic testing be used when screening for cystic fibrosis at birth? What is the relative importance of 'sensitivity' and 'specificity' in the context of newborn screening for CF? Participants were informed that, from approximately 720,000 babies tested each year in the UK, around 200 CF cases are identified. It was explained that a more 'sensitive' approach to testing that includes reporting 'variants of unknown significance' would be likely to minimise the risk of missing babies with true CF but would detect more cases of CFSPID (from approx. 25 pa currently to 80 pa). The more specific approach which would only report combinations of known 'pathogenic variants' would reduce the number of CFSPID cases detected, but may run the risk that a small number of additional babies (<10 pa in addition to the current screening programme) with true CF may not be identified.

The online dialogue workshops were recorded with the consent of the participants. These recordings were transcribed and analysed using NVivo software [8] together with:

- Data from the homework task;
- Results of the Mentimeter [9] online polling questions used live during workshops.

Grounded theory was applied to the analysis of the public dialogue deliberations, in order to gain theoretical insights for the findings [10]. Theories were built from what was heard rather than from testing a preconceived hypothesis. Public dialogue is a qualitative methodology, so the findings do not demonstrate statistically representative analysis, but do allow the exploration of social phenomena through participants sharing their views and experiences [11].

3. Results

Following more than three hours of deliberation and two weeks taken to consider the relative merits of the more 'sensitive' versus more 'specific' approaches, most participants favoured the more 'specific' approach which would identify fewer CFSPID cases.

The reasons offered by those who favoured the more 'specific' approach included: a wish to avoid the uncertainty of a CFSPID designation for more families; an understanding that the increase in the number of CFSPID designations reported would be greater than the number of true CF cases missed; a lack of clarity about the support pathway available for families receiving a CFSPID designation; a recognition that the current CF screening programme does not achieve 100% detection of CF cases; an understanding that if a child with CF were missed at screening, that he/she would be likely to be diagnosed clinically by two years of age and would be unlikely to suffer adverse long-term health consequences.

The reasons offered by those who favoured the more 'sensitive' approach included: a belief that the primary role of a screening programme is to maximise the number of diagnoses of the screened condition; that a CFSPID designation could be helpful in terms of being prepared for identifying CF symptoms if they were to develop later in the child's life; a greater number of CFSPID designations being reported could encourage research; a greater number of CFSPID designations being reported could result in an improved care pathway for those patients and families presented receiving this designation for their baby.

It is important to note that most participants found choosing a preferred approach to the use of wider genomic sequencing in this context hugely challenging. They struggled with the moral dilemma presented by the outcomes of the two approaches: a more 'specific' approach with the risk of missing a true CF case compared with a more 'sensitive' approach leading to a lifetime of uncertainty for those families receiving a CFSPID designation. At the start of the second workshop, 9 of the 18 participants who expressed a preference voted in favour of the more 'sensitive' approach that sought to detect all CF cases, while only 5 preferred a more 'specific' option, and 4 confessed to being unsure. This contrasted with the position at the end of the second workshop where 12 stated a preference for a more 'specific' approach versus 4 who still favoured a more 'sensitive' option; 2 declined to take part.

It is notable that between the first and second workshops, several participants moved in the direction of expressing a preference for 'specificity' while none moved in the direction of 'sensitivity'.

One of the factors cited for choosing a more 'specific' approach was the difference in the number of individuals who may be affected. In the information offered, it was proposed that fewer than 10 babies pa with true CF may be missed compared with approximately 80 families pa who may receive a CFSPID designation for their child. This greater number of families receiving a CFSPID designation, creating uncertainty for their children, was seen as an important outcome to avoid.

The view of the respiratory physician that a child with undiagnosed CF until two years of age would not be significantly harmed in the long term was clearly influential for the participants and it is recognised that this may not be a consensus opinion among medical specialists in the field. It is therefore possible that some or all participants might have expressed a preference for a more 'sensitive' approach to screening if delayed diagnosis were considered to result in long-term harm.

The participants were also strongly influenced by the numerical difference between the low number of potentially missed cases described compared with the greater number expected to receive a CFSPID designation. The indication of a possible lack of comprehensive ongoing support available for the family in receipt of a CFSPID designation also influenced the participants, but to a lesser extent. It remains possible that if different information had been provided, then the views and decisions made by participants might have varied.

As if to emphasise this, some participants commented that if they had received more or different information, they felt that they could easily choose differently.

4. Discussion

The public, patients, professionals, and those responsible for public health policy each approach newborn screening programmes from a range of overlapping viewpoints and priorities. In general, the healthcare professionals and particularly the doctors who care for patients with the disorder often wish to maximise the advantage of the life-changing benefits that screening offers to the children identified, while health policy makers also stress the importance of avoiding a negative impact on the wider population such as the reporting of false positive screening results.

The present study is interesting because it highlights the unique perspective of members of the public without direct experience of CF but with sufficient time to listen to information, question what they have heard, and discuss with one another in order to develop an informed opinion.

Achieving the correct balance between sensitivity and specificity is a well-known issue within screening where typically ensuring that all cases of a particular disorder are identified comes at the cost of either increasing the number of false positive results reported and/or widening the phenotype of those cases identified—not all of whom may benefit from early detection and treatment.

It might reasonably be assumed that the general public view would not tolerate missed cases and indeed during the first workshop, this was the predominant view among the 19 participants who took part in the dialogue. However, it was clear that by the end of the final workshop two weeks later, with time to reflect and discuss within the family, this majority view had changed to one which prized the delivery of unambiguous results to parents over detecting every CF case.

The change in view from the first workshop to the last workshop was particularly notable and emphasises the need for parents to have clear information and sufficient time and information to consider the potential implications of newborn screening when making the right choice for their baby.

A limitation for participants is of course that professional views, such as the concept that a delay in diagnosis of CF until two years of age would not result in significant long-term harm, could be influential and yet may not be shared universally by respiratory physicians treating CF. It also emphasises the difficulty and care needed when helping to inform parents to make decisions on behalf of their children when, as often happens, there is a range of opinion in some crucial areas.

It is particularly interesting that the participants highly prized certainty of outcome in screening linked to clear actions to improve health when compared with approaches that could result in less clarity or long-term uncertainty. This may suggest an important generalisable principle reflecting the public acceptability of new or modified screening programmes, particularly those with a genomic component.

Author Contributions: Investigation, S.K.; Project administration, L.C.; Supervision, H.H.; Writing—original draft, J.R.B. All authors have read and agreed to the published version of the manuscript.

Funding: This research received no external funding.

Informed Consent Statement: Informed consent was obtained from all subjects involved in the study.

Data Availability Statement: This data has not yet been reported.

Acknowledgments: This work was funded by the national Screening Committee and supported by Genomics England and Sciencewise.

Conflicts of Interest: The authors declare no conflict of interest.

References

1. Newborn Blood Spot Screening: Programme Overview-GOV.UK. Last Modified November 2018. Available online: https://www.gov.uk/guidance/newborn-blood-spot-screening-programme-overview (accessed on 11 March 2022).
2. Scotet, V.; Gutierrez, H.; Farrell, P.M. Newborn Screening for CF across the Globe—Where is it worthwhile? *Int. J. Neonatal Screen.* **2020**, *6*, 18. [CrossRef] [PubMed]
3. Cystic Fibrosis Screening Laboratory Handbook-GOV.UK. Last Modified August 2021. Available online: https://www.gov.uk/government/publications/cystic-fibrosis-screening-laboratory-handbook/cystic-fibrosis-screening-laboratory-handbook (accessed on 11 March 2022).
4. Sinclair, G.; McMahon, V.; Schellenberg, A.; Nelson, T.N.; Chilvers, M.; Vallance, H. Performance of a Three-Tier (IRT-DNA-IRT) Cystic Fibrosis Screening Algorithm in British Columbia. *Int. J. Neonatal Screen.* **2020**, *6*, 46. [CrossRef] [PubMed]
5. Baker, M.W.; Atkins, A.E.; Cordovado, S.K.; Hendrix, M.; Earley, M.C.; Farrell, P.M. Improving newborn screening for cystic fibrosis using next-generation sequencing technology: A technical feasibility study. *Genet. Med.* **2015**, *18*, 231–238. [CrossRef] [PubMed]
6. Skov, M.; Baekvad-Hansen, M.; Hougaard, D.M.; Skogstrand, K.; Lund, A.; Pressler, T.; Olesen, H.V.; Duno, M. Cystic fibrosis newborn screening in Denmark: Experience from the first 2 years. *Pediatr. Pulmonol.* **2020**, *55*, 549–555. [CrossRef] [PubMed]
7. Terlizzi, V.; Mergni, G.; Buzzetti, R.; Centrone, C.; Zavataro, L.; Braggion, C. Cystic Fibrosis screen positive inconclusive diagnosis (CFSPID): Experience in Tuscany, Italy. *J. Cyst. Fibros.* **2019**, *18*, 484–490. [CrossRef] [PubMed]
8. Bazeley, P.; Jackson, K. Qualitative Data Analysis with NVivo (Second Edition). In *Qualitative Research in Psychology*; SAGE Publications Ltd.: Thousand Oaks, CA, USA, 2015; Volume 12, pp. 492–494.
9. Hill, L. Mentimeter: A Tool for Actively Engaging Large Lecture Cohorts. *Acad. Manag. Learn. Educ.* **2020**, *19*, 256–258. [CrossRef]
10. Chapman, A.L.; Hadfield, M.; Chapman, C.J. Qualitative research in healthcare: An introduction to grounded theory using thematic analysis. *J. R. Coll. Physicians Edinb.* **2015**, *45*, 201–205. [CrossRef] [PubMed]
11. Isaaca, A.N. An overview of qualitative research methodology for public health researchers. *Int. J. Med. Public Health* **2014**, *4*, 4.

International Journal of
Neonatal Screening

MDPI

Article

Experiences of Families Caring for Children with Newborn Screening-Related Conditions: Implications for the Expansion of Genomics in Population-Based Neonatal Public Health Programs

Lynn Bush [1], Hannah Davidson [2], Shani Gelles [2], Dawn Lea [2] and Laura M. Koehly [2,*]

1 Division of Genetics and Genomics, Boston Children's Hospital and Center for Bioethics, Harvard Medical School, Boston, MA 02115, USA; lynn.bush@childrens.harvard.edu

2 National Human Genome Research Institute, Bethesda, MD 20892, USA; hannah.davidson@nih.gov (H.D.); shani.gelles@nih.gov (S.G.); dawn.lea@nih.gov (D.L.)

* Correspondence: laura.koehly@nih.gov; Tel.: +1-301-451-3999

Abstract: With the expansion of newborn screening conditions globally and the increased use of genomic technologies for early detection, there is a need for ethically nuanced policies to guide the future integration of ever-more comprehensive genomics into population-based newborn screening programs. In the current paper, we consider the lived experiences of 169 family caregivers caring for 77 children with NBS-related conditions to identify lessons learned that can inform policy and practice related to population-based newborn screening using genomic technologies. Based on caregiver narratives obtained through in-depth interviews, we identify themes characterizing these families' diagnostic odyssey continuum, which fall within two domains: (1) medical management implications of a child diagnosed with an NBS-related condition and (2) psychological implications of a child diagnosed with an NBS-related condition. For Domain 1, family caregivers' experiences point to the need for educational resources for both health care professionals that serve children with NBS-related conditions and their families; empowerment programs for family caregivers; training for providers in patient-centered communication; and access to multi-disciplinary specialists. For Domain 2, caregivers' experiences suggest a need for access to continuous, long-term counseling resources; patient navigator resources; and peer support programs. These lessons learned can inform policy recommendations for the benefit of the child, the family, the healthcare system, and society.

Keywords: newborn screening sequencing; newborn genomics; ethics; psychosocial; pediatric rare disease

1. Introduction

As the expansion of population-based newborn screening (NBS) accelerates globally with the increasing integration of genomic technologies, the anticipation of potential implications arising from opportunities and challenges is essential to optimize benefits and mitigate harms [1–11]. This public health endeavor will have a significant influence and impact on many stakeholders [12–14], not the least of whom are the infants receiving a "true-positive" finding and their families. Thus, it is critical to consider the lived experiences of family caregivers who have been navigating the complex landscape of their children's rare conditions that are currently or potentially identifiable through NBS programs. We collectively refer to these disorders as "newborn screening-related conditions," reflecting gene and disease inclusion on the US Recommended Uniform Screening Panel Core and Secondary, NBSTRN-CR Candidates, NC-NEXUS, and others published by experts (i.e., mitochondrial disorders) [15–18].

We also extend the concept of a "diagnostic odyssey" to consider the broader journey that caregivers of children with rare NBS-related conditions can experience in their attempt to understand and manage the uncertain spectrum and evolving course of the newborn's reported screen, presumptive diagnosis, and confirmatory diagnostic results. For even a molecular finding is often not the end of their diagnostic odyssey. We refer to this broader journey as the "diagnostic odyssey *continuum*" (see Bush, Al-Hertani, Bodamer in this Special Issue [19]). Important to this concept is the under-appreciated fact that NBS is a process, not simply a test, and will likely remain a process whether as a "screening" test through current NBS platforms or a genomic "diagnostic" test from the outset. Either way, public health newborn screening programs aim to presymptomatically identify select conditions for which a confirmatory "diagnosis" may be sought, and often diagnosis is an evolving process. Typically, findings are initially communicated in the beginning of the first year of life with the intent that through early identification, negative outcomes for the infant can be averted or mitigated, thereby reducing morbidity and mortality rates for all infants [20,21]. In doing so, beneficence and non-maleficence can be actualized and equitable [9]. However, early signs and symptoms may be missed, the presumptive diagnosis may be a misdiagnosis, or the confirmatory diagnosis may not fully capture the child's condition due to significant variability, resulting in a 'label' that lacks precision. In such cases, families are often on a journey that extends well beyond the initial diagnosis, a journey that continues until a fully realized syndrome is manifest, more precisely identified, and outcomes understood.

Importantly, the heterogeneity in phenotype and genotype-phenotype correlations of many NBS-related conditions (current and proposed) results in prognostic uncertainty which can impact the timespan of the diagnostic odyssey continuum. Long-term follow-up of NBS is key [22,23], yet notably lacking, and could improve understanding of a rare condition's natural history [24]. This is particularly salient as NBS expansion with genomics accelerates and amplifies the need for shared decision-making [25,26] in care management given the level of uncertainty that will accompany the greater magnitude of conditions and carrier statuses identified. While recent studies report opportunities, challenges, and limitations with augmenting, supplementing, and secondary tier use of genomic approaches to characterize this variation [6,27–31], and some professionals are vocal proponents or opponents of primary comprehensive sequencing as part of NBS [32], it is important to seek the voices of caregivers and consider the lived experiences of families who are already caring for children with NBS-related conditions. Such perspectives can contribute to ethically nuanced policy.

From an ethical perspective, the "best interest of the child" [33,34] and the "harm principle" [35] are beacons that guide NBS practices worldwide. However, there is controversy [36] about whether NBS criteria should go beyond the classic 1968 Wilson Jungner [37] World Health Organization (WHO) framework to a broader approach with consideration of parent/family interests and future planning. Andermann and colleagues [38] posited one such screening criteria (also for the WHO) four decades later that they subtitle "for the genomics era" (not necessarily WGS) and more closely parallels contemporary practice involving children. Their framework includes weighing benefits for family interests while not neglecting the child's interests, and is applicable whether sequencing is primary, secondary, confirmatory, or supplemental. Further controversy surrounding inclusion criteria arises from the degree of comprehensiveness, and their potential benefits and harms [32,39,40]. Some commentators note that the incorporation of a genotype-first approach in NBS for an expanding range of conditions may no longer constitute a newborn "screen" and potentially jeopardize a valuable public health program with some parents opting out of consenting. Others argue a more comprehensive genotype-first approach in NBS can shift a learning health care system [41] further from a reactive model to a proactive model, and in turn, improve equitable access to diagnostics and potentially make more actionable diagnoses pre-symptomatically. Doing so, even with less comprehensive panels, may then result in more equitable access to treatments as well as potentially provide greater opportunity for families to make future plans for the child and other family members [42].

With these potential opportunities in mind, and cognizant that many ethical concerns co-exist (see others in this Special Issue), we consider caregiver narratives as they describe their journey through the diagnostic odyssey continuum. The psychosocial implications of their experiences, powerfully articulated from their voices, are particularly timely to help guide an ethically minded approach that is beneficial to the child and that eases the burden for families and minimizes harms in the context of sequencing informed NBS. What we learn from these implications derived through interviews most certainly has ethical implications in the accelerating implementation of genomics in public health NBS programs. Thus, the integration of caregivers' perspectives into policies that guide genomic expansion within population-based NBS has significant value and fosters a family-centered approach to informed decision-making. Moreover, policies that arise from such work can aid in identifying what is required to manage expectations of phenotypes, medical/educational/social needs, outcomes, quality of life, and caregiving responsibilities, while also maximizing benefits and minimizing harm for the family and the child.

The framework of this study is in contrast to the preponderance of research that investigates the ethical and psychological implications of parents receiving false-positive newborn screening results, carrier status, or true positives of single conditions, which typically utilize surveys, focus groups, questionnaires, or interviews that directly inquire about the NBS process. Notably, for previous interview-based NBS studies, relatively small samples were typically engaged. In the current paper, data were obtained from a relatively large sample of caregivers participating in interviews that did not probe specifically about NBS. This study also diverges from most rare disease qualitative research similarly focused on the psychosocial experiences of families in that those studies tend not to then use their findings to generate NBS ethical considerations. In the current paper, we characterize the experiences of caregivers whose children's illnesses are NBS-related conditions and examine their experiences and perspectives in the context of a diagnostic odyssey continuum. We discuss the implications of caregivers' experiences and describe "lessons learned" for guiding ethically nuanced population-based newborn screening expansion involving sequencing in public health programs. Using qualitative analysis of open-ended interviews from a relatively large sample of individuals caring for children with NBS-related conditions, we consider the following questions:

- How does the presumptive diagnosis of a potentially NBS-identifiable condition impact these families' accounts of their diagnostic odyssey?
- How do these caregivers describe the evolution and communication of diagnosis, prognosis, variation, and uncertainty as they navigate the process of understanding the child's condition?
- What meanings and themes arise when these caregivers discuss their experiences with caregiving regarding their past and present reality in the context of a diagnostic odyssey continuum, as well as its impact on future planning?
- What lessons can be learned from the themes identified from these caregiver perspectives to optimize ethically nuanced NBS expansion augmented with sequencing?

The intent of this empirical research is to build upon prior and current efforts in the literature and contribute to the evidence base for developing timely recommendations for guiding the future integration of more comprehensive genomics into NBS. Importantly, in line with ethical principles and a family-centered approach, this work will also inform the identification of caregivers' needs in order to make informed decisions and provide resources that will better support caregivers in their care roles as well as enhance shared decision making. Thus, the lessons learned through caregivers' experiences can help guide policy and practice as it relates to population-based newborn screening with increasing genomic technology in public health programs.

2. Materials and Methods

2.1. Procedures

Data come from the 'Inherited diseases, caregiving, and social networks' protocol (Clinical Trials Identifier NCT01498263), a mixed-methods cross-sectional study that focuses on family caregiving in the context of several rare genetic diseases and undiagnosed conditions. The study was approved by the Institutional Review Boards of the National Human Genome Research Institute and the National Institutes of Health. Participants were recruited through ongoing clinical studies of persons affected by inherited metabolic and mitochondrial conditions and undiagnosed diseases; family meetings and advocacy groups for such rare genetic conditions; and referrals from participating family members.

Following informed consent, eligible participants completed an online survey and semi-structured interview either by telephone or in person. Characteristics of the participant and child were ascertained through both survey and interview. Of note, "child" is used inclusive of those who reached adulthood by the time of the interview. Participant characteristics include age, sex, race/ethnicity, socio-economic status, and kinship tie to the child. Characteristics of the child include age, sex, and diagnosis; in addition, caregivers completed the Children's Habilitation Assessment Tool (CHAT) [43] which provides context for the severity of the child's condition.

Participants also completed a semi-structured interview where they were asked a series of open-ended interview questions assessing their physical and emotional health, experiences with caregiver 'burnout', and the impact of caregiving on family functioning. The semi-structured interview guide (see Supplementary Materials) was derived from a previously published study investigating caregiver health in the context of caring for children with genetic syndromes, learning and attentional disorders, and neurological disorders [44]. All interviews were transcribed verbatim; personally identifiable information of participants, the child, and any family members discussed within the interview was redacted prior to analysis. The current report focuses on a subset of participants who are family caregivers of children with a newborn screening-related condition (those currently or potentially identifiable through NBS), specifically 169 participants from 77 families.

2.2. Sample Characteristics

Family caregivers of children with NBS-related conditions were, on average, 42 years of age, and approximately 70% of these caregivers were parents of these children. Two-thirds self-identified as female (66.9%) and the majority reported being married (82.2%). Slightly more than 10% had some high school or a diploma, while just under a quarter had an associate degree or technical training; most caregivers completed a bachelor's degree (42.6%), and one-fifth had post-graduate training. Slightly more than twenty percent of caregivers reported an annual household income of USD 50,000 or less, while about forty percent reported an annual household income of at least USD 100,000. The majority of caregivers identified as non-Hispanic or Latino (90%) and White (84%) (see Table 1).

The children with NBS-related conditions were, on average, 10 years of age; a few were over 18 years of age when their family caregiver was interviewed. About a third of the children were female (36.4%) and the majority (80.5%) were diagnosed with an organic acidemia. Based on the CHAT [43], care needs were largely in the life skills domain, with disability scores for social skills and behavior falling in the mid to lower ranges, respectively (see Table 1). Higher scores are indicative of greater support required for activities of daily living in the respective domain.

Table 1. Caregiver and child socio-demographic characteristics.

Participant Characteristics (N = 169)		M (SD) or % (N)
Gender		
	Female	66.9% (N = 113)
	Male	33.1% (N = 56)
Age		M = 43.3 years (SD = 12.7)
Marital status		
	Married/living as married	82.2% (N = 139)
	Never married	7.1% (N = 12)
	Divorced or separated	5.3% (N = 9)
	Widowed	0.6% (N = 1)
	NA	4.7% (N = 8)
Kinship		
	Mother	44.4% (N = 75)
	Father	26% (N = 44)
	Sibling	3.6% (N = 6)
	Grandparent	14.2% (N = 24)
	Aunt/uncle	5.9% (N = 10)
	Other kin	1.2% (N = 2)
	Non-kin	4.7% (N = 8)
Education Level		
	Middle school/some high school	1.2% (N = 2)
	High school graduate/GED	10.1% (N = 17)
	Associate degree/technical training	22.5% (N = 38)
	Bachelor degree	42.6% (N = 72)
	Post-graduate degree	20.7% (N = 35)
	NA	3.0% (N = 5)
Income Level		
	>USD 200,000	11.8% (N = 20)
	USD 100,001 to USD 200,000	28.4% (N = 48)
	USD 50,000 to USD 100,000	29.6% (N = 50)
	USD 20,001 to USD 50,000	16.0%(N = 27)
	<USD 20,000	4.8% (N = 8)
	Don't know	5.8% (N = 10)
	NA	3.6% (N = 6)
Race		
	White	84% (N = 142)
	Black or African-American	3.5% (N = 6)
	Asian	3.0% (N = 5)
	Mixed race	3.0% (N = 5)
	Other	4.1% (N = 7)
	NA	2.4% (N = 4)

Table 1. *Cont.*

Participant Characteristics (*N* = 169)		M (SD) or % (*N*)
Ethnicity		
	Hispanic or Latino	5.3% (*N* = 9)
	Non-Hispanic or Latino	90.0% (*N* = 152)
	NA	4.7% (*N* = 8)
	Child Characteristics (N = 77)	**M (SD) or % (*N*)**
Gender		
	Female	36.4% (*N* = 28)
	Male	63.6% (*N* = 49)
Age		M = 10.3 years (SD = 7.8 years)
Diagnosis Category		
	Organic acidemia	80.5% (*N* = 62)
	Fatty acid oxidation disorder	5.2% (*N* = 4)
	Carbohydrate metabolism disorder	1.3% (*N* = 1)
	Lipid storage disorder	3.9% (*N* = 3)
	Mitochondrial disorder	3.9% (*N* = 3)
	Undiagnosed condition	5.2% (*N* = 4)
Childhood Activities of Daily Living		
	Life skills [Range: 0–20]	M = 12.9 (SD = 6.7)
	Social skills [Range: 0–16]	M = 7.6 (SD = 5.5)
	Behavioral [Range: 0–24]	M = 3.3 (SD = 4.0)

2.3. Analysis

Families who referenced caring for children with NBS-related disorders were identified after multiple readings of the open-ended transcripts (LB). NVivo 12 Plus Version 12.6.0.959 (64 bit), QSR International, Melbourne, Australia [45], a qualitative data analysis software program, was used to facilitate coding and analysis. A preliminary iterative codebook was developed after an initial round of coding (SG and HD); 52 participant transcripts, from 25 families, were double coded to identify recurrent themes related to the proposed research questions, organized by overarching themes and more specific motifs. Inter-rater reliability was assessed, and these preliminarily coded transcripts were reviewed to identify additional codes and revise initial codes. The remaining transcripts (117 participants from 52 families) were randomly divided between two coders (SG and HD) for single coding according to the established codebook. Coders met to further refine existing codes and identify sub-codes throughout this second phase of analysis. After reaching saturation, codes were shared with the research team at-large (SG, HD, LK, DL, LB). Coders (SG, HD, LK, LB) grouped salient codes into broader thematic categories in accordance with research questions. Aspects of grounded theory and inductive qualitative analysis were used to help coders avoid preconceptions and to find unanticipated themes and commonalities within the corpus of data [46,47]. Participant unique identification numbers follow quotes used to illustrate identified themes; the first three digits of each identification number denote the family, followed by three digits that denote the family caregiver.

3. Results

3.1. Domain 1. Medical Management Implications of a Child Diagnosed with NBS-elated Condition: "there's so much, still, that's unknown" (747000)

Caregiver responses highlighted the multi-faceted challenges arising from their experiences of diagnoses for rare diseases. They describe their experiences as an odyssey that often move families into a caregiving role filled with uncertainty. One component of this uncertainty was expressed as being related to how much is unknown about the rare conditions affecting the child and the limited understanding of such conditions within the medical community. These unknowns made their challenging caregiving roles ever more complex. Family caregivers were acutely aware of how much there is still to learn, for both themselves and medical professionals:

> *"There was a lot of unknowns, a lot of unknowns. What is his condition? And what's it all going to mean?"* (747001)

> *"– we had a doctor tell us one time that if it has hooves it's probably a horse and not a zebra. It's like, well, we were the zebra. Like [child], you know, didn't have reflux, he had a metabolic disease . . . "* (119000)

> *"We were really worried initially about [the child]'s, like, physical health. Like, there wasn't very much research on his disorder and what there was, kind of, was very dire and like, 'Oh, he could have these medical crises at any second.'"* (702000)

Many of these caregivers also expressed that in addition to the rarity of these conditions, the phenotypic variability within conditions compounded their challenges with ongoing uncertainties. A medically named diagnosis does not capture the lived experience or prognosis of the individual child and family.

> *"We just don't even have any clue what the outcome's going to be like in this . . . The spectrum is so wide."* (116001)

> *"When you read things online, it can be, like, sort of, like, worst-case scenarios . . . when I first read about [condition] when he first got diagnosed, like, this could be true, but this hasn't turned out to be true for him or the majority of other patients we know."* (126004)

The rarity of such conditions, and phenotypic variation within, reportedly shaped these families' diagnostic odyssey continuum—that is, how they inform themselves about the child's condition following a presumptive diagnosis and subsequent modifications to the diagnosis, act as patient advocates, interface with the medical community, and approach treatment-related decisions.

3.1.1. "And then the next day we heard, '[condition]', and it has just been a whirlwind since then." (140000)

While the odyssey from the unknown to a "screen" to a "diagnosis" for current NBS conditions typically begins at birth with the heelstick, for most of our participants the diagnostic odyssey continuum did not end at the point of the first reported finding.

> *" . . . neurologist at the hospital—he said something I'll never forget . . . 'as soon as something like this happens, all they [sic parents] think about is, 'Is my baby going to die? . . . You just need to be aware of where your mind goes when you look at your child. Especially when they're at the doctor, or you're getting new and different news about the diagnosis.' And our geneticist in [city] told us that he—because I asked him point-blank, 'Okay, so what's the lifespan for a kid who has this?' At the time, we didn't know his mutation. He told us maybe 11 or 12 years old."* (112000)

> *"– when he was in the hospital as a brand-new newborn, ... I said, 'Man, let's keep things in perspective. The baby next to us has to get a liver transplant,' and that, like, things were much worse for them than they were for us. And then, eight months later, there we were, getting a liver transplant."* (126004)

As described, in some cases, the child's clinician incorrectly considered the initial results to be a 'false positive', *"It's too rare of a disease. He doesn't have this disease. This was a false positive."* (119000), extending experiences of uncertainty as families awaited a conclusive result. For several, the child experienced a medical crisis before results were disclosed.

> *"Well, it was caught in the screening. However, I think it took too long, because she was 7 days old when we got the call that something was abnormal on the screening, but she was already sick by then, and they—all they said was, 'Abnormal.' So, we took her to the pediatrician. They did more bloodwork and, I think, got urine and stool samples, something like that, and sent it off and told us – . . . told us to keep feeding her. Well—but it was the next day that we were in the ER . . . I mean, it was newborn screening-detected, so that's great. That probably saved her life. She might have been a SIDS baby otherwise. But . . . knowing about it sooner would—could have possibly prevented the metabolic crisis."* (140000)

> *" . . . but then his dad was like, "We'll just wait until the doctor contacts us, or like contacts us, and like, you know, they'll handle it", but they didn't, and then he had like seizures and he had to keep him in NICU."* (148000)

Given caregivers' limited understanding of such rare diseases, there is a reliance on the medical team, who may also have limited understanding of and limited experience with these rare conditions. Yet, healthcare professionals don't always recognize, or share, that the confirmation testing following an initial screen and consultation process can be lengthy. Such delays not only can have significant medical implications for the child, but they also have the potential to impact patient–provider relationships moving forward. This time period is pivotal in shaping how caregivers interface with the medical community.

> *"– all of the initial testing where . . . we were kind of naive and, like, we didn't know, like, of course we were going to go along with what the doctor said, and like, it's kind of like they tested the same thing four times just to make sure."* (745000)

> *"Yeah, well, that's the thing. Like, I don't feel like—now, in our first year it was a lot of new information thrown at us all the time. He had 86 doctor's appointments in 10 months."* (401000)

3.1.2. "– just make sure you learn as much as you can" (150001)

As these caregivers entered the world of rare diseases, they speak about learning and processing information that encompasses both the intricacies of their child's condition, as well as the nuances of the health care system. Many considered developing a literacy in this world as being paramount to providing effective care for their child. Said one parent:

> *"It's pretty overwhelming. Like, it's pretty, like wow, like this is intense, you know, to not only be in—like to be the one that's, you know, helping to keep these kids alive, but like to like, have all this medical stuff that you have to do along with it. So, it's definitely a learning curve, like you learn a lot of information that no one else understands, unless you run into someone who understands it."* (110000)

Caregivers describe a vast range of resources used to build their knowledge base, ranging from the more professional and academic (including keeping up to date on emergent research and primary literature) to the more informal, such as parent Facebook groups. They spoke of the necessity of building this knowledge base as being rooted in the rarity of the conditions themselves:

> *"Well, I was the one up on the internet, you know, up on the computers trying to research—he was detected through newborn screening that [child] had [condition] . . . And no one at the hospital where he was born had—knew what this was . . . So, even though we were in a big city hospital with all these great doctors, no one had heard of this . . . condition."* (747000)

However, the available sources for information gathering can yield mixed results: caregivers note both the necessity to keep up to date with information, and also acknowledge that it is imperative to *"take the things you read with a grain of salt"* (126004) since some of the sources were outdated or did not address phenotypic variability within the condition.

3.1.3. "like, become informed, because you're going to have to be an advocate when your child has a rare disease" (126004)

As a result of extensive information gathering, caregivers stressed the need to become expert advocates for their child, ever cognizant of the gaps between the care system they and the patient must navigate and the state of the science on their child's condition:

> *"Recognize that if you want your child to have the best care, you're going to have to really do that research and, like, stick up for things, because many doctors have only seen one or two cases of this in their career."* (126004)

Many acknowledge that stepping into the role of expert advocate requires caregivers to develop considerable information-gathering and organizational skills:

> *"– we take the time to go see a doctor four to five hours away, we have a list of questions ... then we have time for other questions that may arise spontaneously ... But I think the organization and the openness in conversation and planning ahead has helped."* (112000)

3.1.4. "finding those right doctors ... is the most important thing" (116001)

For many of these families, an imperative action in the initial time frame and long-term is building an effective, knowledgeable, and cohesive care team. In addition to gathering information and advocating for their child, caregivers also need to identify health care providers that have the appropriate expertise and patient-centered communication skills. For many, locating such experts is challenging, often requiring trial and error and out-of-state travel:

> *"I went to [advocacy conference] in 20##. That's where I actually met [child's specialist]. He was speaking there ... And I'm a little shy, so <unintelligible> I walked up to him and I said, you know, 'Are you taking new patients?' And I almost made an appointment right there. So, that was how we connected with him and we've been very happy with [hospital's] team."* (116000)

> *"The best advice I can give is make sure you find a doctor that will listen to you ... She could look at him and tell, like, "Okay, something's not right." Or she can smell him and tell that something's not right ... – just know your kid."* (150001)

Family caregivers' interviews reveal that often, building an optimal care team is impacted by prior experiences with healthcare providers who have limited knowledge of treating patients with rare conditions. In some cases, such experiences are noted to have resulted in negative health outcomes due to medical crises. In other cases, narratives of such experiences seem to dehumanize the child. In all, how the medical community interacts with patients and families affected by rare NBS-related conditions shapes caregivers' perceptions of the health care system—including feelings of medical mistrust—adding further complexity to building an effective care team for the child and family.

> *"I think like a big thing with me is dealing with, like, trust with doctors because when [child] was diagnosed, the doctor said, 'He doesn't have [condition]. There's no way he has [condition]. It's too rare of a disease ... Like he—you know, he doesn't have it.' So then he ended up having it. So now, like, if, you know, there's a health issue that arises and the doctors say we don't have it, I don't believe them and I don't trust them, you know."* (119000)

> *"He's a person with feelings and experiences and day-to-day life, you know, that have to be taken into consideration. And they just kind of view him as, like, 'Wow, this is exciting. Like, once in a lifetime we get to see one like this.' You know, stuff like that. We've had people—doctors—say that to us. And I find that to be very offensive and*

(laughs) detrimental to the relationship ... But because they had no ability to care for him personally, you know, we kind of eliminated them from the repertoire of people we had to see ... And I always have thought here that they're goal is not just to, you know, learn about this science experiment, but they're goal is to give [child] the best quality of life he can have." (141000)

While healthcare professionals and caregivers strive to bring their knowledge, experience, and unique skillsets to the table and are mindful of the best interests of the child, their ability to optimally work together can be significantly influenced by how they communicate with each other.

" ... trying to be assertive, as well as respectful, and get heard, like, can be really hard things when you're dealing with, like, the medical community and you don't have any kind of degree you feel, like—and you're, also, just trying to learn it through, like, a psychosocial component of that, too. Because different medical doctors have different personalities and, like, different triggers, right? Like, if I say something one way to one doctor, it's going to rub him the wrong way. And, then, he has a perception of me. And, then, like, I don't know. Like, you hope that they hold you with as much grace as you try to hold with them." (747000)

3.1.5. "Unfortunately, the situation isn't such what ... we have this treatment and that treatment. It's so specific and so specific to our own family ... " (700001)

For many of these caregivers, uncertainty related to the child's health outcomes was depicted as being inextricably tied to challenges with disease management and treatment options, which are often limited and individualized due to the rarity of such conditions and the phenotypic variation expressed within specific diagnostic categories. These factors present further complexity as caregivers navigate an expanding healthcare system due to the evolution of the condition, diagnosis, or therapeutics, each impacting care decisions for their child that must be (re)evaluated.

" ... So, I called Dr. [X], and I said, 'What do we do? What are our options?' He said, 'Well, we could do a liver and kidney transplant when he's about three months old.' And at that time, and still, kind of still actually, there's still lots of problems that go on with transplants. You don't just give someone a transplant, and they live 80 years, and they're perfectly fine. I mean, you do have stories like that. Don't get me wrong. But when you have [condition], there's still other problems that are associated with these kids, so it doesn't just all of a sudden, rainbows come out and the sun's shining and you don't have any more problems. It's not like that." (100000)

Caregivers are often called upon to make difficult and emergent decisions as they experience the push and pull of balancing potentially invasive interventions and their child's quality of life, especially when information is limited or outcomes are unknown. To help them make informed decisions—decisions that are often described as temporally challenging—caregivers speak of needing to increase their literacy regarding the rare disease (often through their lived experience) as well as the potential interventions or treatment(s) for their child while building a knowledgeable care team. However, doing so (even when they have a medically named diagnosis) does not always lead to a clear understanding of the child's prognosis, care, and treatment or prevent deterioration in health outcomes.

"I mean, when he was age zero to three, before that liver transplant, every day was, like, brutal. He was so volatile from a health perspective ... .in hindsight, I think we thought, at the time, the G tube represented failure to some degree. But I think as time went on, and his issues became more clear, and the reality of things became more clear, you know, we kind of pulled the ripcord and got that G tube put in ... .We probably should have done that sooner, but, you know, you live and learn or whatever. And then, the liver just changed everything ... I mean, he, you know, we were at the shore, you know, watching him run down the boardwalk, you know, and unfortunately, that stroke robbed him of

that kind of stuff. And you know, the biggest—the shame of it—of everything he went through and all the issues he faces and that damn stroke, like, robbed him of, and created challenges for him on a day-to-day basis that don't seem like they're going to be able to be significantly mitigated." (135001)

The interviews also highlight that new genomic technologies offer these caregivers hope that such treatment interventions, and associated decisions, are just around the corner or at least on the horizon.

"It's not like it's something that everybody has and they're going to be looking— . . . for a cure. It's the way that you're going to solve this disease–the only way you're going to cure this is that there's going to be some—somebody's going to come with some breakthrough in like genetic sequencing or something or being able to change, you know, change the genome around, or you know, make those kind of changes that can be generic for every kind of disease." (116001)

"We are very positive . . . We think that, "Okay, this will work out.' He have a [sic] deafness, we got cochlear implant for him. He's losing his vision. We are hoping, and we are very positive, that someday they will come up with something where his vision problem will be solved. Some genetic modification or some gene therapy or something." (134001)

3.2. Domain 2. Psychosocial Implications of a Child Diagnosed with NBS-Related Condition: "We just don't even have any clue what the outcome's going to be like in this." (116001)

In addition to navigating the child's medical care, these caregivers report that they are also coping with the myriad of intricacies when caring for a potentially medically fragile child where the outcomes may be uncertain. As one caregiver stated:

"And when you have a child with an inborn error of metabolism, every day is unknown. There are worst case scenarios that are very real, and possible, and even sometimes probable." (722000)

Indeed, the caregivers point to the fact that—"everybody develops different" (115000)—and this variability was noted to have a broad impact on these caregivers' experiences. Importantly, as caregivers connect with each other, they spoke of gaining an understanding of this variation and developing a support system that they were able to leverage as they navigated their caregiving role:

"But it was a relief many ways to meet other families whose children were not severely—I mean, there were some who had more severe parents [sic patients] but some whose kids seemed pretty normal, so that was a lot better than, you know, what the doctors that we currently had, the picture they were painting." (116000)

"I went to some parent group when he was in—early on, and they were like, [the child] will—he will do his own thing. It will be his own path, and there's no—there are no marks for this road. You don't have any benchmarks . . . It's just a different perspective once you recognize he won't ever fit in this normal box, so it's kind of freeing that way." (149000)

The uncertainty, both in terms of how the condition manifests symptomatically for the child, as well as for the child's future, also impacts family caregivers' psychosocial adjustment. Caregivers' reports describe adjustments related to integrating the child's diagnosis and medical management into the caregiver's day to day activities; the process of acceptance, which requires them to adjust their perceptions and feelings about the child's abilities and future outlook; and how caregivers plan for an uncertain future, both for themselves and the child.

3.2.1. "... We're kind of in a battle rhythm ... we know for the most part what we're dealing with." (126001)

Following a presumptive diagnosis of an NBS-related condition, many of these caregivers describe learning a new "battle rhythm" in an effort towards integrating disease management into everyday life. Caregivers report that although the day-to-day activities associated with disease management initially overtake their lives, they are able to adjust to, redefine, and create their 'new normal'. Narratives show that this adjustment may be in the form of feeling capable to address a crisis that may arise, and through gaining a different perspective with respect to what it means to have a good enough or an optimal quality of life:

> *"Getting used to just kind of living with the uncertainty, and living with that, you know, being ready to, you know, change tactic at a moment's notice."* (138001)

> *"And try to adjust your life. You don't have to live in a cave and not travel anywhere and, you know, – this family said the doctors told us that, you know, she needs to stay home and not leave because if it gets too cold they could die. Well, yeah, they can. But is it worth living your life that way? ... For us, you know, [the child] needs to ride rollercoasters. So what if she shouldn't because she's got problems with her heart and stuff? If she died on a rollercoaster, that would be great because she would go out happy."* (131000)

3.2.2. "And you learn to appreciate what you have and not what you don't" (126001)

Adjustments in the caregiver's roles are reflected in daily activities, and also in their perceptions, feelings, and expectations as expressed in the interviews. They tell stories whereby this coping process involves acknowledging the feelings, good and bad, that come with caring for a child with an NBS-related condition, and accepting what one can control and what one can't:

> *"And actually, life becomes normal and a lot of the time you don't think about it. When you get used to it it's just your life and our life is normal. And you have feelings in the beginning that you shouldn't be afraid of, to express. If you feel like you wish you wouldn't have had that child, allow yourself to feel it. Allow yourself to feel everything because you have to work through all those feelings."* (107000)

> *"people need to be as educated as they can about the disease process so that they can try to minimize any problems. But then, at the same time, you have to embrace that there's a lot of things outside of our control."* (127000)

> *"And you know, certainly, I've accepted some realities over time, and adjusted what I thought 'good' looked like."* (135001)

3.2.3. "fear of the unknown, fear of the unknown future" (119001)

While caregivers shared stories across a continuum of hope, optimism, and expectations that new discoveries will allow the child seriously affected by the NBS-related rare condition to live independently, they also reported on the psychological toll related to their fears of the future and the process of acceptance:

> *"– you kind of have this whole future planned out in your head for them, and then, when you get this diagnosis, it's just like—almost like a punch in the stomach. Like, you don't—everything becomes uncertain, unstable, and it's very—I mean, it's heartbreaking."* (740000)

> *"– you don't know when something bad can happen, so I'm always thinking the worst. I don't really know. Like, I don't—I don't know if my kids are going to go to college. I don't know if my kids are going to, like, have families."* (146000)

> *"I think when [child] was younger I had so many goals and so many, I don't know, things in mind for him or hopes and stuff. And it was so painful when, I guess, things kind of would slowly but—it's interesting because I think when he was really tiny, like a little*

baby, I think part of me already knew how bad things were going to be at some point. And I didn't want to like accept that, so I kept hoping things were going to change or get better, or he wouldn't be as bad as I guess I thought. And I think it has turned out to be as bad as I feared (laughs)—very early on. But, I don't know, I feel like that's almost part of the coping that you like—you come to accept that little by little, rather than just—because it's too much. Like it's too overwhelming to try to accept the depth of how bad things will be. Like at—all at once, you know?" (141000)

4. Discussion

Narratives from retrospective in-depth interviews with this relatively large sample of family caregivers of children with NBS-related conditions provide rich empirical data describing their evolving journey and the challenges they experience as they navigate a landscape replete with unknowns, uncertainty, and variability. These caregiver stories contribute valuable 'lessons learned' that can inform ethically minded integration of genomics within a population-based newborn public health program—implementation that fosters respect for informed shared decision making—by bringing to light a constellation of challenges that largely fall within two domains. The first domain focuses on their critical caregiving role that necessitates developing medical expertise, advocating for the child with the rare condition, and navigating the healthcare system; whilst the second highlights psychosocial aspects of adjusting to and coping with their caregiving role. These domains reflect both problem-focused coping as they attempt to manage their child's condition and emotion-focused coping as caregivers realign their expectations of what is important for their own and their child's lives.

Given the inherent characteristics of the majority of NBS-related conditions—notable phenotypic variability, prognostic uncertainty, and a wide range of gene variants with low phenotypic correlation in concert with current limited knowledge of rare diseases by health care professionals and others—we anticipate that many of the significant challenges expressed by these family caregivers will persist for other families as more conditions are identified with population-based genome approaches. We acknowledge that the challenges identified here are not all new and there are prior and current efforts to address them. However, many of the challenges raised by family caregivers in these interviews highlight that they have not yet been sufficiently met. Thus, there is a very real need to further mitigate the challenges that caregivers of children with rare diseases experience in order for a more sequence-informed NBS to be realized, including complementary to biochemical assessments. Based on the domains and themes identified from the narratives and perspectives of these family caregivers, we share several points of consideration to optimize ethically nuanced NBS expansion augmented with sequencing, with the hope that such lessons learned can potentially further inform policy recommendations for the benefit of the child, the family, the healthcare system, and society.

4.1. Domain 1. Medical Management Implications of a Child Diagnosed with NBS-Related Condition

The provision of up-to-date enhanced **educational resources for pediatricians and other primary healthcare professionals (and students)** regarding the increasing number of rare conditions that are potentially NBS-identifiable with genomic technologies will be essential to reduce incorrect assumptions of false-positive results and minimize the expressed negative impact when a presumptive diagnosis is initially communicated to families. In addition, there is a need to educate healthcare professionals about the screening to the diagnostic process and address incorrect assumptions about screening and confirmatory testing, including realistic expectations of repeat screening and the speed of results. This in turn may help alter the experience of losing trust in the healthcare system while on their diagnostic odyssey and beyond, including understanding their child's condition and seeking treatment.

Readily accessible and appropriately vetted **educational resources for families** regarding rare conditions that are potentially NBS identifiable with genomic technologies is an imperative to minimize the expressed negative impact when a presumptive diagnosis is communicated to families and thus help alter the experience on their diagnostic odyssey. We recommend provisions of responsibly vetted educational resources, including a general web link to help families locate IRB-approved government registered clinical trials and designated centers of excellence and/or clinical researchers recognized to have expertise in this specialized space.

Empowerment programs that help **family caregivers build capabilities** to advocate for the child, both in terms of treatment and intervention, but also to improve quality of life. Caregivers will take on the role of patient advocate for the child, and thus building communication and advocacy skills, along with literacy, early in the caregiving career will help caregivers interface with the healthcare system and improve treatment and care provided to the child. Due to the range of experiences, baseline literacy, and time constraints that caregivers have, it is imperative that these programs be developed and implemented through an equity and access lens.

Training in the principles and practice of **patient-centered communication** [48–50] **for providers**, which has long been identified as a fundamental physician competency. Components of patient-centered communication include (1) responding to emotions; (2) managing uncertainty; (3) enabling disease- and treatment-related behaviors; (4) exchanging information; (5) shared decision making; and (6) fostering healing relationships [51]. Improved patient–provider communication can help to build trust, and in turn, reinforce caregivers' capabilities to advocate and care for the child.

Ease of access to **multi-disciplinary specialists**, both in person and virtual/remote, to help with the diagnostic odyssey and acute and chronic long-term care management, and to improve more realistic understanding and expectation of the condition as its manifestations evolve. Equitable access to specialist care and advice may have a positive impact not only on the child's health but may also help families adjust to shifting 'new normal' and plans for the future.

4.2. Domain 2. Psychosocial Implications of a Child Diagnosed with NBS-Related Condition

The affordable and accessible provision of **continuous, long-term counseling resources** (genetic counseling, psychology, social work) for families to support, better understand, and cope with the diagnostic odyssey continuum and the evolution of the child's condition as increasing numbers of rare disorders become NBS identifiable with genomic technologies. These resources will be essential to minimize the expressed negative impact when a presumptive diagnosis is communicated to families and play an integral role to assuage the experience of adjusting to the "whirlwind" of their child's condition and the evolving caregiver roles during the diagnostic odyssey continuum.

Accessible **patient navigator resources and complex care programs with transition services** for families who have children with rare conditions that are potentially NBS identifiable using genomic technologies. This is imperative to minimize the expressed negative impact of attempting to navigate healthcare systems and manage conditions after a presumptive diagnosis is communicated to families and thus help alter the experience beyond the initial diagnostic odyssey.

Peer support programs, including mentoring programs facilitated by clinicians trained in psychosocial services, that connect families with shared experiences. Such programs provide an opportunity for caregivers whose children have relatively similar needs and/or prognoses to learn from each other and foster support for each other as they navigate psychosocial challenges related to the uncertainty surrounding the child's diagnosis, disease course, and potential therapeutics [52].

Keeping in mind the two domains described here, it is important to consider that they are intertwined. With a lens towards ethical tenets of non-maleficence, beneficence, autonomy, and justice/fairness [53] for the family as well as the infant/child, this data from psychosocial research offers considerations that emphasize respecting key stakeholder informed decision making and empathically managing expectations related to prognostic certainty, outcome, quality of life, and care. Central to these considerations is an ethical framework grounded in the harm principle [35] and the best interests of the child [33,34]. Care team interactions can be sources of stress and strain for caregivers, thereby impacting caregivers' psychosocial well-being and the well-being of the child. Thus, identifying and implementing best practices to help families navigate the healthcare system can alleviate some of the associated strain. Provider interactions that are empathic and bi-directional exchanges provide an opportunity for open communications such that healthcare providers and caregivers can learn from each other and be equal partners in care decisions for the child. For example, providers who are empathically direct about the assumptions underlying diagnostic testing and the length of the diagnostic odyssey help families gain knowledge and understanding about the process. Moreover, caregivers who feel comfortable openly discussing their concerns and experiences can educate providers to fully appreciate what it means to care for a child with a rare condition.

Fundamentally, such practices demonstrate respect for persons, a key characteristic of the principle of autonomy, and shared decision making, particularly when children are involved [25]. These ethical considerations can, and should, be addressed through the provision of improved education, communication, support, and equitable access from before the screening process to the initial diagnostic label to evolving symptomatology, care, treatment, and future planning for all involved. "So long as the child is part of a viable family, his [sic] own interests are merged with those of the other members" [33]. With this acknowledgment, the voices of family caregivers in this study resonate and deserve to be heard, with strategies implemented to address their concerns as genomic expansion evolves within population-based NBS. To do less is ethically unjustifiable.

5. Limitations

As the promise of genomic integration into NBS becomes realized, it is important to consider the experiences of caregivers in informing best practices for translation into a population-based screening program, and future research should include a more broadly diverse group of caregivers than the scope this study could offer. Here, we provide recommendations that stem from the narratives provided by caregivers of children with NBS-related conditions. Importantly, those who provided their perspective through in-depth qualitative interviews were referred to this research through ongoing natural history protocols at the National Institutes of Health and through related advocacy groups. Participants largely identified as non-Hispanic and White and had completed post-secondary education. The majority of children receiving care were diagnosed with a number of inborn metabolic disorders. Thus, the results herein should be interpreted with this in mind and may not be generalizable to the rare disease community as a whole or to the general population for which NBS as a public health measure serves. Despite this, these findings are based on a large sample, and caregivers provided rich narratives regarding their journey through the diagnostic odyssey continuum with themes that other caregivers have expressed, and others may experience. Finally, the scope of ethical considerations and NBS details considered here were purposefully limited in accordance with this Special Issue's aim to minimize redundancy of the ethical-psychosocial aspects raised and the associated scholarship presented within this collection.

6. Conclusions

The promise of expanding population-based newborn screening to include ever more increasing degrees of molecular sequencing may be realized in the near future. For some, these new technologies may shorten the diagnostic odyssey and may lessen the diagnostic odyssey continuum, whereas for others there may be a lengthier diagnostic odyssey continuum due to greater identification of conditions that may never manifest as disease. However, in either case, greater integration of genomics into public health NBS programs will likely not change most of the experiences reported herein without multi-faceted efforts to seriously address these challenges and the ethical considerations raised.

Supplementary Materials: The Supplementary Materials is available online at https://www.mdpi.com/article/10.3390/ijns8020035/s1.

Author Contributions: Conceptualization, L.B. and L.M.K.; data curation, L.B., H.D. and D.L.; formal analysis, L.B., H.D., S.G. and L.M.K.; funding acquisition, L.M.K.; investigation, H.D., D.L. and L.M.K.; methodology, L.B., H.D. and L.M.K.; resources, L.M.K.; supervision, L.M.K.; validation, D.L.; writing—original draft, L.B., H.D., S.G., D.L. and L.M.K.; writing—review and editing, L.B., H.D., S.G., D.L. and L.M.K. All authors have read and agreed to the published version of the manuscript.

Funding: This research was supported by the Intramural Research Program of the National Human Genome Research Institute, National Institutes of Health [ZIAHG200395 PI: Koehly].

Institutional Review Board Statement: The study was conducted in accordance with the Declaration of Helsinki, and approved by the Institutional Review Board of the National Human Genome Research Institute and the National Institutes of Health, USA (12HG0022, approved July, 2015).

Informed Consent Statement: Informed consent was obtained from all subjects involved in the study.

Data Availability Statement: The data that support the findings of this study are available from the corresponding author upon reasonable request.

Acknowledgments: The authors thank Peter McGuire, Cynthia Tifft, and Charles Venditti for referring participants into this study. We thank the participants and their families for sharing their experiences with us as part of this study.

Conflicts of Interest: The authors declare no conflict of interest.

References

1. Adhikari, A.N.; Gallagher, R.C.; Wang, Y.; Currier, R.J.; Amatuni, G.; Bassaganyas, L.; Chen, F.; Kundu, K.; Kvale, M.; Mooney, S.D.; et al. The role of exome sequencing in newborn screening for inborn errors of metabolism. *Nat. Med.* **2020**, *26*, 1392–1397. [CrossRef] [PubMed]
2. van Campen, J.C.; Sollars, E.S.; Thomas, R.C.; Bartlett, C.M.; Milano, A.; Parker, M.D.; Dawe, J.; Winship, P.R.; Peck, G.; Grafham, D.; et al. Next generation sequencing in newborn screening in the United Kingdom National Health Service. *Int. J. Neonatal Screen.* **2019**, *5*, 40. [CrossRef] [PubMed]
3. Chinnery, P.F. Shortening the diagnostic odyssey—The impact of whole genome sequencing in the NHS. *BMJ* **2021**, *375*, n2683. [CrossRef] [PubMed]
4. Bergougnoux, A.; Lopez, M.; Girodon, E. The role of extended CFTR gene sequencing in newborn screening for cystic fibrosis. *Int. J. Neonatal Screen.* **2020**, *6*, 23. [CrossRef] [PubMed]
5. Trier, C.; Fournous, G.; Strand, J.M.; Stray-Pedersen, A.; Pettersen, R.D.; Rowe, A.D. Next-generation sequencing of newborn screening genes: The accuracy of short-read mapping. *NPJ Genom. Med.* **2020**, *5*, 36. [CrossRef]
6. Currier, R.; Puck, J.M. SCID newborn screening: What we've learned. *J. Allergy Clin. Immunol.* **2021**, *147*, 417–426. [CrossRef]
7. Puck, J.M. Lessons for sequencing from the addition of severe combined immunodeficiency to newborn screening panels. *Hastings Cent. Rep.* **2018**, *48* (Suppl. S2), S7–S9. [CrossRef]
8. Woerner, A.C.; Gallagher, R.C.; Vockley, J.; Adhikari, A.N. The use of whole genome and exome sequencing for newborn screening: Challenges and opportunities for population health. *Front. Pediatr.* **2021**, *9*, 663752. [CrossRef]
9. Powell, C.M. What genomic sequencing can offer universal newborn screening programs. *Hastings Cent. Report.* **2018**, *48* (Suppl. S2), S18–S19. [CrossRef]
10. Lund, A.M.; Wibrand, F.; Skogstrand, K.; Bækvad-Hansen, M.; Gregersen, N.; Andresen, B.S.; Hougaard, D.M.; Dunø, M.; Olsen, R.K.J. Use of molecular genetic analyses in Danish routine newborn screening. *Int. J. Neonatal Screen.* **2021**, *7*, 50. [CrossRef]
11. Scarpa, M.; Bonham, J.R.; Dionisi-Vici, C.; Prevot, J.; Pergent, M.; Meyts, I.; Mahlaoui, N.; Schielen, P.C. Newborn screening as a fully integrated system to stimulate equity in neonatal screening in Europe. *Lancet Reg. Health Eur.* **2022**, *13*, 100311. [CrossRef] [PubMed]
12. Azzopardi, P.J.; Upshur, R.E.; Luca, S.; Venkataramanan, V.; Potter, B.K.; Chakraborty, P.K.; Hayeems, R.Z. Health-care providers' perspectives on uncertainty generated by variant forms of newborn screening targets. *Genet. Med.* **2020**, *22*, 566–573. [CrossRef] [PubMed]
13. Goldenberg, A.J.; Ponsaran, R.; Gaviglio, A.; Simancek, D.; Tarini, B.A. Genomics and newborn screening: Perspectives of public health programs. *Int. J. Neonatal Screen.* **2022**, *8*, 11. [CrossRef]

14. Genomics England; Hopkins van Mil. *Implications of Whole Genome Sequencing for Newborn Screening: A Public Dialogue*; London, UK. 2021. Available online: https://s3.eu-west-2.amazonaws.com/ge-production-s3/documents/public-dialogue-wgs-for-nbs-final-report.pdf (accessed on 9 May 2022).
15. Milko, L.V.; O'Daniel, J.M.; DeCristo, D.M.; Crowley, S.B.; Foreman, A.K.M.; Wallace, K.E.; Mollison, L.F.; Strande, N.T.; Girnary, Z.S.; Boshe, L.J.; et al. An age-based framework for evaluating genome-scale sequencing results in newborn screening. *J. Pediatr.* **2019**, *209*, 68–76. [CrossRef] [PubMed]
16. Ceyhan-Birsoy, O.; Machini, K.; Lebo, M.S.; Yu, T.W.; Agrawal, P.B.; Parad, R.B.; Holm, I.A.; McGuire, A.; Green, R.C.; Beggs, A.H.; et al. A curated gene list for reporting results of newborn genomic sequencing. *Genet. Med.* **2017**, *19*, 809–818. [CrossRef] [PubMed]
17. Health Resources and Services Administratio. Recommended Uniform Screening Panel. 2020. Available online: https://www.hrsa.gov/advisory-committees/heritable-disorders/rusp/index.html (accessed on 14 February 2022).
18. Newborn Screening Translational Research Network. NBS Condition Resource (NBS-CR). 2020. Available online: https://www.nbstrn.org/tools/nbs-cr (accessed on 14 February 2022).
19. Bush, L.; Al-Hertani, W.; Bodamer, O. The Complex Ethical and Psychosocial Landscape of Genomics in the Neonatal Period. in preparation.
20. Levy, H.L. Ethical and psychosocial implications of genomic newborn screening. *Int. J. Neonatal Screen.* **2021**, *7*, 2. [CrossRef]
21. Howell, R.R. Ethical issues surrounding newborn screening. *Int. J. Neonatal Screen.* **2021**, *7*, 3. [CrossRef]
22. Berry, S.A.; Lloyd-Puryear, M.A.; Watson, M.S. Long-term follow-up of newborn screening patients. *Genet. Med.* **2010**, *12*, S267–S268. [CrossRef]
23. Wasserstein, M.P. Long-term follow-up in newborn screening: The role of collaboration. *Genet. Med.* 2016. [CrossRef]
24. Holm, I.A. Using newborn sequencing to advance understanding of the natural history of disease. *Hastings Cent. Rep.* **2018**, *48* (Suppl. S2), S45–S46. [CrossRef] [PubMed]
25. Opel, D.J. A push for progress with shared decision-making in pediatrics. *Pediatrics* **2017**, *139*, e20162526. [CrossRef] [PubMed]
26. Lewis, M.A.; Paquin, R.S.; Roche, M.I.; Furberg, R.D.; Rini, C.; Berg, J.S.; Powell, C.M.; Bailey, D.B. Supporting parental decisions about genomic sequencing for newborn screening: The NC NEXUS Decision Aid. *Pediatrics* **2016**, *137* (Suppl. S1), S16–S23. [CrossRef] [PubMed]
27. Berg, J.S.; Agrawal, P.B.; Bailey, D.B.; Beggs, A.H.; Brenner, S.E.; Brower, A.M.; Cakici, J.A.; Ceyhan-Birsoy, O.; Chan, K.; Chen, F.; et al. Newborn sequencing in genomic medicine and public health. *Pediatrics* **2017**, *139*, e20162252. [CrossRef]
28. Roman, T.S.; Crowley, S.B.; Roche, M.I.; Foreman, A.K.M.; O'Daniel, J.M.; Seifert, B.A.; Lee, K.; Brandt, A.; Gustafson, C.; DeCristo, D.M.; et al. Genomic sequencing for newborn screening: Results of the nc nexus project. *Am. J. Hum. Genet.* **2020**, *107*, 596–611. [CrossRef] [PubMed]
29. Ceyhan-Birsoy, O.; Murry, J.B.; Machini, K.; Lebo, M.S.; Timothy, W.Y.; Fayer, S.; Genetti, C.A.; Schwartz, T.S.; Agrawal, P.B.; Parad, R.B.; et al. Interpretation of genomic sequencing results in healthy and ill newborns: Results from the babyseq project. *Am. J. Hum. Genet.* **2019**, *104*, 76–93. [CrossRef]
30. Wojcik, M.H.; Zhang, T.; Ceyhan-Birsoy, O.; Genetti, C.A.; Lebo, M.S.; Yu, T.W.; Parad, R.B.; Holm, I.A.; Rehm, H.L.; Beggs, A.H.; et al. Discordant results between conventional newborn screening and genomic sequencing in the BabySeq Project. *Genet. Med.* **2021**, *23*, 1372–1375. [CrossRef]
31. Currier, R.J. Single-gene sequencing in newborn screening: Success, challenge, hope. *Hastings Cent. Rep.* **2018**, *48* (Suppl. S2), S37–S38. [CrossRef]
32. Biesecker, L.G.; Green, E.D.; Manolio, T.; Solomon, B.D.; Curtis, D. Should all babies have their genome sequenced at birth? *BMJ* **2021**, *375*, n2679. [CrossRef]
33. Goldstein, J.; Freud, A.; Solnit, A.J. *Before the Best Interests of the Child*; Free Press: New York, NY, USA, 1979.
34. Ross, L.F.; Swota, A.H. The best interest standard: Same name but different roles in pediatric bioethics and child rights frameworks. *Perspect. Biol. Med.* **2017**, *60*, 186–197. [CrossRef]
35. Diekema, D.S. Parental refusals of medical treatment: The harm principle as threshold for state intervention. *Theor. Med. Bioeth.* **2004**, *25*, 243–264. [CrossRef] [PubMed]
36. Cornel, M.C.; Rigter, T.; Jansen, M.E.; Henneman, L. Neonatal and carrier screening for rare diseases: How innovation challenges screening criteria worldwide. *J. Community Genet.* **2021**, *12*, 257–265. [CrossRef] [PubMed]
37. Wilson, J.M.G.; Jungner, G. *Principles and Practice of Screening for Disease*; World Health Organization: Geneva, Switzerland, 1968.
38. Andermann, A.; Blancquaert, I.; Beauchamp, S.; Déry, V. Revisiting Wilson and Jungner in the genomic age: A review of screening criteria over the past 40 years. *Bull. World Health Organ.* **2008**, *86*, 317–319. [CrossRef] [PubMed]
39. Genomics England. New Public Dialogue Finds Support for the Use of Whole Genome Sequencing in Newborn Screening—Providing that the Right Safeguards and Resources are in Place. 2021. Available online: https://www.genomicsengland.co.uk/public-dialogue-genomics-newborn-screening/ (accessed on 9 May 2022).
40. Johnston, J.; Lantos, J.D.; Goldenberg, A.; Chen, F.; Parens, E.; Koenig, B.A.; NSIGHT Ethics and Policy Advisory Board. Sequencing newborns: A call for nuanced use of genomic technologies. *Hastings Cent. Rep.* **2018**, *48* (Suppl. S2), S2–S6. [CrossRef] [PubMed]
41. Solomon, M.; Bonham, A. (Eds.) *Ethical Oversight of Learning Health Care Systems*; Wiley-Blackwell: Malden, MA, USA, 2013.

42. National Center for Advancing Translational Sciences (NCATS) (US). *Gene-Targeted Therapies: Early Diagnosis and Equitable Delivery (Day 1)*; NIH Videocast; NCATS: Bethesda, MD, USA, 2021. Available online: https://videocast.nih.gov/watch=41968 (accessed on 21 October 2021).
43. State of Maine; Department of Health and Human Services; Children's Behavioral Health Services. Children's Habilitation Assessment Tool (CHAT). 2011. Available online: https://www.maine.gov/future/sites/maine.gov.dhhs/files/documents/ocfs/cbhs/provider/word/chat.doc (accessed on 14 January 2016).
44. Murphy, N.A.; Christian, B.; Caplin, D.A.; Young, P.C. The health of caregivers for children with disabilities: Caregiver perspectives. *Child Care Health Dev.* **2007**, *33*, 180–187. [CrossRef]
45. QSR International, Ltd. Nvivo 12 Plus Version 12.6.0.959 (64 bit). Melbourne, Australia, 2018. Available online: https://www.qsrinternational.com/nvivo-qualitative-data-analysis-software/home (accessed on 9 May 2022).
46. Halverson, C.M.E.; Clift, K.E.; McCormick, J.B. Was it worth it? Patients' perspectives on the perceived value of genomic-based individualized medicine. *J. Community Genet.* **2016**, *7*, 145–152. [CrossRef]
47. Corbin, J.M.; Strauss, A.L.; Strauss, A.L. *Basics of Qualitative Research: Techniques and Procedures for Developing Grounded Theory*, 3rd ed.; Sage Publications, Inc.: Los Angeles, CA, USA, 2008.
48. King, A.; Hoppe, R.B. "Best practice" for patient-centered communication: A narrative review. *J. Grad. Med. Educ.* **2013**, *5*, 385–393. [CrossRef]
49. Hashim, M.J. Patient-centered communication: Basic skills. *Am. Fam. Physician* **2017**, *95*, 29–34.
50. Boissy, A.; Windover, A.K.; Bokar, D.; Karafa, M.; Neuendorf, K.; Frankel, R.M.; Merlino, J.; Rothberg, M.B. Communication skills training for physicians improves patient satisfaction. *J. Gen. Intern. Med.* **2016**, *31*, 755–761. [CrossRef]
51. Epstein, R.M.; Street, R.L., Jr. *Patient-Centered Communication in Cancer Care: Promoting Healing and Reducing Suffering*; NIH Publication No. 07-6225; National Cancer Institute: Bethesda, MD, USA, 2007. Available online: https://cancercontrol.cancer.gov/sites/default/files/2020-06/pcc_monograph.pdf (accessed on 9 May 2022).
52. Koehly, L.M.; Ashida, S.; Sumrall, S.; Hyman, S. Malfeasant, nonfeasant, and uplifting caregiving interactions and behaviors in the care of children with rare genetic or undiagnosed conditions. (In review)
53. Beauchamp, T.L.; Childress, J.F. *Principles of Biomedical Ethics*, 6th ed.; Oxford University Press: New York, NY, USA, 2009.

International Journal of
Neonatal Screening

MDPI

Article

Parental Preferences about Policy Options Regarding Disclosure of Incidental Genetic Findings in Newborn Screening: Using Videos and the Internet to Educate and Obtain Input

Michael H. Farrell [1], Katherine E. Mooney [2], Anita Laxova [3] and Philip M. Farrell [4,*]

[1] Departments of Internal Medicine and Pediatrics, University of Minnesota Medical School, Minneapolis, MN 55455, USA
[2] Department of Medicine, University of Wisconsin School of Medicine and Public Health, Madison, WI 53792, USA
[3] Department of Pediatrics, University of Wisconsin School of Medicine and Public Health, Madison, WI 53792, USA
[4] Departments of Pediatrics and Population Health Sciences, University of Wisconsin School of Medicine and Public Health, CSC Room K4/948, 600 Highland Avenue, Madison, WI 53792, USA
* Correspondence: pmfarrell@wisc.edu; Tel.: +1-608-345-2308; Fax: +1-608-263-2820

Abstract: Our objective was to develop and test a new approach to obtaining parental policy guidance about disclosure of incidental findings of newborn screening for cystic fibrosis (CF), including heterozygote carrier status and the conditions known as CFTR-related metabolic syndrome (CRMS) and/or cystic fibrosis screen positive inconclusive diagnosis, CFSPID. The participants were parents of infants up to 6 months old recruited from maternity hospitals/clinics, parent education classes and stores selling baby products. Data were collected using an anonymous, one-time Internet-based survey. The survey introduced two scenarios using novel, animated videos. Parents were asked to rank three potential disclosure policies—Fully Informed, Parents Decide, and Withholding Information. Regarding disclosure of information about Mild X (analogous to CRMS/CFSPID), 57% of respondents ranked Parents Decide as their top choice, while another 41% ranked the Fully Informed policy first. Similarly, when considering disclosure of information about Disease X (CF) carrier status, 50% and 43% gave top rankings to the Fully Informed and Parents Decide policies, respectively. Less than 8% ranked the Withholding Information policy first in either scenario. Data from value comparisons suggested that parents believed knowing everything was very important even if they became distressed. Likewise, parents preferred autonomy even if they became distressed. However, when there might not be enough time to learn everything, parents showed a slight preference for deferring decision-making. Because most parents strongly preferred the policies of full disclosure or making the decision, rather than the withholding option for NBS results, these results can inform disclosure policies in NBS programs, especially as next-generation sequencing increases incidental findings.

Keywords: cystic fibrosis; incidental findings; CFTR-related metabolic syndrome; cystic fibrosis screen positive inconclusive diagnosis; newborn screening; next generation sequencing; policy

1. Introduction

1.1. Cystic Fibrosis Newborn Screening

Cystic fibrosis (CF) newborn screening (NBS) has been performed in the United States for over 30 years [1], and in some European regions such as Veneto, Italy for almost 50 years [2]. The protocols have changed over time, especially during the past decade with nationwide programs underway [3,4]. The original protocols used a first tier of immunoreactive trypsinogen (IRT) analysis followed by a second IRT [5], and later a DNA-based test was introduced for the p.Phe508del (F508del) variant of the cystic fibrosis transmembrane conductance regulator (*CFTR*) gene [6]. Subsequently, the DNA tier was expanded to between 23 and 372 pathogenic variants [7–9]. When a single *CFTR* variant is detected in the DNA tier, sweat testing is essential because in up to 10% of such cases a second, undetected *CFTR* variant may be present to cause the disease [6]. NBS also produces incidental findings (IFs), namely detection of more babies who are heterozygote carriers [8–10], and others have a condition known as CFTR-related metabolic syndrome (CRMS) or CF screen positive, inconclusive diagnosis (CFSPID) [11,12]. Many IFs lack significance for the child's health and may lead to misconceptions, emotional complications, and biomedical risks because of unnecessary tests or treatments [13,14]. NBS policy has been crafted by public health experts and sometimes informed by bioethics commentary, surveys of parents, and advocacy by laboratory methodologists [1,15–17]. Many variations in CF NBS algorithms have resulted from these efforts [3], rarely with input by parents.

1.2. Next Generation Sequencing in Newborn Screening

Next-generation sequencing (NGS) technologies [8,9] are now available and will help to increase NBS sensitivity, i.e., the percentage of CF cases identified. However, NGS also produces more IFs. Thus, the application of NGS may lead to more psychosocial complications. NBS programs are looking for ways to mitigate harm as they increase the benefits through NGS.

Thus, the pivotal introduction of NGS with its unprecedented technology has reinvigorated the longstanding debate about whether NBS programs should notify parents about IFs, given that the risk/benefit ratio is uncertain [14,18]. CF carrier status and CRMS/CFSPID are unlike most NBS results as they do not require immediate medical attention, although these conditions are often disclosed with counseling in the neonatal period. However, some programs do not ensure that IFs are disclosed. In fact, at least one country (Norway) by law does not reveal *CFTR* carrier status discovered through NBS [4]. In the USA, many IF results are returned to the primary care provider who may lack sufficient time, knowledge or counseling skill [19,20], and may not even know the family because of inaccurate or insufficient labeling of dried blood spot specimens [21,22]. Therefore, parents can become anxious or confused about the implications of the results, as has been noted after NBS and other community screening programs [23,24]. Infants with CRMS/CFSPID may also have had biomedical complications of tests or treatments, which might have been unnecessary [11,12]. Since NGS and the increased number of IFs may cause a change in the balance of risks and benefits of NBS, it is important to re-examine policies and responsibilities for reporting results.

1.3. Policy Options for Disclosure

After reviewing the limited literature on this topic, we decided that it would be important to obtain fresh perspectives from new parents about potential policies. We were aware of three potential policy options for communicating IFs, namely Fully Informed, Withhold Information, and Parents Decide (see descriptions in Table 1). We sought to develop a survey instrument to gather parents' policy advice about two research questions: (1) how should NBS programs communicate with parents about single-variant NBS results that are consistent with being a carrier?; (2) how should NBS programs communicate with parents about one or two mutations consistent with a mild version of the screened disease, which has minor health significance compared to the full disease (e.g., CRMS/CFSPID)? Our hypotheses were based on three decades of NBS follow-up experience and especially our recent studies [21,23–26], suggesting parents would wish to know about IFs even if the information was complex and potentially stressful and even if the condition was mild.

Table 1. Disclosure Policy Definitions and Associated Advantages, Disadvantages, and Added Values.

Policy	Definition	Advantages (Benefits)	Disadvantages	Added Value [a]
Fully Informed	Incidental findings always disclosed to parents	No information is withheld from parents	Requires more time that could be devoted to other health care needs Potential for confusion, misconceptions, emotional stress	Being fully informed
Withholding Information	Incidental findings with very minimal or no risk to health are withheld from parents	Reduces parental confusion and risk of emotional problems	Parents not consulted about information that is part of them and their family	Reducing emotional stress
Parents Decide	Parents are counseled just prior to results communication, and then make a decision about how much information to receive about incidental genetic findings	Parents are in control of the screening results that affect their baby and can determine if they want full details if they are willing to risk emotional distress	Requires more time that could be devoted to other health care needs Curiosity may lead to the parents asking questions about details they don't actually want or need to know	Autonomy is preserved (freedom of choice) [b]

[a] Values associated with policies were not directly presented to participants. [b] Preserving the principle of autonomy is ethically sound.

2. Materials and Methods

2.1. Design

The study used an anonymous online survey that contained three animated video clips, each of which explained some background information necessary for understanding the questions. The survey was hosted by Qualtrics (Provo, Utah and Seattle, Washington, DC, USA). Participants could complete the survey using a computer, smartphone, or iPad with Internet access. IRB approval was obtained from Aurora Health Care in Milwaukee, Wisconsin, the University of Wisconsin School of Medicine and Public Health, and Meriter Hospital in Madison Wisconsin. Parents were recruited to take the survey predominantly in Madison, after an initial effort had limited success in Milwaukee. Consent was obtained online from each participant before they began the survey.

2.2. Methodologic Elements to Support the Objectives

To increase the utility of the study for policy making, we included several innovations in the design. These resulted from sequential quality improvement efforts to create a user-friendly, unbiased survey of parental opinions during the first six postpartum months.

2.2.1. Embedded Explanatory Videos

Preference and opinion surveys often present several sentences of background information to read before asking questions. During our survey instrument's development, we became concerned about the amount of text that would be needed before asking key questions. We therefore created three animated video clips embedded between sections of the survey (Figures 1–3). The videos featured an animated character, Nurse Maria, who explained the basics of NBS and presented different scenarios for disclosure of NBS results. The videos were scripted in stages to support a careful order of survey questions, as described below. Each video lasted about 5 min. The language was assessed and determined to be appropriate for those with an eighth-grade education.

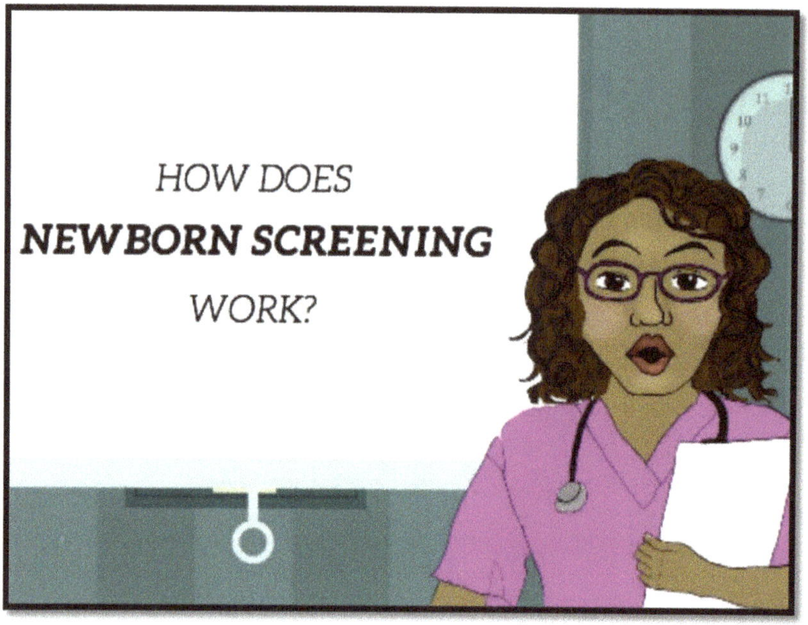
HOW DOES
NEWBORN SCREENING
WORK?

Figure 1. Still Image from the introductory video featuring "Nurse Maria" and explaining. the process and benefits of newborn screening Full video available at https://www.youtube.com/watch?v=2qeBX0FDp_I&t=3s [last accessed on 25 July 2022].

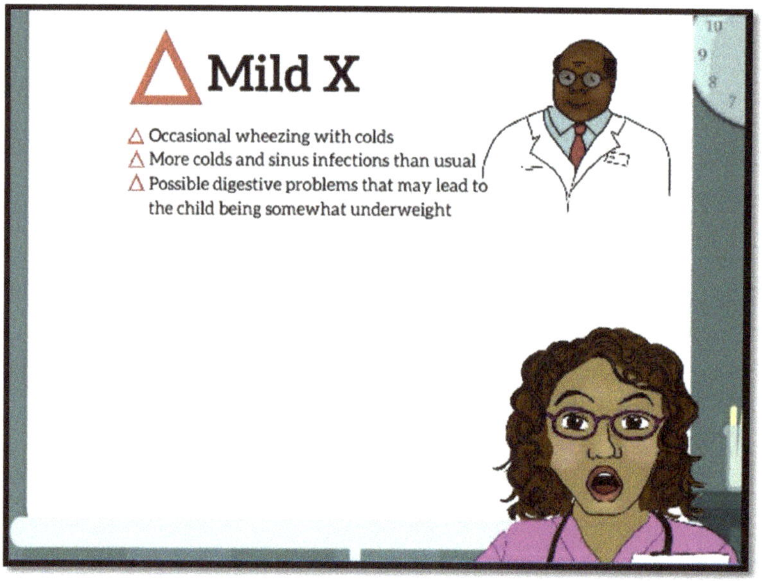
Mild X
Occasional wheezing with colds
More colds and sinus infections than usual
Possible digestive problems that may lead to the child being somewhat underweight

Figure 2. Still Image from the second video depicting symptoms of "Mild X" (analogous to CRMS/CFSPID). Full video available at https://www.youtube.com/watch?v=3HiFPywnCb0 [last accessed on 25 July 2022].

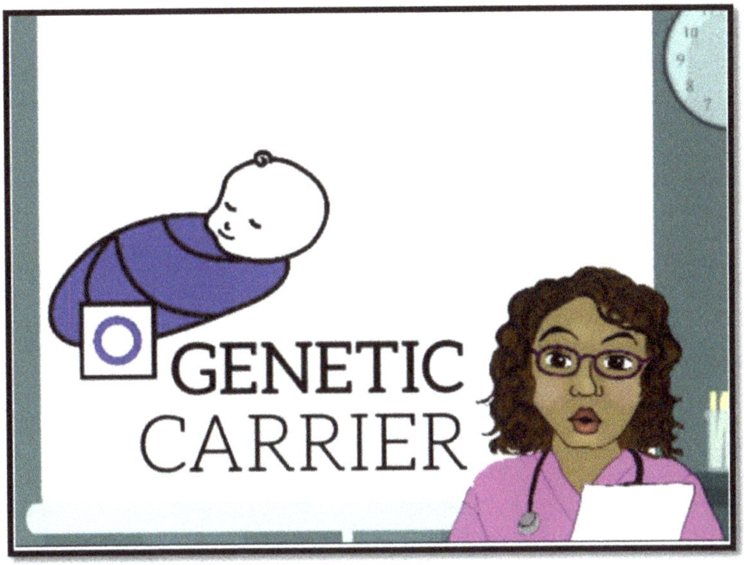

Figure 3. Still image from the third video detailing the meaning of carrier status. for "Disease X". Full video available at https://www.youtube.com/watch?v=Y572EiX_hWY [last accessed on 25 July 2022].

The video's script and graphics were drafted and vetted with a variety of parents and NBS educators so that they would be accessible to participants regardless of prior education and medical experience. The animations were revised and pilot tested before routine use in this study. All videos were uploaded to YouTube for embedding within the Qualtrics webtool. To our knowledge, this is the first time an Internet-based educational video has been used in an NBS-related survey.

2.2.2. Substitution of a Generic Disease X instead of CF

Our experience with previous surveys suggested that community respondents would have varied knowledge about CF, and we grew concerned that this heterogeneity might have an unpredictable influence on summarizing analyses. We therefore substituted for CF a fictitious "Disease X" with symptoms and implications that are very similar to CF. We also felt that the Disease X substitution would be useful for generalizing the study to other genetic conditions included on NBS panels. We developed explanations for autosomal recessive carrier status for Disease X and also created an analog for CRMS/CFSPID called "Mild X".

2.2.3. Vignettes and Complementary Modes for Preference Questions

We considered a variety of approaches to the vignettes and questions and settled on a method from experimental psychology called an imagination exercise, in which respondents would be presented with a vignette and asked to imagine themselves in the position of a character in the story. The first vignette asked the respondent to imagine that at the same time her/his baby was born, a best friend named Tonya had a baby (Natalie) who was diagnosed with Mild X. Tonya conveys to the respondent all the information about Disease X and Mild X, and then the Nurse Maria character explains about the three policies in Table 1. After the video, the parents were asked to rank the three policies in relation to this scenario. Policies had to be ranked in different positions (first, second, third), but parents were given the option to leave policies unranked.

Next, the respondents were asked "Do you think MOST parents would share your opinion about the policies?" and given two options; "Yes, I think more than half of all parents would share my opinion" and "No, I think that one of the other two policies would be better for most parents *(you will be asked which policy in the next question)*". Respondents who selected the latter choice were given the policies again and asked "Which policy do you think would be best for most parents of infants with a Mild X result?"

The second vignette reprised the Tonya and Natalie story, but with Natalie diagnosed with genetic carrier status for Disease X, and Nurse Maria explaining carrier status using an animated Punnett square. After the video, respondents were given the same ranking task for placing themselves in Tonya's position and whether more than half of all parents would share their opinion, and if not then another ranking task for "most parents". After respondents were asked about their own preferences and their opinions about "most parents", we used three slider questions to compare how important different values were to each other such as autonomy compared with deferring to a clinician expert.

2.3. Sample and Recruitment

Eligible participants were parents of infants up to six months of age regardless of medical history. Fluency in English was required. The study began with a plan to recruit two samples of parents in the state of Wisconsin, beginning with one phase in Milwaukee and then proceeding to another in Madison. The Milwaukee recruiting strategy used fliers at a maternity hospital and clinics that served a poor urban population that is mostly African American. However, due to limited resources for recruiting, the Milwaukee phase served primarily as a pilot testing effort while resulting in six respondents. The Madison phase used recruiting fliers distributed in person at a popular store selling products for infants and at parent education classes located at a hospital with a large and diverse obstetrical population. Participants were told that the survey would take approximately 20 min to complete. As a gratuity for participation, respondents were offered a $10 retail gift card. The contact information for sending the gift card was obtained in a separate survey that was not linked to the subjects' responses on the survey questions.

2.4. Data Management and Statistical Analyses

During the final analyses, descriptive statistics were derived for both parent and child characteristics and frequency information from items evaluating experience with NBS. The proportion of parents ranking each policy first, second, and third was obtained separately for the Mild X and Disease X carrier status scenarios and was reported with Wilson 95% confidence intervals. Descriptive statistics were reported for the continuous value comparison variables and one-way ANOVA was used to evaluate differences in value scores between parents who ranked the Fully Informed, Withhold, and Parents Decide policies first. Statistical significance was determined using two-tailed tests with $\alpha = 0.05$. All data were analyzed using JMP software (SAS Institute, Cary, NC, USA).

3. Results

3.1. Sample Characteristics

A total of 213 surveys were started, including 11 in the Milwaukee phase and 202 in the Madison phase. Of those, 35% (4 and 81, respectively) were excluded because the participant stopped early, or generated a response that was too incomplete for analysis, or completed the survey in under 1000 s, suggesting that the subject didn't watch the entire duration of the video clips. Although these responses contributed some information, we decided as a stringent quality control requirement to accept only complete responses. The final sample included 128 respondents (60.1% of surveys begun). The median duration for the included surveys was 1406 s (IQR = 1007 s), not counting four outliers who left the survey open for more than 30,000 s.

The mother was the respondent in 81.3% of surveys. The median respondent age was 33, while the median infant age was 2 months. Further descriptive data are shown in

Table 2. In general, this was a well-educated sample of white married women. However, their knowledge about NBS was limited; 20% of respondents knew nothing or very little about NBS, despite their infant having been screened only a few months before, and 66% wished that they had known more. Thus, information on NBS policy options was new to this group, which we considered an advantage in this survey.

Table 2. Sample Characteristics for 128 Respondents.

Characteristic	N	(%)
Married or stable relationship	123	(96.1)
First-time parent	93	(72.7)
Infant born >2 weeks before due date	19	(14.8)
NICU stay >2 days	11	(8.6)
Race and/or ethnicity of respondent		
White	112	(87.5)
Non-White	11	(8.6)
Missing response	5	(3.9)
Education		
High school	11	(9)
Undergraduate degree	62	(48.4)
Postgraduate degree	52	(40.6)
Missing response	3	(2.3)
Health literacy (need help reading ...)		
never	86	(67.2)
rarely	28	(21.9)
sometimes	8	(6.3)
often	1	(0.8)
always	1	(0.8)
not answered	4	(3.1)

3.2. *Reaction to Animated Video Survey Format*

Reactions to the Nurse Maria videos were favorable among those who finished the survey, with 92% of respondents agreeing or strongly agreeing that they liked the videos, and 98% agreeing or strongly agreeing that the "videos explained things in a way that was easy to understand". Similarly, 98% agreed or strongly agreed that "the videos were better than reading several long paragraphs". In view of the well-educated nature of the sample, these responses are a significant finding of this study.

3.3. *Disclosure Preferences*

Parents' rankings of NBS disclosure policies were analyzed separately for both the Mild X and Carrier X scenarios, and for each of two questions: "If you had been in (the vignette), which of the three policies would you have preferred for yourself and your baby?" and "What do you think would be best for most parents of infants with (condition in the vignette)?" The proportion of respondent rankings for these four analyses are shown in Figure 4 where the top-ranked policies are compared (error bars are Wilson confidence intervals). As seen in Figure 4, the Withholding Information policy was obviously less popular than the other two policies. It was more challenging to compare the Fully Informed and Parents Decide policies, but there appeared to be a marginal trend favoring Parent Decide. Several other analyses shed additional light on this situation.

As shown in Figure 4, respondents began by describing what they would have wanted in the Mild X vignette for themselves and their infants. The next three vignettes allowed us to investigate how respondents changed their preferences in different situations. Between 10–25% of parents changed a preference when asked about the Carrier X vignette, or when opining about what would be best for other parents. Five parents (4.2%) who began with a Fully Informed or Parents Decide preference for Mild X answered that Withholding Information would be better for other parents. Nine parents (7.6%) who began with Fully

Informed or Parents Decide for Mild X answered that Withholding Information would be better for themselves in the Carrier X vignette.

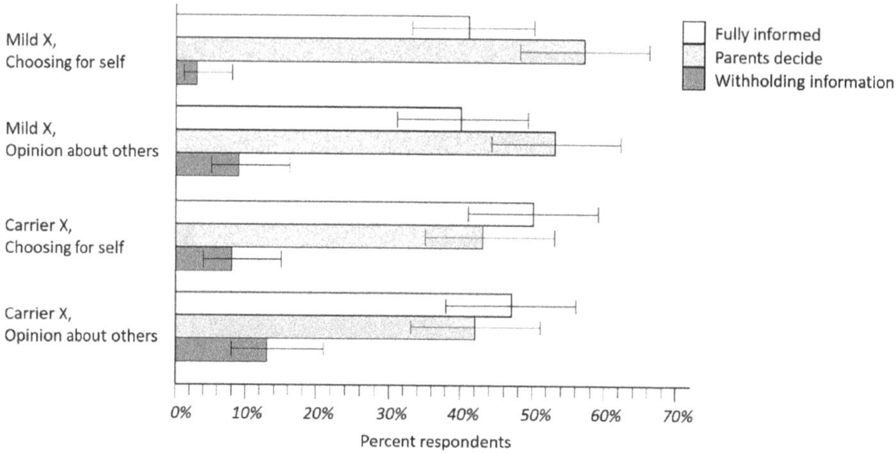

Figure 4. Rankings of disclosure policies for Mild X and Disease X carrier status. Results shown are from respondents asked to rank their preferences for disclosure of policy options that could be implemented by caregivers for either a Mild X condition analogous to CRMS/CFSPID or Disease X like CF. The intent of this exercise was to learn what parents preferred and what they were opposed to as well: clearly, the Withholding Information policy option.

Respondents' preferences for the individual policies are compared with the data in Table 2 and other variables obtained through the survey. Respondents who had reported being the primary caregiver for the baby were more likely to vote for the Parents Decide policy ($p = 0.006$, Wilcoxon) or full disclosure policy ($p = 0.035$, Wilcoxon). Respondents with newer infants were less likely to vote in favor of the Parents Decide policy ($r = -0.19$, $p < 0.035$). A vote in favor of the Withholding Information policy was less likely for parents who recalled being told about the NBS result.

3.4. Value Comparison

Table 3 and Figure 5 depict the three value comparison questions with the latter showing the median (interquartile range) responses for the sample indicated. When comparing the importance of being Fully Informed to reducing emotional distress (Comparison A), parents gave preference to autonomy at the risk of becoming unnecessarily alarmed (Figure 5A). Likewise, when weighing the importance of autonomy in decision-making versus reducing emotional distress (Comparison B), parents preferred the statement consistent with autonomy (Figure 5B). However, when choosing between autonomous decision-making without all pertinent details or allowing someone who is knowledgeable to make decisions (Comparison C), parents showed a slight preference for deferring to someone who knows all necessary information (Figure 5C).

We also explored value scores based on which policy parents ranked first for the Mild X and Disease X carrier status scenarios. All ANOVA results showed significant differences in mean value scores between first-rank policy groups except for Comparison C value scores between first-rank policy groups for Disease X carrier status. For Comparison A (comparing the importance of being fully informed to reducing emotional distress), parents who ranked the Fully Informed policy first most strongly favored being fully informed, followed by those who ranked the Parents Decide policy first, and finally by those who ranked the withhold option first. This pattern was present for first-rank policy groups from both the Mild X and Disease X carrier scenarios. For Mild X, all Hochberg's GT2 post-hoc tests were significant except the Withholding and Parents Decide groupings for

Mild X. Similarly, in Comparison B (comparing the importance of autonomy in decision-making versus reducing emotional distress), parents who gave the Fully Informed policy a first-place ranking most strongly favored autonomy, followed by those who ranked the Parents Decide policy first, and finally by those who ranked the withhold policy first. For Disease X carrier status, all Hochberg's GT2 post-hoc tests were significant except the Fully Informed and Parents Decide groupings. Compared to those who favored Fully Informed and Parents Decide, parents who ranked Withholding Information first in either scenario had average value scores closest to the withholding statement in Comparisons A and B. Even so, the Withholding Information group averages did not reflect a strong affinity for the withholding statement and tended to indicate a neutral attitude or even slight preference for the opposing statement. Regarding Comparison C (choosing between autonomous decision-making without all pertinent details or allowing someone who is knowledgeable to make decisions), the average value scores for all groups were near the midpoint, with the exception of the Parents Decide groups that slightly favored deferring decision-making to someone else. There were no significant differences in Comparison C value scores for Mild X first-rank policy groups.

Table 3. Value Score Results for First-rank Policy Groups.

	First-Rank Policy Group			*p*-Value *
	Fully Informed	**Withholding Information**	**Parents Decide**	
Comparison A (comparing the importance of being fully informed to reducing distress)				
Mild X scenario				
mean (std. dev.)	0.28 (0.33)	0.76 (0.78)	0.58 (0.44)	<0.001 *
median (IRQ)	0.17 (0.42)	0.73 (1.55)	0.48 (0.52)	
Disease X carrier status scenario				
mean (std. dev.)	0.32 (0.38)	0.96 (0.61)	0.55 (0.38)	<0.001 *
median (IRQ)	0.19 (0.40)	1.0 (0.92)	0.47 (0.44)	
Comparison B (comparing the importance of autonomy in decision-making versus reducing emotional distress)				
Mild X scenario				
mean (std. dev.)	1.61 (0.50)	0.76 (0.74)	1.37 (0.46)	<0.001 *
median (IRQ)	1.76 (0.63)	0.58 (1.10)	1.40 (0.61)	
Disease X carrier status scenario				
mean (std. dev.)	1.51 (0.56)	1.03 (0.40)	1.45 (0.43)	0.015 *
median (IRQ)	1.69 (0.71)	1.05 (0.66)	1.46 (0.58)	
Comparison C (comparing autonomous Decision-making without all details to allowing experts to make decisions)				
Mild X scenario				
mean (std. dev.)	0.97 (0.62)	0.95 (0.83)	1.27 (0.51)	0.008 *
median (IRQ)	1.01 (1.00)	1.01 (1.60)	1.33 (0.61)	
Disease X carrier status scenario				
mean (std. dev.)	1.04 (0.61)	1.08 (0.61)	1.25 (0.54)	0.092
median (IRQ)	1.13 (1.01)	1.23 (0.92)	1.33 (0.65)	

* One-way ANOVA.

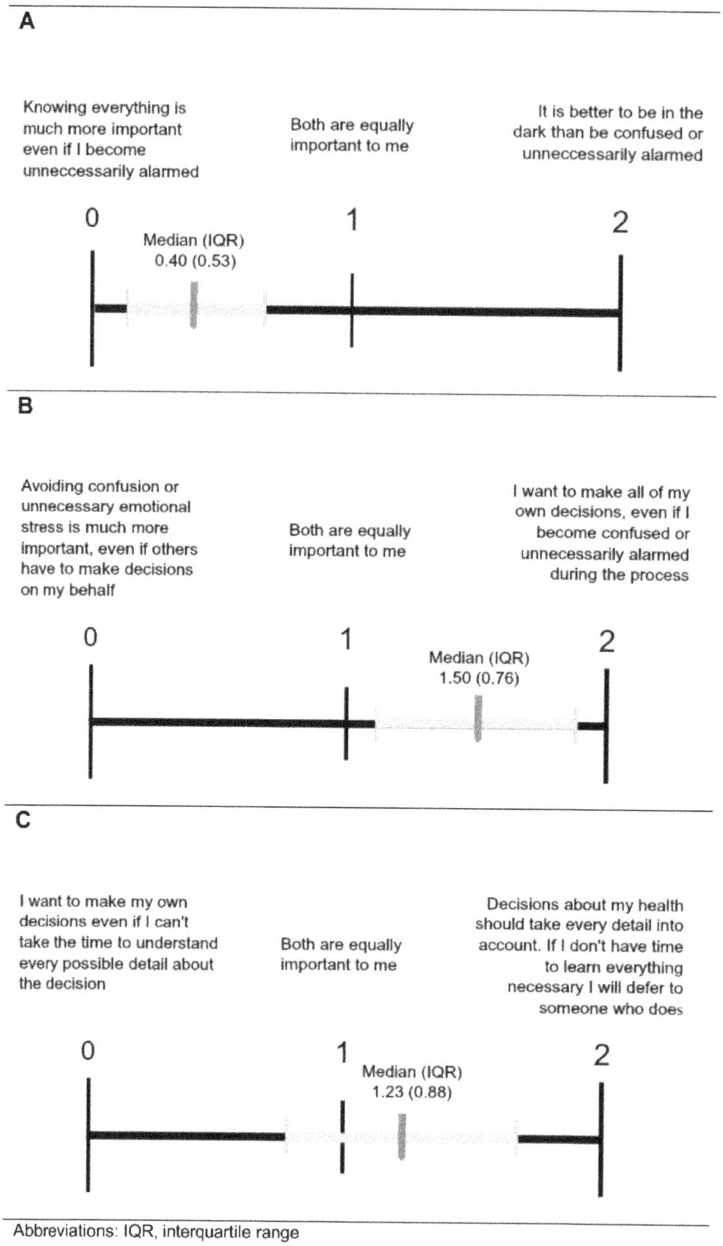

Figure 5. Comparisons of values associated with Fully Informed (**A**), Parents Decide (**B**), and Withholding policies (**C**). Results from parents given value comparison questions to express their views about the importance of the three policy options that may be associated with stress. Values are as described in Figure 3.

4. Discussion

There are three main options for policy regarding informing parents about IFs after newborn screening (Table 1), each with its advantages/benefits, disadvantages, and potential value for society. It is ideal for screening policy decisions to incorporate parental perceptions, but the literature provides a mixture of views, along with varying designs and sample populations [15,25–34]. This study examined preferences for disclosure of NBS results among generally well-educated parents who recently experienced the NBS process, thus seeking their policy preferences in an ideal timeframe when NBS might be fresh in their minds.

In this sample, the policy of withholding IFs (for the purpose of reducing unnecessary distress) was unpopular for both scenarios, although this strategy is often advocated for among clinicians. Applying this policy in NBS as in Norway [4] can be challenged, particularly when there are benefits to knowing your genetic status [23].

In reaction to videos describing a Mild X condition analogous to CRMS/CFSPID, many parents favored policies that kept them fully informed or allowed them to determine whether to receive IFs. This confirms the wisdom of clinical practice recommendations that encourage full disclosure about this condition and the importance of longitudinal follow-up evaluations [11,12,35]. Although incidental findings related to CF were the focus of this study, the generic nature of the video contents might allow these preferences to be informative for disclosure of NBS results beyond CF. If further supported by future study and commentary, the onus would be on NBS programs and their funding providers to mitigate harm following disclosure.

Distinguishing parents' preferences between the Fully Informed and Parents Decide policies is challenging. In the case of Mild X, more parents ranked the Parents Decide policy option first than ranked the Fully Informed policy first, but for Disease X carrier status, the Fully Informed option was slightly more popular than the Parents Decide policy as a top choice. This may mean that parents believe universal disclosure is less critical for Mild X (CRMS/CFSPID) than for Disease X/CF carrier status, but further study is warranted before such a conclusion could be made. However, the notion that parents may have different preferences for different categories of incidental findings raises the possibility of hybrid policies where certain results are always disclosed, and others are optional.

The value comparison results were largely consistent with policy preferences; parents favored autonomy and being fully informed at the risk of experiencing emotional distress. While we did not probe participants about why they were willing to endure distress, others have reported a sense of obligation or duty among parents in similar situations [31]. Interestingly, even the small number of parents who ranked the Withholding Information policy first did not strongly endorse the withhold statements in value comparison questions. This suggests that perhaps those who favor the withhold policy have high regard for being fully informed and maintaining autonomy but are influenced by other factors to choose the Withholding Information option. Given concerns about the capacity of NBS programs and practitioners to prepare parents to make informed decisions about IFs, we gave special attention to time and resource limitations in value comparison C. Statements in this comparison were written to reflect the possibility that there may not be time to teach parents all relevant information before a health decision needs to be made. On one end, parents could choose to maintain autonomy without all pertinent details, and on the other end, they could defer the health decision to someone who knows all the details. After favoring autonomy in Comparison B, this sample was more inclined to defer decision-making in Comparison C, indicating that knowledge, rather than personal control alone, was important to them. This is a positive indication that parents will understand the difficulties inherent to teaching/learning about IFs as the era of NGS evolves. Although one might argue that parents should not be the sole determinants of the child's interest in learning about IFs, practical considerations have led to the parent-child dyad as being responsible for this information transfer. In fact, counseling resource limitations make it difficult to engage professional experts in this aspect of NBS follow up communications.

Our study was successful in employing a novel video survey design to deliver complex genetic and clinical information to the public. Thus, it adds to the previous NBS-related research on parental preferences by providing survey methodology that is more user-friendly than reading "several long paragraphs". Nearly all parents found the contents understandable and more engaging than a conventional written survey format. Although technical expertise is required for video design and creation, this model should be considered for future studies with non-medical populations and perhaps for parent education in association with NBS rather than the traditional brochures. In connection with this, the first video that can be accessed through Figure 1 provides a succinct, 2-min explanation of all aspects of the NBS process.

A limitation of this study is the use of a convenience sample made up mostly of American mothers from a single community that selects for those willing and able to attend a voluntary class in the middle of the day. The sample was disproportionately white, well-educated, and married, all of which limit the generalizability of our results. The homogeneity of the sample was identified during preliminary analyses, after which the research team explored adding more recruitment sites that traditionally serve low-income and minority populations, such as public health departments administering the Special Supplemental Nutrition Program for Women, Infants, and Children (WIC). Unfortunately, we were unable to secure new collaborations. Past research on adults regarding their desire to learn about IFs discovered in genetic testing, including carrier status, has found little association between sociodemographic and literacy factors and preference for disclosure [32–34]. Therefore, our results may be similar with a more diverse population, although this remains a topic for further study.

Despite these limitations in generalizability, our study extends previous observations about parental preferences [15,26–30] by its comparison of reactions to information disclosure about a potentially severe disease such as CF (Disease X) with a mild condition such as CRMS/CFSPID, and by incorporating three policy options into the survey, in addition to contributing a user-friendly video survey option to the range of methodologies available. Although there was less interest in the Parents Decide disclosure option with Disease X, the respondents clearly were opposed to withholding information on carrier status, even if the condition is mild. Policymakers need to keep this in mind as NGS-based screening expands, requiring both ethical [18,23] and practical issues [17] need to be addressed. Thus, another implication of our study is that valuable parental input can be obtained about policy options with user-friendly, efficient methods prior to widespread implementation of NGS. Although some may argue that parental input should not be considered in formulating disclosure policies about IFs from screening tests, people participating in healthcare systems have a right to be engaged in the sharing of health-related, relevant knowledge, and NBS is a hybrid of public health and healthcare. The strong preference for autonomy that was identified in this survey underscores the importance of that ethical principle.

Author Contributions: M.H.F. conceptualized and designed the survey questions and video scripts, contributed to data collection and analysis, drafted sections of the manuscript, and then reviewed, extensively revised, and approved the manuscript. K.E.M. visited and communicated with recruitment sites, performed data collection, cleaning and analyses, drafted the initial manuscript, reviewed, revised, and approved the manuscript. A.L. participated in the design of the study, supervised data collection as well as its analysis and interpretation, and reviewed, revised, and approved the manuscript after drafting sections on methodology. P.M.F. secured partnerships with recruitment sites after participating in the final design, drafted sections of the initial manuscript, and then reviewed and revised the manuscript. All authors have read and agreed to the published version of the manuscript.

Funding: This study was supported by grants from The Legacy of Angels Foundation and the Cystic Fibrosis Foundation.

Institutional Review Board Statement: IRB approval was obtained from Aurora Health Care in Milwaukee, Wisconsin, the University of Wisconsin School of Medicine and Public Health in Madison, and Meriter Hospital in Madison.

Informed Consent Statement: Consent was obtained from each participant before they began the survey.

Acknowledgments: We thank Nadia Ahmad, who contributed to the survey design and script for the animated videos, and Megan Wells for creating the videos. We are also grateful to Lori Hughes, Sue Ellen Dolan, and Laurel Rice and Gregory Bills for facilitating access to the Meriter Hospital Mother-Baby Hour program. We also appreciate Sarah Smith's willingness to allow recruitment at the Happy Bambino store in Madison. We wish to acknowledge the funding received from The Legacy of Angels Foundation through a grant awarded to Mei Baker, Philip Farrell, and Michael Farrell, as well as the Cystic Fibrosis Foundation for a Student Traineeship awarded to Katherine Mooney during her medical school education.

Conflicts of Interest: The authors declare no conflict of interest.

Financial Disclosure: The authors have no financial relationships relevant to this article to disclose.

Abbreviations

cystic fibrosis	CF
CFTR-related metabolic syndrome	CRMS
cystic fibrosis screen positive inconclusive diagnosis	CFSPID
newborn screening	NBS
next generation sequencing	NGS
incidental findings	IFs
confidence interval	CI

References

1. Grosse, S.D.; Boyle, C.A.; Botkin, J.R.; Comeau, A.M.; Kharrazi, M.; Rosenfeld, M.; Wilfond, B.S.; CDC. Newborn screening for cystic fibrosis: Evaluation of benefits and risks and recommendations for state newborn screening programs. *Morb. Mortal. Wkly. Rep. Recomm. Rep.* **2004**, *53*, 1–36.
2. Pederzini, F.; Armani, P.; Barbato, A.; Borgo, G.; Castellani, E.; Girella, M.; Manfrini, G.; Olivieri, D.; Righetti, G.; Zamboni, C.; et al. Newborn screening for cystic fibrosis. The methods compared on 229,626 newborns tested in 8 years in the Veneto Region. *Riv. Ital. Pediatr.-Ital. J. Pediatrics* **1983**, *9*, 445–457.
3. Scotet, V.; Gutierrez, H.; Farrell, P.M. Newborn screening for CF across the globe—Where is it worthwhile? *Int. J. Neonatal Screen* **2020**, *6*, 18. [CrossRef] [PubMed]
4. Lundman, E.; Gaup, H.J.; Bakkeheim, E.; Olafsdottir, E.J.; Rootwelt, T.; Storrøsten, O.T.; Pettersen, R.D. Implementation of newborn screening for cystic fibrosis in Norway. Results from the first three years. *J. Cyst. Fibros.* **2016**, *15*, 318–324. [CrossRef]
5. Hammond, K.B.; Abman, S.H.; Sokol, R.J.; Accurso, F.J. Efficacy of statewide neonatal screening for cystic fibrosis by assay of trypsinogen concentrations. *N. Engl. J. Med.* **1991**, *325*, 769–774. [CrossRef]
6. Gregg, R.G.; Wilfond, B.S.; Farrell, P.M.; Laxova, A.; Hassemer, D.; Mischler, E.H. Application of DNA analysis in a population-screening program for neonatal diagnosis of cystic fibrosis (CF): Comparison of screening protocols. *Am. J. Hum. Genet.* **1993**, *52*, 616–626.
7. Comeau, A.M.; Parad, R.B.; Dorkin, H.L.; Dovey, M.; Gerstle, R.; Haver, K.; Lapey, A.; O'Sullivan, B.P.; Waltz, D.A.; Zwerdling, R.G.; et al. Population-based newborn screening for genetic disorders when multiple mutation DNA testing is incorporated: A cystic fibrosis newborn screening model demonstrating increased sensitivity but more carrier detections. *Pediatrics* **2004**, *113*, 1573–1581. [CrossRef]
8. Sicko, R.J.; Stevens, C.F.; Hughes, E.E.; Leisner, M.; Ling, H.; Saavedra-Matiz, C.A.; Caggana, M.; Kay, D.M. Validation of a custom next-generation sequencing assay for cystic fibrosis newborn screening. *Int. J. Neonatal Screen* **2021**, *7*, 73. [CrossRef]
9. Baker, M.W.; Atkins, A.E.; Cordovado, S.K.; Hendrix, M.; Earley, M.C.; Farrell, P.M. Improving newborn screening for cystic fibrosis using next-generation sequencing technology: A technical feasibility study. *Genet. Med.* **2016**, *18*, 231–238. [CrossRef]
10. Hughes, E.E.; Stevens, C.F.; Saavedra-Matiz, C.A.; Tavakoli, N.P.; Krein, L.M.; Parker, A.; Zhang, Z.; Maloney, B.; Vogel, B.; DeCelie-Germana, J.; et al. Clinical sensitivity of cystic fibrosis mutation panels in a diverse population. *Hum. Mutat.* **2016**, *37*, 201–208. [CrossRef]
11. Ren, C.L.; Borowitz, D.S.; Gonska, T.; Howenstine, M.S.; Levy, H.; Massie, J.; Milla, C.; Munck, A.; Southern, K.W. Cystic fibrosis transmembrane conductance regulator-related metabolic Syndrome and cystic fibrosis screen positive, inconclusive diagnosis. *J. Pediatrics* **2017**, *181S*, S45–S51. [CrossRef] [PubMed]
12. Munck, A.; Mayell, S.J.; Winters, V.; Shawcross, A.; Derichs, N.; Parad, R.; Barben, J.; Southern, K.W.; ECFS Neonatal Screening Working Group. cystic fibrosis screen positive, inconclusive diagnosis (CFSPID): A new designation and management recommendations for infants with an inconclusive diagnosis following newborn screening. *J. Cyst. Fibros.* **2015**, *14*, 706–713. [CrossRef] [PubMed]
13. Berg, J.S.; Agrawal, P.B.; Bailey DBJr Beggs, A.H.; Brenner, S.E.; Brower, A.M.; Cakici, J.A.; Ceyhan-Birsoy, O.; Chan, K.; Chen, F.; Currier, R.J.; et al. Newborn Sequencing in Genomic Medicine and Public Health. *Pediatrics* **2017**, *139*, e20162252. [CrossRef] [PubMed]

14. Howard, H.C.; Knoppers, B.M.; Cornel, M.C.; Wright Clayton, E.; Sénécal, K.; Borry, P. Whole-genome sequencing in newborn screening? A statement on the continued importance of targeted approaches in newborn screening programmes. *Eur. J. Hum. Genet.* **2015**, *23*, 1593–1600. [CrossRef] [PubMed]
15. Ulph, F.; Cullinan, T.; Qureshi, N.; Kai, J. Parents' responses to receiving sickle cell or cystic fibrosis carrier results for their child following newborn screening. *Eur. J. Hum. Genet.* **2015**, *23*, 459–465. [CrossRef] [PubMed]
16. Castellani, C.; Duff, A.J.A.; Bell, S.C.; Heijerman, H.G.M.; Munck, A.; Ratjen, F.; Sermet-Gaudelus, I.; Southern, K.W.; Barben, J.; Flume, P.A.; et al. ECFS best practice guidelines: The 2018 revision. *J. Cyst. Fibros.* **2018**, *17*, 153–178. [CrossRef]
17. CLSI. *Newborn Screening for Cystic Fibrosis*, 2nd ed.; CLSI Guideline NBS05; Clinical and Laboratory Standards Institute: Wayne, PA, USA, 2019.
18. Goldenberg, A.J.; Sharp, R.R. The ethical hazards and programmatic challenges of genomic newborn screening. *JAMA* **2012**, *307*. [CrossRef]
19. Farrell, M.; Certain, L.; Farrell, P. Genetic counseling and risk communication services of newborn screening programs. *Arch. Pediatrics Adolesc. Med.* **2001**, *155*, 120–126. [CrossRef]
20. Farrell, M.H.; Christopher, S.A. Frequency of high-quality communication behaviors used by primary care providers of heterozygous infants after newborn screening. *Patient Educ. Couns.* **2013**, *90*, 226–232. [CrossRef]
21. La Pean, A.; Farrell, M.H.; Eskra, K.L.; Farrell, P.M. Effects of immediate telephone follow-up with providers on sweat chloride test timing after cystic fibrosis newborn screening identifies a single mutation. *J. Pediatrics* **2013**, *162*, 522–529. [CrossRef]
22. Christopher, S.A.; Collins, J.L.; Farrell, M.H. Effort required to contact primary care providers after newborn screening identifies sickle cell trait. *J. Natl. Med. Assoc.* **2012**, *104*, 528–534. [CrossRef]
23. Farrell, P.M.; Langfelder-Schwind, E.; Farrell, M.H. Challenging the dogma of the healthy heterozygote: Implications for newborn screening policies and practices. *Mol. Genet. Metab.* **2021**, *134*, 8–19. [CrossRef] [PubMed]
24. Ciske, D.J.; Haavisto, A.; Laxova, A.; Rock, L.Z.M.; Farrell, P.M. Genetic counseling and neonatal screening for cystic fibrosis: An assessment of the communication process. *Pediatrics* **2001**, *107*, 699–705. [CrossRef] [PubMed]
25. La Pean, A.; Collins, J.L.; Christopher, S.A.; Eskra, K.L.; Roedl, S.J.; Tluczek, A.; Farrell, M.H. A qualitative secondary evaluation of statewide follow-up interviews for abnormal newborn screening results for cystic fibrosis and sickle cell hemoglobinopathy. *Genet. Med.* **2012**, *14*, 207–214. [CrossRef] [PubMed]
26. Collins, J.L.; La Pean, A.; O'Tool, F.; Eskra, K.L.; Roedl, S.J.; Tluczek, A.; Farrell, M.H. Factors that influence parents' experiences with results disclosure after newborn screening identifies genetic carrier status for cystic fibrosis or sickle cell hemoglobinopathy. *Patient Educ. Couns.* **2013**, *90*, 378–385. [CrossRef]
27. Lang, C.W.; McColley, S.A.; Lester, L.A.; Ross, L.F. Parental understanding of newborn screening for cystic fibrosis after a negative sweat-test. *Pediatrics* **2011**, *127*, 276–283. [CrossRef]
28. Fernandez, C.V.; Bouffet, E.; Malkin, D.; Jabado, N.; O'Connell, C.; Avard, D.; Knoppers, B.M.; Ferguson, M.; Boycott, K.M.; Sorensen, P.H.; et al. Attitudes of parents toward the return of targeted and incidental genomic research findings in children. *Genet. Med.* **2014**, *16*, 633–640. [CrossRef]
29. Harris, E.D.; Ziniel, S.I.; Amatruda, J.G.; Clinton, C.M.; Savage, S.K.; Taylor, P.L.; Huntington, N.L.; Green, R.C.; Holm, I.A. The beliefs, motivations, and expectations of parents who have enrolled their children in a genetic biorepository. *Genet. Med.* **2012**, *14*, 330–337. [CrossRef]
30. Ziniel, S.; Savage, S.K.; Huntington, N.; Amatruda, J.; Green, R.C.; Weitzman, E.R.; Taylor, P.; Holm, I.A. Parents' preferences for return of results in pediatric genomic research. *Public Health Genom.* **2014**, *17*, 105–114. [CrossRef]
31. Christensen, K.D.; Savage, S.K.; Huntington, N.L.; Weitzman, E.R.; Ziniel, S.I.; Bacon, P.L.; Cacioppo, C.N.; Green, R.C.; Holm, I.A. Preferences for the return of individual results from research on pediatric biobank samples. *J. Empir. Res. Hum. Res. Ethics* **2017**, *12*, 97–106. [CrossRef]
32. Anderson, J.A.; Meyn, M.S.; Shuman, C.; Shaul, R.Z.; Mantella, L.E.; Szego, M.J.; Bowdin, S.; Monfared, N.; Hayeems, R.Z. Parents perspectives on whole genome sequencing for their children: Qualified enthusiasm? *J. Med. Ethics* **2017**, *43*, 535–539. [CrossRef]
33. Rini, C.; Khan, C.M.; Moore, E.; Roche, M.I.; Evans, J.P.; Berg, J.S.; Powell, B.C.; Corbie-Smith, G.; Foreman, A.K.M.; Griesemer, I.; et al. The who, what and why of research participants' intentions to request a broad range of secondary findings in a diagnostic genomic sequencing study. *Genet. Med.* **2018**, *20*, 760–769. [CrossRef]
34. Haga, S.B.; O'Daniel, J.M.; Tindall, G.M.; Lipkus, I.R.; Agans, R. Public attitudes towards ancillary information revealed by pharmacogenetic testing under limited information conditions. *Genet. Med.* **2011**, *13*, 723–728. [CrossRef]
35. Barben, J.; Castellani, C.; Munck, A.; Davies, J.C.; de Winter-de Groot, K.M.; Gartner, S.; Kashirskaya, N.; Linnane, B.; Mayell, S.J.; McColley, S.; et al. Updated guidance on the management of children with cystic fibrosis transmembrane conductance regulator-related metabolic syndrome/cystic fibrosis screen positive, inconclusive diagnosis (CRMS/CFSPID). *J. Cyst. Fibros.* **2021**, *20*, 810–819. [CrossRef]

International Journal of
Neonatal Screening

MDPI

Article

Public and Healthcare Provider Receptivity toward the Retention of Dried Blood Spot Cards and Their Usage for Extended Genetic Testing in Hong Kong

Kiran Moti Belaramani [1,†], Cheuk Wing Fung [1], Anne Mei Kwun Kwok [1], Shing Yan Robert Lee [2], Eric Kin Cheong Yau [3], Ho Ming Luk [4], Chloe Miu Mak [5], Matthew Chun Wing Yeung [5] and Olivia Miu Yung Ngan [6,7,*,†]

1 Metabolic Medicine Unit, Department of Paediatrics and Adolescent Medicine, Hong Kong Children's Hospital, Hong Kong, China
2 Department of Paediatrics and Adolescent Medicine, Pamela Youde Nethersole Eastern Hospital, Hong Kong, China
3 Department of Paediatrics and Adolescent Medicine, Princess Margaret Hospital, Hong Kong, China
4 Clinical Genetics Service Unit, Hong Kong Children's Hospital, Hong Kong, China
5 Newborn Screening Laboratory, Division of Chemical Pathology, Department of Pathology, Hong Kong Children's Hospital, Hong Kong, China
6 Medical Ethics and Humanities Unit, School of Clinical Medicine, LKS Faculty of Medicine, University of Hong Kong, Hong Kong, China
7 Centre for Medical Ethics and Law, Faculty of Law and LKS Faculty of Medicine, University of Hong Kong, Hong Kong, China
* Correspondence: olivianl@hku.hk
† These authors contributed equally to this work.

Abstract: Dried blood spot (DBS) cards from newborn screening (NBS) programs represent a wealth of biological data. They can be stored easily for a long time, have the potential to support medical and public health research, and have secondary usages such as quality assurance and forensics, making it the ideal candidate for bio-banking. However, worldwide policies vary with regard to the duration of storage of DBS cards and how it can be used. Recent advances in genomics have also made it possible to perform extended genetic testing on DBS cards in the newborn period to diagnose both actionable and non-actionable childhood and adult diseases. Both storage and secondary uses of DBS cards raise many ethical, clinical, and social questions. The openness of the key stakeholders, namely, parents and healthcare providers (HCPs), to store the DBS cards, and for what duration and purposes, and to extended genetic testing is largely dependent on local cultural–social-specific factors. The study objective is to assess the parents' and HCPs' awareness and receptivity toward DBS retention, its secondary usage, and extended genetic testing. A cross-sectional, self-administrated survey was adopted at three hospitals, out of which two were public hospitals with maternity services, between June and December 2022. In total, 452 parents and 107 HCPs completed and returned the survey. Overall, both HCPs and parents were largely knowledgeable about the potential benefits of DBS card storage for a prolonged period and its secondary uses, and they supported extended genetic testing. Knowledge gaps were found in respondents with a lower education level who did not know that a DBS card could be stored for an extended period ($p < 0.001$), could support scientific research ($p = 0.033$), and could aid public health research, and future policy implementation ($p = 0.030$). Main concerns with regard to DBS card storage related to potential privacy breaches and anonymity (Parents 70%, HCPs 60%). More parents, compared to HCPs, believed that storing DBS cards for secondary research does not lead to a reciprocal benefit to the child ($p < 0.005$). Regarding extended genetic testing, both groups were receptive and wanted to know about actionable childhood- and adult-onset diseases. More parents (four-fifths) rather than HCPs (three-fifths) were interested in learning about a variant with unknown significance ($p < 0.001$). Our findings report positive support from both parents and HCPs toward the extended retention of DBS cards for secondary usage and for extended genetic testing. However, more efforts to raise awareness need to be undertaken in addition to addressing the ethical concerns of both parents and HCPs to pave the way forward toward policy-making for DBS bio-banking and extended genetic testing in Hong Kong.

Keywords: newborn screening; inborn error of metabolism; inherited metabolic diseases; dried blood spots; residual dried blood spots; extended genetic testing; biobank; survey; Hong Kong

1. Introduction

The advances in high-resolution tandem mass spectrometry in the 1990s led to a paradigm shift in expanded newborn screening (NBS) based on dried blood spot (DBS) cards [1]. Currently, NBS using a heel prick test, collecting a few drops of blood from the baby's heel on filter paper, is widely available in many regions and countries [2]. The residual DBS cards can be stored for long periods, and storing these materials represents a wealth of biological data. It offers an excellent opportunity for secondary analytic uses to improve current screening programs, facilitate laboratories' quality control and assurance, forensics, and expand biomedical research [3–6]. Studies have also shown that dried bloodspots can also aid disease treatment via early detection of genetic and infectious diseases. DNA is stable in DBS for prolonged periods, making it the ideal candidate to aid early diagnosis of genetic conditions using expanded genetic screening. Studies have shown that DBS cards can aid the diagnosis of congenital cytomegalovirus and neonatal herpes simplex virus infection. Other potential maternally transmissible conditions that could be diagnosed using DBS cards include HIV, Hepatitis B, and C. In utero exposure to potentially toxic environmental agents such as lead, mercury, and dichlorodiphenyldichloroethylene (DDE) are also measurable on DBS cards and could aid diagnosis and etiologic studies of birth defects and developmental disabilities in relation to environmental agent epidemiology [7–9].

Storing DBS cards for secondary usage raises clinical, ethical, and social considerations. The most frequently discussed concern is informed consent. A pre-requisite for informed consent is knowledge. Locally, Mak et al. have shown that parents have a deficient knowledge of DBS cards and NBS programs [10]. Van Teeffelen et al. have shown that 81.8% of parents were unaware of the DBS card screening, storage, and use policies in the Netherlands [11]. On the other hand, Tarini et al. showed that parents in the United States (US) demonstrated high trust and support toward storing DBS cards [12], and they were willing to give out their child's DBS cards only if explicit consent was obtained through an opt-in approach [13–15]. Another significant issue is data privacy breaches. Studies showed fears about misusing information for purposes that deviate from their original intended use, driving discrimination by employment, insurance, or medical treatment, inequitable access to healthcare services, and potential bias against individuals [16,17]. However, some medical geneticists argued that these are negligible concerns, as most research uses involve de-identified or anonymized bio-samples [18]. Some evidence suggests that deliberative consent procedures encourage research participation, helping parents understand the process and purpose of the secondary use of DBS samples for research and empowering their need for control over the use of their samples. Other apprehensions about DBS card storage include unauthorized access to information, unclear research purposes, and the absence of data management and governance [16,19].

The rapid development of next-generation sequencing is leading to an evolution in NBS, using DNA material on the DBS card to discover disease genes and diseases at an early age [20]. This technology can be used as a primary screen, especially for those early-onset actionable disorders that lack a good biochemical marker or follow-up testing after an abnormal primary screen. However, on the downside, extended genetic testing can also provide provisional positive or inconclusive information about an individual's future health, which can significantly impact their lives and the lives of their family members. Studies have shown that although parents were often optimistic about receiving their child's health information and felt it would be a parental obligation to ensure a healthy life, their initial affective responses toward an inconclusive test result were often ones of distress, shock, and anxiety, mainly due to their inadequate knowledge of screened-for conditions and genetics [21,22].

Policies worldwide vary regarding how and when to consent for biospecimen storage and its secondary uses because of the sensitive information that can be derived from the DBS card [2]. In Hong Kong, there is a DBS-based opt-in NBS program covering 26 inherited metabolic diseases (IMD) and severe combined immunodeficiency which has been available to all newborns at all eight public hospitals with maternity services since 2020 and 2021, respectively. Parents are given information about the NBS program in both the antenatal and postnatal period through the display of videos and distribution of education pamphlets to help them understand the newborn screening program prior to the attainment of written consent. In the current framework, DBS samples will be archived for six months except for quality assurance purposes, and no research purposes will be served. The optimal policy governing NBS technologies is contextually dependent, and empirical research on this topic among the general public and medical professionals is limitedly reported in the local context. The specific study objective is to describe the knowledge, attitudes, and practices toward the storage and secondary use of DBS, including extended genetic testing among parents and healthcare providers (HCPs) in Hong Kong.

2. Materials and Methods

2.1. Sampling and Recruitment

A cross-sectional, self-administrated survey was adopted at three hospitals, including two public hospitals with maternity services, between June and December 2022 (The survey questionnaires are included in the Supplementary Materials). The study population comprised parents and HCPs.

Parents were recruited using convenience sampling. They were initially approached while they attended the pediatric service outpatient clinic at three public hospitals. The researcher ensured that parents were fully informed about the study. Basic background information on the concepts of the DBS card and its potential were included in the study information leaflet during recruitment. After obtaining written consent, they received a hard copy or an e-copy of the survey. HCPs, including doctors, nurses, dieticians, laboratory technicians, and those in other fields relating to clinical services, were invited to participate in the study using snowballing sampling. The study was emailed to every member of the department. A survey package, including an informed consent form and a paper questionnaire, was also distributed to the HCPs' office mailbox. Anyone who was incompetent in Chinese or English, or refused to consent, was excluded from the study.

The completed survey questionnaires were either submitted online, returned by mail using a self-addressed stamped envelope, or collected on-site. A reminder was also sent two weeks after the initial email. No incentives for survey participation were provided.

2.2. Survey Measures

The survey consists of two main themes, along with demographic information. The first theme aims to gather views on the awareness of NBS for uncommon disorders and assess knowledge, attitudes, and practices toward the storage of DBS cards. A vignette is provided to ensure survey respondent has an equal understanding the study context (Box 1).

Box 1. Description of Newborn Screening with Dried Blood Spots Card.

Shortly after the baby infant is born, a health professional will perform a heel prick to collect a few drops of blood on a special card. The Card will be sent to the laboratory for the screening of some rare but serious conditions which could be picked up and treated early with benefit the affected babies in the long run. The information also benefits the paediatric population and other scientific research.

At present, the card is kept for 6 months after the test has been performed for quality assurance purposes and will then be discarded. Other countries, the card will be kept longer (a few years or twenty years or more) for other research purposes.

The domain of questions includes several key areas:

(1) The source of information, which is evaluated by assessing various sources of knowledge, such as discussions with healthcare professionals, media, leaflets, colleagues, and online forums.
(2) Knowledge about the potential benefits of storing a DBS card is assessed by presenting participants with 11 true or false statements. These statements have been developed based on a thorough review of the NBS literature and position statements. A higher score indicates a better understanding of the advantages of storing a DBS card.
(3) Attitudes toward DBS card storage are assessed by examining concerns relating to privacy breaches, data sharing among institutions, linking research information to medical records, lack of immediate individual benefits, and serving secondary research purposes. Each item is rated on a 5-point Likert scale, ranging from 0 (not concerned at all) to 5 (extremely concerned).
(4) Practices are assessed by evaluating participants' interest in storing their child's sample after the NBS on a 1-to-10 Likert scale (1 indicating not supportive, and 10 indicating extremely supportive). Additionally, participants are asked how long they believe the DBS card should be stored.

The second theme of the study focused on exploring the inclination toward opting for extended genetic testing after reading the vignette (Box 2). To achieve this, a set of eight scenarios were presented to parents, inquiring whether they would like to receive the results of the extended genetic testing for their child. Similarly, HCPs were asked if they would disclose this information to parents, and both groups responded with a simple "Yes" or "No". The study also delved into the factors that influence the interest of parents and HCPs in extended genetic testing, which were measured using a 5-point Likert scale, with 1 indicating "not important at all" and 5 indicating "extremely important". Finally, the participants were asked to express their level of interest in extended genetic testing, either for their child or as an offering, on a scale of 1 to 10, where 1 represents no interest at all, and 10 represents an extremely high level of interest.

Box 2. Description of Extended Genetic Testing.

It is possible to study a person's entire genome extracted from DBS card. This process is called extended genetic sequencing. It may give you information about a person's risk of having different diseases both in the present and in the future, including childhood diseases such as epilepsy and adult-onset diseases breast cancer or diabetes.
Imagine that you have a recently born baby. Newborn Screening program now offers you the chance to get extended genetic sequencing done for your baby. You would receive the results and would not have to pay for the testing. You can decide whether or not you want the information to be a part of your child's medical record.

2.3. Data Analysis

Descriptive statistics were applied. Analyses specifically focused on the differences between parents and healthcare professionals. Chi-square and t-test were used to compare these two groups. Statistical significance was considered if the p-value was less than 0.05. Data were analyzed using SPSS (Version 28; SPSS, Inc., Chicago, IL, USA).

3. Results

3.1. Demographics Characteristics

A total of 452 parents and 107 HCPs completed and returned the survey. Table 1 describes their demographic characteristics. Among 452 parents, the majority were female (74.3%), Hong Kong Chinese (86.9%), had no religious affiliation (70.4%), had two or more children (56.2%), and did not work in a healthcare-related industry (90.5%). Around three-fifths attained post-secondary school education (62.0%), which is similar to the educational attainment of the general population reported in the 2022 census [23]. Around 62.4% of respondents earned more than the median monthly household income (HKD 29,100) [24].

Over 93.8% of respondents were not part of a consanguineous marriage. There were 161 (35.6%) parents who were taking care of a child with a disease, of whom 40 (8.8%) were suffering from cardiac disease, 21 (4.7%) from hematological disorders, 16 (3.5%) from respiratory diseases, 15 (3.3%) from neonatal diseases, 14 (3.1%) from endocrine diseases, 9 (2.0%) neurological diseases, and 8 (1.8%) from inherited metabolic diseases.

Table 1. Demographics of survey respondents.

	All (*n* = 559)	Healthcare Providers (*n* = 107)	Parents (*n* = 452)	Chi/t	*p*-Value
	n (%)	*n* (%)	*n* (%)		
Age					
mean (SD)	36.8 (6.57)	39.39 (10.33)	36.17 (5.18)	3.06	<0.001
Gender				ns	ns
Female	412 (73.7%)	76 (71%)	336 (74.3%)		
Male	147 (26.3%)	31 (29%)	116 (25.7%)		
Ethnicity				15.6	<0.001
Hong Kong Chinese	500 (89.5%)	107 (100%)	393 (86.9%)		
Mainland Chinese	32 (5.7%)	-	32 (7.1%)		
Other	27 (4.8%)	-	27 (6%)		
Religion				31.25	<0.001
None	370 (66.2%)	52 (48.6%)	318 (70.4%)		
Christian	111 (19.8%)	39 (36.4%)	72 (15.9%)		
Catholic	39 (7.1%)	12 (11.2%)	27 (6%)		
Buddhist	26 (4.6%)	4 (3.8%)	22 (4.8%)		
Other	13 (2.3%)	-	13 (2.9%)		
Do you work in a health-care related field?					
No	-	-	409 (90.5%)	-	-
Yes	-	-	43 (9.5%)	-	-
Profession					
Doctor	-	34 (31.8%)	-	-	-
Nurse	-	36 (33.6%)	-	-	-
Laboratory Technician	-	5 (4.7%)	-	-	-
Others	-	32 (29.9%)	-	-	-

Table 1. *Cont.*

	All (n = 559)	Healthcare Providers (n = 107)	Parents (n = 452)	Chi/t	p-Value
	n (%)	n (%)	n (%)		
Years of Experience in NBS					
Mean (SD)	-	5.49 (7.35)	-		
Highest Education				89.55	<0.001
Upper Secondary or lower	174 (31.1%)	2 (1.9%)	172 (38.0%)		
Post-Secondary	78 (14.0%)	3 (2.8%)	75 (16.6%)		
Tertiary	197 (35.2%)	47 (43.9%)	150 (33.2%)		
Master or above	110 (19.7%)	55 (51.4%)	55 (12.2%)		
Family Income				89.55	<0.001
Below HKD 19,999	93 (16.7%)	3 (2.8%)	90 (19.9%)		
HKD 20,000–29,999	81 (14.5%)	1 (0.9%)	80 (17.7%)		
HKD 30,000–39,999	89 (15.9%)	6 (5.6%)	83 (18.4%)		
HKD 40,000–49,999	37 (6.6%)	4 (3.7%)	33 (7.3%)		
Above HKD 50,000	259 (46.3%)	93 (87.0%)	166 (36.7%)		
Consanguinity					
No	-	-	424 (93.8%)	-	-
Yes	-	-	24 (5.3%)	-	-
Not Sure	-	-	4 (0.9%)	-	-
Kid Number					
1	-	-	198 (43.8%)	-	-
2	-	-	202 (44.7%)	-	-
3 or above	-	-	52 (11.5%)	-	-
Diagnosed Disease					
None	-	-	291 (64.4%)	-	-
Cardiac Diseases	-	-	40 (8.8%)	-	-
Haematology	-	-	21 (4.7%)	-	-
Respiratory	-	-	16 (3.5%)	-	-
Neonatology	-	-	15 (3.3%)	-	-
Endocrine Diseases	-	-	14 (3.1%)	-	-
Neurology	-	-	9 (2.0%)	-	-
Metabolic Diseases	-	-	8 (1.8%)	-	-
Others	-	-	38 (8.4%)	-	-

ns = not significant.

Among 107 HCPs, the majority were female (71%), Hong Kong Chinese (100%), had no religious affiliation (48.6%), and attained post-secondary school education (98.1%). About one-third were doctors (31.8%) and nurses (33.6%). The remaining were allied health professionals, including dietitians, physiotherapists, occupational therapists, and laboratory technicians (34.6%) involved in healthcare provision to patients with uncommon diseases such as IMD. The average number of years of experience/involvement in NBS practice was 5.49 (SD = 7.35).

3.2. Awareness of Newborn Screening for Uncommon Disorders

In terms of sources of information, some parents have obtained NBS-related information from more than one medium. Among 452 parents, 237 (52.4%) have heard about NBS, where they rely on health providers as the most credible source of information (61.2%), followed by hospital brochures (37.1%) and online platforms and media (13.9%). Of those 237 responding parents who have heard about NBS, 139 (58.7%) have taken part in an NBS program for uncommon diseases, 56 parents (23.6%) have not taken part in any screening program, and 42 (17.7%) are uncertain.

Among 107 HCPs, 93 (86.9%) have heard of NBS, where they receive test information from colleagues (84.9%), hospital brochures (36.6%), and academic research papers (19.4%). Of those 93 responding HCPs who have heard about NBS, 47 (50.5%) are involved in NBS, performing various duties including informing parents of test results (34%), drawing blood tests (21.3%), providing consultation (19.1%), conducting laboratory analysis (12.8%), hosting educational sessions (6.4%), and facilitating consent procedure (6.4%).

Overall, most parents who have participated in NBS (97.9%), and all HCPs who are involved in NBS (100%), find NBS for uncommon disorders useful.

3.3. Knowledge about the Potential Benefits of Storing Dried Blood Spot Cards

Figure 1 describes the knowledge about potential benefits of storing a DBS card. Overall, healthcare professionals demonstrated a higher understanding when compared to parents, with a mean of 10.2 and 9.43 correct answers out of 11 items, respectively ($p < 0.001$). While most parents (95.1%) acknowledged that their consent is required to keep their child's DBS card, and that the DBS card supports scientific research (93.8%), identifies rare and serious conditions in babies (93.6%), provides diagnostic purposes (92.7%), aids disease treatment (91.4%), contains genetic material (90.3%) and can be connected to personal medical record (82.1%), fewer parents knew that the DBS card could be stored for a long time (66.6%) or be used for forensic purposes (63.3%). Among HCPs, 99.1% knew that DBS cards could be used to identify rare and serious conditions in babies, and 96.3% acknowledged that their consent is required to keep their child's DBS card. They were aware that DBS card could be used in scientific research (97.2%), quality assurance (95.3%), aid disease treatment (96.3%), and contains genetic material (90.7%). Around one-sixth did not know that the DBS can be connected to personal medical records (15.9%), stored for a long time (14.0%), and be used for forensic purposes (13.1%) or diagnostic purposes (13.1%).

Subgroup analysis showed that lack of prior exposure to NBS for uncommon disorders and lower educational background contribute to the knowledge gaps. Compared with those who had heard of NBS for uncommon diseases, those who had not heard about the test were not aware of the use of DBS for identifying rare and severe conditions ($p = 0.009$), forensic purposes ($p = 0.024$), supporting the development of individual-specific disease treatment ($p = 0.03$). Respondents who attained an education level below secondary schools did not know the DBS card could be stored for an extended period ($p < 0.001$), support scientific research ($p = 0.033$), and aid public health research and future policy implementation ($p = 0.030$). No significant difference was observed by any other demographics.

3.4. Concerns and Views about Storing Dried Blood Spot Cards

Regarding concerns about DBS card storage (see Figure 2), about half of the parents (51.3%) and HCPs (58.9%) were not concerned about sharing DBS among academic institutions. Over 70% of parents and 60% of HCPs demonstrated considerable concerns about potential privacy breaches and anonymity. Compared to their lower-educated counterparts, the more educated expressed statistically significant concerns about the DBS being linked with personal or medical records ($p = 0.005$) or privacy breaches ($p < 0.001$). While over 70% of HCPs expressed no concern with regard to the DBS being used for secondary research, more parents (50.5%) than HCPs (25.2%) were of the opinion that the DBS secondary research does not benefit their child and are thus more reluctant to store the card for public health or scientific research purposes ($p < 0.005$). Pearson correlations reveal a negative relationship between knowledge of keeping DBS and concerns about altruistic benefits (correlation coefficient = -0.125, $p = 0.003$).

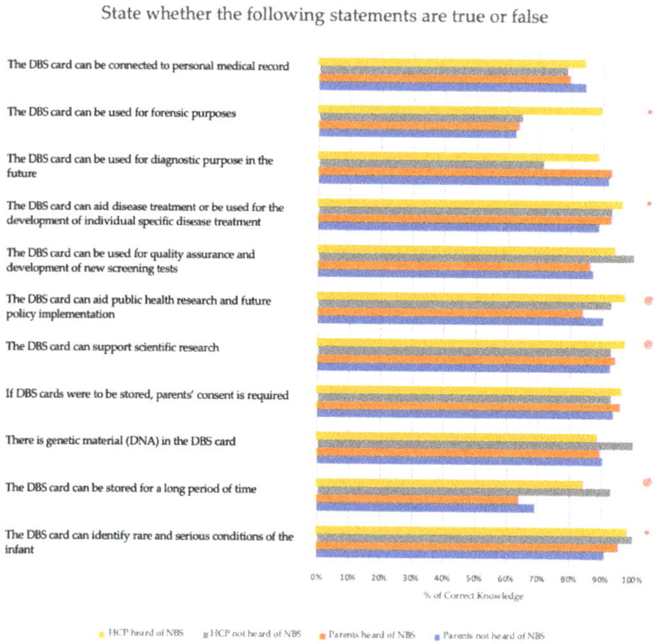

Figure 1. Knowledge about potential benefits of storing dried blood spot cards. * denotes statistically significant differences according to awareness of NBS; @ denotes statistically significant differences according to education level.

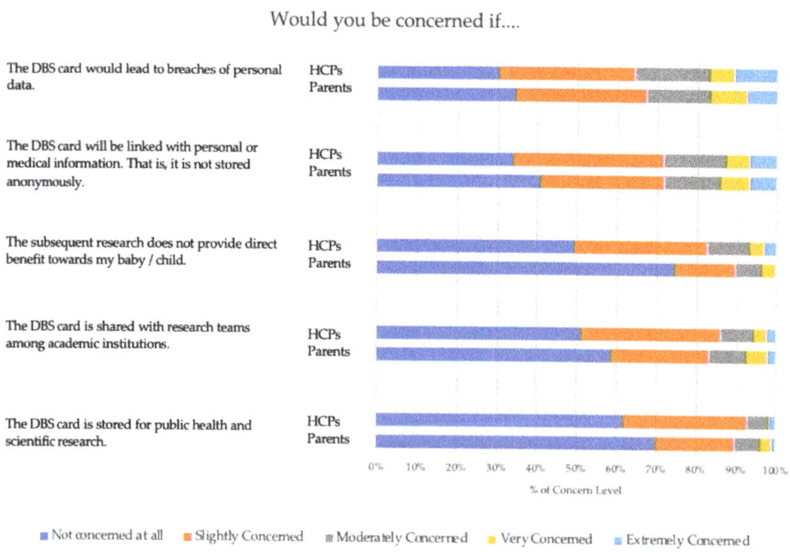

Figure 2. Concerns about storing dried blood spot cards. HCPs = healthcare providers.

Table 2 shows views about storing DBS cards. Most parents and HCPs (72.3%) showed interest in storing DBS cards for longer than six months, which is the current protocol in public hospitals. Of these, 21.1% support storage for up to 2 years, 15.9% support it for up to 5 years, 17.9% support it for up to 18 years, and 17.4% support storing the DBS card infinitely. The only significant difference is observed by education groups: respondents who obtained post-secondary education or higher were more supportive of longer storage of more than six months (77.7%) than their lower-educated counterparts (61.3%). Overall, on a scale of 1 (do not support) to 10 (strongly support), parents (mean = 8.13) and HCPS (mean = 8.26) supported the public policy in DBS card storage. No significant difference was observed by other demographics.

Table 2. Views toward storing dried blood spots.

	All (*n* = 559)	Healthcare Providers (*n* = 107)	Parents (*n* = 452)	Chi/t	*p*-Value
	n (%)	*n* (%)	*n* (%)		
How long do you think DBS should be stored?					
Up to 6 months	155 (27.7%)	29 (27.2%)	126 (27.9%)	ns	ns
Up to 2 years	118 (21.1%)	23 (21.5%)	95 (21%)	ns	ns
Up to 5 years	89 (15.9%)	24 (22.4%)	65 (14.4%)	ns	ns
Up to 18 years	100 (17.9%)	21 (19.6%)	79 (17.5%)	ns	ns
Indefinitely	97 (17.4%)	10 (9.3%)	87 (19.2%)	ns	ns
Do you support DBS storage? (1 as not interested at all; 10 as extremely interested)					
mean (SD)	8.15 (1.66)	8.26 (1.70)	8.13 (1.65)	ns	ns

ns = not significant.

3.5. Interest in Opting for Extended Genetic Testing

Table 3 shows the assessment of interest in opting for extended genetic testing. Around 31% of parents and 43.9% of HCP have heard of extended genetic testing in NBS. The top two conditions in extended genetic testing that parents and HCPs are interested in learning are, respectively, a childhood-onset disease with treatment (87.4% and 90.7%) and a condition listed on the current medical recommended screening panel (85.6% and 87.9%). While around 77.9% of parents are interested in learning about a variant with unknown clinical implications, only three-fifths (57%) of HCPs agreed with the early disclosure of the variant (Chi = 19.5, $p < 0.001$).

When asked about the major factor driving their interest in extended genetic testing from a scale of 1 (not important at all) to 5 (very important), parents identified the potential usefulness of genetic extended testing to help shorten the diagnosis time (mean = 3.57), identify new disease genes and diagnose individuals with rare disorders (mean = 3.54) as important factors. In contrast, HCPs, put greater emphasis on the accuracy of test results (mean = 4.32) and access to existing treatment (mean = 4.31).

Overall, on a scale of 0 (do not support) to 10 (strongly support), parents (mean = 7.87) and HCPS (mean = 7.64) supported extended genetic testing. No significant difference found between parents who have a child with a disease and other demographics.

Table 3. Interest in opting for extended genetic testing.

	All (*n* = 559) *n* (%)	Healthcare Providers (*n* = 107) *n* (%)	Parents (*n* = 452) *n* (%)	Chi	*p*-Value
If you were the parent, would you wish to receive the following information with regard to your child/If you were a healthcare provider, would you wish to disclose the following information to parents?					
A childhood-onset disorder is a condition with treatment	492 (88.0%)	97 (90.7%)	395 (87.4%)	ns	ns
A condition list on the current medical recommended screening panel	481 (86.0%)	94 (87.9%)	387 (85.6%)	ns	ns
Increase risk for an adult-onset disease	467 (83.5%)	83 (77.6%)	384 (85.0%)	ns	ns
The newborn is a carrier for the condition but will not develop it	470 (84.1%)	93 (86.9%)	377 (83.4%)	ns	ns
An adulthood-onset disorder is a condition with treatment	466 (83.4%)	94 (87.9%)	372 (82.3%)	ns	ns
A childhood-onset disorder is a condition with NO available treatment	456 (81.6%)	91 (85.0%)	365 (80.8%)	ns	ns
A variant that has unknown clinical implications	413 (73.9%)	61 (57.0%)	352 (77.9%)	19.5	<0.001
An adulthood-onset disorder is a condition with NO available treatment	421 (75.3%)	81 (75.7%)	340 (75.2%)	ns	ns
What is the factor(s) impacting your interest in extended genetic testing? (1 is not important at all; 5 is extremely important)					
	mean (SD)	mean (SD)	mean (SD)	t	*p*-value
Shorten the diagnosis time in future	3.69 (1.17)	4.20 (0.884)	3.57 (1.19)	6.11	<0.001
Identify new disease genes and diagnose individuals with rare disorders	3.66 (1.16)	4.14 (0.976)	3.54 (1.17)	5.45	<0.001
Access to existing treatment for affected individuals	3.68 (1.15)	4.31 (0.862)	3.53 (1.16)	7.84	<0.001
Accuracy of the test results/sequencing results	3.67 (1.19)	4.32 (0.938)	3.52 (1.20)	7.52	<0.001
Access to specialist follow-up for affected individuals	3.64 (1.15)	4.18 (0.92)	3.51 (1.17)	6.38	<0.001
Impinge on the child's right to an open future	3.58 (1.19)	4.06 (0.96)	3.47 (1.21)	5.37	<0.001
Diagnosing susceptibility to adult-onset disease during the newborn period	3.35 (1.18)	3.45 (1.27)	3.32 (1.16)	ns	ns
How interested would you be in obtaining your child's extended genetic testing? (1 as not interested at all; 10 as extremely interested)					
mean (SD)	7.83 (1.85)	7.64 (1.87)	7.87 (1.85)	ns	ns

ns = not significant.

4. Discussion

DBS unquestionably provides us with an easy way to store a wealth of data that can be used for many secondary purposes and extended genetic testing. The sensitive information it holds has resulted in many debates amongst experts worldwide regarding the duration of storage, secondary usage, and research policies and how and when to consent to DBS storage and its secondary uses. This has resulted in variable global policies. There, however, is a trend to store DBS cards for a prolonged period of time and to use them for biobanking. In New Zealand [25], some states in the US, such as Minnesota [26,27], and Victoria in Australia [28], DBS cards are stored indefinitely. In Denmark, the residual DBS cards are stored at the Danish Newborn Screening Biobank indefinitely [29]. The United Kingdom stores DBS cards for 5 years [30].

The opt-in NBS for inherited metabolic diseases and severe combined immunodeficiency for newborns born in public hospitals is funded by the Hong Kong Government. DBS samples were collected for NBS purposes and archived for six months after reporting except for quality assurance purposes. The issues about DBS storage and its secondary use are yet to be explored. Ethical questions and consenting logistics remain challenges. However, before moving on, it is essential to know the receptivity of our key stakeholders, i.e., the parents and HCPs in Hong Kong, toward the retention of DBS cards and their secondary usage, including extended genetic testing, and this was the purpose of our study.

Our study has shown that the awareness of NBS locally is still low, with only 52.4% of parents and 86.9% of HCPs being aware of NBS. In the Netherlands, 98.5% of mothers were aware of NBS [11], and in Australia, 93% of mothers had heard of NBS [31]. Having said that, our study includes parents who have (58.7%) heard of NBS had taken part in in NBS, and this may account for the difference. Our figures are more comparable to a Japanese study examining mothers and an American study examining the general public regarding their awareness of NBS, and these studies showed that only 57% and 55%, respectively, were aware of NBS [13,32]. Another reason for the low awareness is that NBS has only been established territory wide in Hong Kong in the last five years, and it will take the public more time to become more aware of NBS.

This lack of awareness is also reflected in the lack of knowledge about DBS storage. Only 66.6% of parents and 86% of HCPs were aware that DBS could be stored for a long time. Despite not knowing about the prolonged storage of DBS, parents were generally aware that DBS contains genetic material (90.3%), could be used for quality assurance (86.9%) and scientific and public health research (93.8%), and was connected to personal medical record (82.1%), but few (63.3%) knew that it could be used to for forensic purposes. Lack of knowledge and awareness may be the reason that Hui et al. [16] noted the lack of support of local parents in using DBS to trace victims (69%) or suspects of crimes (52%), while they were more supportive of using DBS for quality control (85%) and health-related research (75%). This is in contrast to the Dutch population, where NBS has been established since 1974, and the population is highly supportive of using DBS to help trace suspects of serious crimes, with a rating mean of 3.63 on a 5-point scale [11]. In contrast to parents, our HCPs (86.9%) were more aware of DBS's secondary uses and forensics uses of DBS (86.9%). Thus, our frontline HCPs should be recruited as collaborative partners to help fill the knowledge gap of the parents since our respondents (61.2%) considered HCPs to be the most credible source of information.

The concerns of both HCPs (65.4%) and parents (69.5%) relating to the storage of DBS with regard to breaches of personal data are very reasonable concerns to have, considering the sensitivity of information the DBS contains about an individual. This concern only reiterates that strict data protection policies need to be put into place to gain the trust of our parents and HCPs if prolonged DBS storage is to be considered in Hong Kong.

Interestingly, the parents (50.5%) in Hong Kong did not seem to be as altruistic as our HCP (25.2%) when it came to research, and they were concerned that the research did not directly benefit their child/baby. Bombard et al. [1] showed that among Canadian citizens, 77% supported anonymous research. Further analysis revealed that Canadian citizens' acceptance of or discomfort with a routinised approach to research with stored samples varied along axes of trust, concern for harm, and individual versus collective interests. There is a need for a more focus group-based research locally to understand parent's motivations for supporting and the reservations to use DBS for secondary research.

An important issue that our study did not discuss extensively is consent. Storage policies are an opt-out option in New Zealand, Minnesota (US), Denmark, and the United Kingdom. In New Zealand, Denmark, and Minnesota (US), the secondary use of DBS, including research, is mentioned on the leaflet for NBS or the website for NBS. In the United Kingdom, no consent for de-identifiable blood spots is necessary. Victoria in Australia uses an opt-in approach, and written consent for the de-identified secondary use and health research is taken during the NBS consent. Denmark has a clear policy and states the purpose of storage for the (1) diagnosis and treatment of congenital disorders, including documentation, repeat testing, quality assurance, statistics, and improvement of screening methods; (2) diagnostic use later in infancy after informed consent; (3) legal use after a court order; and (4) the possibility of research projects after approval by the Scientific Ethical Committee System in Denmark, The Danish Data Protection Agency and the NBS-Biobank Steering Committee. Hui et al. showed that Hong Kong parents prefer the opt-in approach rather than the opt-out approach [16]. More research is required to understand local preferences.

Regarding the length of storage of DBS, keeping their concerns aside, 17.5% of parents and 19.6% of HCPs were willing to store the DBS up to 18 years of age, and 19.2% of parents and 9.3% of HCPs were supportive of storing the DBS indefinitely. Overall, 72.3%

of parents and HCPs supported storing DBS beyond the current 6-month practice, and this is a promising start for any bio-banking future in Hong Kong.

In the US, various projects are underway to test the usefulness of whole-exome sequencing (WES) or whole-genome sequencing (WGS) as a tool in newborn sequencing—Babyseq project [33], NC Nexus [34], etc. The United Kingdom National Health Service is also exploring the benefits of next-generation sequencing in newborn screening [35]. All of these programs have discovered the benefits of extended genetic testing in NBS, including the reduction in false-positive and false-negative rates [36], the discovery of conditions not identified by MS/MS newborn screening [34,37], and even shortening time to diagnosis [38]. Extended genetic testing in NBS is the future that will radically change the face of health screening worldwide. Goldenberg et al. showed that 74% of parents were interested in WGS in newborns [39]. This is similar to our results in which 78.1% of parents and 73.4% of HCPs supported extended genetic testing in NBS.

However, apart from identifying medically actionable childhood-onset disease, it can also identify actionable adult-onset disease. This may have a huge psychological impact on the individual and their family members regarding the uncertainty of the time of onset of the disease. Extended genetic testing can also detect non-actionable conditions and conditions of unknown significance. Our parents (90.7%) and HCPs (87.4%) were more interested in knowing about actionable conditions and less about non-actionable conditions. This is different from the Western population, where Lewis et al. showed that with regard to non-actionable conditions, parents preferred to learn about disorders with more severe manifestations, even though this may result in increased distress [40]. Our parents and HCPs were well aware that a genetic diagnosis alone is inadequate, and thus, the factors which will influence their interest in extended genetic testing include the accuracy of test results, access to specialist follow-up and waiting time length, and access to existing treatment without any impingement on an open future. These are all important factors for a society to consider before embarking on including extended genetic screening in their NBS program. More small group analysis is required to comprehend better the societal and ethical preferences of local HCPS and parents.

5. Conclusions

In conclusion, the establishment of DBS-based NBS in Hong Kong started in 2015. The issues of DBS storage and secondary usages, including extended genetic testing, need to be further explored, hoping to be in line with other countries. Our study shows that addressing the clinical, ethical, and social concerns of HCPs and parents is paramount to making the leap forward. Thus, more research is needed to understand the local preferences and views. In the meantime, we will continue to engage our HCPs to enhance the education of parents about NBS and DBS storage and its secondary uses in order to fill the knowledge gap and conduct more research to understand local preferences.

6. Strengths and Limitations

There are several limitations to the current study. First, this was a cross-sectional assessment of attitudes toward the retention of DBS cards and their usage for extended genetic testing. We compared groups of parents and HCPs, but the results should be interpreted carefully at the community level as sociodemographic and professional characteristics observed individual variances. Second, the study did not report the baseline knowledge of medical genetics, which may have affected respondents' views of extended genetic testing. Third, the sample consisted of those who responded to our survey and are willing to participate in a study in the public sector only, and we have no private sector data for comparison. Finally, the survey instrument's closed-ended questionnaire structure did not allow additional ethical concerns to be raised. Thus, the data do not fully describe the ethical considerations in the sample population but rather their views about predetermined issues.

Supplementary Materials: The survey questionnaires can be downloaded at: https://www.mdpi.com/article/10.3390/ijns9030045/s1.

Author Contributions: Conceptualization, K.M.B. and O.M.Y.N.; methodology, O.M.Y.N.; validation, O.M.Y.N.; formal analysis, K.M.B. and O.M.Y.N.; data curation, O.M.Y.N.; writing—original draft preparation, K.M.B. and O.M.Y.N.; writing—review and editing, C.W.F., A.M.K.K., E.K.C.Y., S.Y.R.L., H.M.L., C.M.M. and M.C.W.Y.; supervision, C.W.F., A.M.K.K., E.K.C.Y., S.Y.R.L. and H.M.L.; project administration, K.M.B., E.K.C.Y., S.Y.R.L. and O.M.Y.N.; funding acquisition, K.M.B. and O.M.Y.N. All authors have read and agreed to the published version of the manuscript.

Funding: This research is supported by the Health and Medical Research Fund from the Health Bureau of the Government of the Hong Kong Special Administrative Region. The funder has no role in the research project design or data interpretation.

Institutional Review Board Statement: The study was conducted in accordance with the Declaration of Helsinki and approved by the Hong Kong Children's Hospital Research Ethics Committee [HKCH-REC-2020-028], Kowloon West Cluster Research Ethics Committee [KW/EX21-036(157-01), and Hong Kong East Cluster Research Ethics Committee [HKECREC-2021-005].

Informed Consent Statement: Informed consent was obtained from all subjects involved in the study.

Data Availability Statement: The data supporting this study's findings are available on reasonable request from the corresponding author.

Acknowledgments: We would like to express our sincere thanks for the support from the Hong Kong Children's Hospital research team, parents, and healthcare providers participating in the study. We especially thank the anonymous reviewers for their careful reading of our manuscript and their many insightful suggestions.

Conflicts of Interest: The authors declare no conflict of interest.

References

1. Bombard, Y.; Miller, F.A.; Hayeems, R.Z.; Carroll, J.C.; Avard, D.; Wilson, B.J.; Little, J.; Bytautas, J.P.; Allanson, J.; Axler, R.; et al. Citizens' values regarding research with stored samples from newborn screening in Canada. *Pediatrics* **2012**, *129*, 239–247. [PubMed]
2. Loeber, J.G.; Platis, D.; Zetterström, R.H.; Almashanu, S.; Boemer, F.; Bonham, J.R.; Borde, P.; Brincat, I.; Cheillan, D.; Dekkers, E.; et al. Neonatal screening in Europe revisited: An ISNS perspective on the current state and developments since 2010. *Int. J. Neonatal Screen.* **2021**, *7*, 15. [CrossRef]
3. Olney, R.S.; Moore, C.A.; Ojodu, J.A.; Lindegren, M.L.; Hannon, W.H. Storage and use of residual dried blood spots from state newborn screening programs. *J. Pediatr.* **2006**, *148*, 618–622. [CrossRef] [PubMed]
4. Lei, K.; Zhao, Y.; Sun, L.; Liang, H.; Luo, R.; Sun, X.; Tao, Y.; Chen, L.; Zhang, L.; Li, A.; et al. A pilot screening of high-risk Gaucher disease children using dried blood spot methods in Shandong province of China. *Orphanet J. Rare Dis.* **2018**, *13*, 48. [CrossRef] [PubMed]
5. Reuser, A.J.; Verheijen, F.W.; Bali, D.; van Diggelen, O.P.; Germain, D.P.; Hwu, W.-L.; Lukacs, Z.; Mühl, A.; Olivova, P.; Piraud, M.; et al. The use of dried blood spot samples in the diagnosis of lysosomal storage disorders—Current status and perspectives. *Mol. Genet. Metab.* **2011**, *104*, 144–148. [PubMed]
6. Chace, D.H.; DiPerna, J.C.; Mitchell, B.L.; Sgroi, B.; Hofman, L.F.; Naylor, E.W. Electrospray tandem mass spectrometry for analysis of acylcarnitines in dried postmortem blood specimens collected at autopsy from infants with unexplained cause of death. *Clin. Chem.* **2001**, *47*, 1166–1182. [CrossRef] [PubMed]
7. Barbi, M.; Binda, S.; Primache, V.; Tettamanti, A.; Negri, C.; Brambilla, C. Use of Guthrie cards for the early diagnosis of neonatal herpes simplex virus disease. *Pediatr. Infect. Dis. J.* **1998**, *17*, 251–252. [CrossRef] [PubMed]
8. Chaudhuri, S.N.; Butala, S.J.M.; Ball, R.W.; Braniff, C.T. Pilot study for utilization of dried blood spots for screening of lead, mercury and cadmium in newborns. *J. Expo. Sci. Environ. Epidemiol.* **2009**, *19*, 298–316. [CrossRef] [PubMed]
9. Tuaillon, E.; Kania, D.; Pisoni, A.; Bollore, K.; Taieb, F.; Ngoyi, E.N.O.; Schaub, R.; Plantier, J.-C.; Makinson, A.; Van De Perre, P. Dried blood spot tests for the diagnosis and therapeutic monitoring of HIV and viral hepatitis B and C. *Front. Microbiol.* **2020**, *11*, 373. [CrossRef] [PubMed]
10. Mak, C.; Lam, C.W.; Law, C.Y.; Siu, W.; Kwong, L.; Chan, K.; Chow, K.; Lee, K.; Chan, W.; Chan, A. Parental attitudes on expanded newborn screening in Hong Kong. *Public Health* **2012**, *126*, 954–959. [PubMed]
11. Van Teeffelen, S.R.; Douglas, C.M.W.; van El, C.G.; Weinreich, S.S.; Henneman, L.; Radstake, M.; Cornel, M.C. Mothers' views on longer storage of neonatal dried blood spots for specific secondary uses. *Public Health Genom.* **2016**, *19*, 25–33. [CrossRef] [PubMed]

12. Tarini, B.A.; Goldenberg, A.; Singer, D.; Clark, S.; Butchart, A.; Davis, M. Not without my permission: Parents' willingness to permit use of newborn screening samples for research. *Public Health Genom.* **2010**, *13*, 125–130. [CrossRef] [PubMed]
13. Botkin, J.R.; Rothwell, E.; Anderson, R.; Stark, L.; Goldenberg, A.; Lewis, M.; Burbank, M.; Wong, B. Public attitudes regarding the use of residual newborn screening specimens for research. *Pediatrics* **2012**, *129*, 231. [CrossRef] [PubMed]
14. Rothwell, E.; Anderson, R.; Goldenberg, A.; Lewis, M.H.; Stark, L.; Burbank, M.; Wong, B.; Botkin, J.R. Assessing public attitudes on the retention and use of residual newborn screening blood samples: A focus group study. *Soc. Sci. Med.* **2012**, *74*, 1305–1309. [CrossRef] [PubMed]
15. Hendrix, K.S.; Meslin, E.M.; Carroll, A.E.; Downs, S.M. Attitudes about the use of newborn dried blood spots for research: A survey of underrepresented parents. *Acad. Pediatr.* **2013**, *13*, 451–457. [CrossRef] [PubMed]
16. Hui, L.L.; Nelson, E.A.S.; Deng, H.B.; Leung, T.Y.; Ho, C.H.; Chong, J.S.; Fung, G.P.; Hui, J.; Lam, H.S. The view of Hong Kong parents on secondary use of dried blood spots in newborn screening program. *BMC Med. Ethics* **2022**, *23*, 105. [CrossRef] [PubMed]
17. Rothwell, E.W.; Anderson, R.A.; Burbank, M.J.; Goldenberg, A.J.; Lewis, M.H.; Stark, L.A.; Wong, B.; Botkin, J.R. Concerns of newborn blood screening advisory committee members regarding storage and use of residual newborn screening blood spots. *Am. J. Public Health* **2011**, *101*, 2111–2116. [CrossRef] [PubMed]
18. Benkendorf, J.; Goodspeed, T.; Watson, M.S. Newborn screening residual dried blood spot use for newborn screening quality improvement. *Genet. Med.* **2010**, *12*, S269–S272. [CrossRef]
19. Ngan, O.M.Y.; Li, C.K. Ethical Issues of Dried Blood Spot Storage and Its Secondary Use after Newborn Screening Programme in Hong Kong. *Hong Kong J. Paediatr.* **2020**, *25*, 8–15.
20. Chace, D.H.; Kalas, T.A.; Naylor, E.W. Use of tandem mass spectrometry for multianalyte screening of dried blood specimens from newborns. *Clin. Chem.* **2003**, *49*, 1797–1817. [PubMed]
21. Tluczek, A.; McKechnie, A.C.; Lynam, A. When the cystic fibrosis label does not fit: A modified uncertainty theory. *Qual. Health Res.* **2010**, *20*, 209–223. [CrossRef] [PubMed]
22. Pruniski, B.; Lisi, E.; Ali, N. Newborn screening for Pompe disease: Impact on families. *J. Inherit. Metab. Dis.* **2018**, *41*, 1189–1203. [CrossRef]
23. Hong Kong SAR Government, Census and Statistics Department. Population Estimates. Available online: https://www.censtatd.gov.hk/en/scode459.html (accessed on 2 May 2023).
24. Population and Household Statistics Analysed by District Council District 2022 Edition. Available online: https://www.censtatd.gov.hk/en/wbr.html?ecode=B11303012022AN22&scode=500 (accessed on 2 May 2023).
25. How the Process Works. Available online: https://www.nsu.govt.nz/pregnancy-newborn-screening/newborn-metabolic-screening-programme-heel-prick-test/how-process-works (accessed on 2 May 2023).
26. Newborn Screening Materials and Resources: Education Materials and Forms. Available online: https://www.health.state.mn.us/people/newbornscreening/materials/education.html (accessed on 2 May 2023).
27. Blood Spots and Test Results: Retention Practices. Available online: https://www.health.state.mn.us/people/newbornscreening/program/retention.html (accessed on 2 May 2023).
28. Newborn Bloodspot Screening. Available online: https://www.health.vic.gov.au/sites/default/files/2021-12/newborn-screening-policy-and-guidelines.pdf (accessed on 2 May 2023).
29. Nørgaard-Pedersen, B.; Hougaard, D.M. Storage policies and use of the Danish Newborn Screening Biobank. *J. Inherit. Metab. Dis.* **2007**, *30*, 530–536. [CrossRef] [PubMed]
30. Newborn Blood Spot Cards Explained. Available online: https://www.nhs.uk/conditions/baby/newborn-screening/blood-spot-cards-explained/ (accessed on 2 May 2023).
31. Davey, A.; French, D.; Dawkins, H.; O'Leary, P. New mothers' awareness of newborn screening, and their attitudes to the retention and use of screening samples for research purposes. *Genom. Soc. Policy* **2005**, *1*, 41. [CrossRef]
32. Fujii, C.; Sato, Y.; Harada, S.; Kakee, N.; Gu, Y.-H.; Kato, T.; Shintaku, H.; Owada, M.; Hirahara, F.; Umehashi, H.; et al. Attitude to extended use and long-term storage of newborn screening blood spots in Japan. *Pediatr. Int.* **2010**, *52*, 393–397. [CrossRef] [PubMed]
33. Ceyhan-Birsoy, O.; Murry, J.B.; Machini, K.; Lebo, M.S.; Yu, T.W.; Fayer, S.; Genetti, C.A.; Schwartz, T.S.; Agrawal, P.B.; Parad, R.B.; et al. Interpretation of genomic sequencing results in healthy and ill newborns: Results from the BabySeq Project. *Am. J. Hum. Genet.* **2019**, *104*, 76–93. [CrossRef] [PubMed]
34. Roman, T.S.; Crowley, S.B.; Roche, M.I.; Foreman, A.K.M.; O'daniel, J.M.; Seifert, B.A.; Lee, K.; Brandt, A.; Gustafson, C.; DeCristo, D.M.; et al. Genomic sequencing for newborn screening: Results of the NC NEXUS project. *Am. J. Hum. Genet.* **2020**, *107*, 596–611. [PubMed]
35. Van Campen, J.C.; Sollars, E.S.A.; Thomas, R.C.; Bartlett, C.M.; Milano, A.; Parker, M.D.; Dawe, J.; Winship, P.R.; Peck, G.; Grafham, D.; et al. Next generation sequencing in newborn screening in the United Kingdom National Health Service. *Int. J. Neonatal Screen.* **2019**, *5*, 40. [CrossRef]
36. Huang, X.; Wu, D.; Zhu, L.; Wang, W.; Yang, R.; Yang, J.; He, Q.; Zhu, B.; You, Y.; Xiao, R.; et al. Application of a next-generation sequencing (NGS) panel in newborn screening efficiently identifies inborn disorders of neonates. *Orphanet J. Rare Dis.* **2022**, *17*, 66. [CrossRef]

37. Veldman, A.; Kiewiet, M.B.G.; Heiner-Fokkema, M.R.; Nelen, M.R.; Sinke, R.J.; Sikkema-Raddatz, B.; Voorhoeve, E.; Westra, D.; Dollé, M.E.T.; Schielen, P.C.J.I.; et al. Towards next-generation sequencing (NGS)-based newborn screening: A technical study to prepare for the challenges ahead. *Int. J. Neonatal Screen.* **2022**, *8*, 17. [CrossRef]
38. Kingsmore, S.F.; Smith, L.D.; Kunard, C.M.; Bainbridge, M.; Batalov, S.; Benson, W.; Blincow, E.; Caylor, S.; Chambers, C.; Del Angel, G.; et al. A genome sequencing system for universal newborn screening, diagnosis, and precision medicine for severe genetic diseases. *Am. J. Hum. Genet.* **2022**, *109*, 1605–1619. [CrossRef] [PubMed]
39. Goldenberg, A.J.; Dodson, D.S.; Davis, M.M.; Tarini, B.A. Parents' interest in whole-genome sequencing of newborns. *Genet. Med.* **2014**, *16*, 78–84. [CrossRef] [PubMed]
40. Lewis, M.A.; Stine, A.; Paquin, R.S.; Mansfield, C.; Wood, D.; Rini, C.; Roche, M.I.; Powell, C.M.; Berg, J.S.; Bailey, D.B. Parental preferences toward genomic sequencing for non-medically actionable conditions in children: A discrete-choice experiment. *Genet. Med.* **2018**, *20*, 181–189. [CrossRef] [PubMed]

International Journal of
Neonatal Screening

Article

Australian Public Perspectives on Genomic Newborn Screening: Risks, Benefits, and Preferences for Implementation

Fiona Lynch [1,2], Stephanie Best [3,4,5], Clara Gaff [6,7,8], Lilian Downie [6,8,9], Alison D. Archibald [6,8,9], Christopher Gyngell [1,8], Ilias Goranitis [4,10], Riccarda Peters [10], Julian Savulescu [1,2,11], Sebastian Lunke [9,12], Zornitza Stark [4,8,9] and Danya F. Vears [1,2,8,13,*]

1 Biomedical Ethics Research Group, Murdoch Children's Research Institute, Parkville, VIC 3052, Australia; fiona.lynch@mcri.edu.au (F.L.); christopher.gyngell@mcri.edu.au (C.G.); jsavules@nus.edu.sg (J.S.)
2 Melbourne Law School, The University of Melbourne, Melbourne, VIC 3052, Australia
3 Sir Peter MacCallum Cancer Centre Department of Oncology, University of Melbourne, Melbourne, VIC 3052, Australia; stephanie.best@petermac.org
4 Australian Genomics, Melbourne, VIC 3052, Australia; ilias.goranitis@unimelb.edu.au (I.G.); zornitza.stark@vcgs.org.au (Z.S.)
5 Department of Health Services Research, Peter MacCallum Cancer Centre, Melbourne, VIC 3052, Australia
6 Murdoch Children's Research Institute, Parkville, VIC 3052, Australia; clara.gaff@melbournegenomics.org.au (C.G.); lilian.downie@vcgs.org.au (L.D.); alison.archibald@vcgs.org.au (A.D.A.)
7 Melbourne Genomics, Melbourne, VIC 3052, Australia
8 Department of Paediatrics, Faculty of Medicine, Dentistry and Health Sciences, The University of Melbourne, Melbourne, VIC 3052, Australia
9 Victorian Clinical Genetics Services, Murdoch Children's Research Institute, Parkville, VIC 3052, Australia; sebastian.lunke@vcgs.org.au
10 Melbourne School of Population and Global Health, The University of Melbourne, Melbourne, VIC 3052, Australia; riccarda.peters@unimelb.edu.au
11 Centre for Biomedical Ethics, Yong Loo Lin School of Medicine, National University of Singapore, Singapore 117597, Singapore
12 Department of Pathology, The University of Melbourne, Melbourne, VIC 3052, Australia
13 Centre for Biomedical Ethics and Law, Department of Public Health and Primary Care, KU Leuven, 3000 Leuven, Belgium
* Correspondence: danya.vears@mcri.edu.au

Abstract: Recent dramatic reductions in the timeframe in which genomic sequencing can deliver results means its application in time-sensitive screening programs such as newborn screening (NBS) is becoming a reality. As genomic NBS (gNBS) programs are developed around the world, there is an increasing need to address the ethical and social issues that such initiatives raise. This study therefore aimed to explore the Australian public's perspectives and values regarding key gNBS characteristics and preferences for service delivery. We recruited English-speaking members of the Australian public over 18 years of age via social media; 75 people aged 23–72 participated in 1 of 15 focus groups. Participants were generally supportive of introducing genomic sequencing into newborn screening, with several stating that the adoption of such revolutionary and beneficial technology was a moral obligation. Participants consistently highlighted receiving an early diagnosis as the leading benefit, which was frequently linked to the potential for early treatment and intervention, or access to other forms of assistance, such as peer support. Informing parents about the test during pregnancy was considered important. This study provides insights into the Australian public's views and preferences to inform the delivery of a gNBS program in the Australian context.

Keywords: newborn screening; bioethics; genomic sequencing; qualitative; public views

1. Introduction

Newborn bloodspot screening (NBS) is a highly successful population screening initiative in many parts of the world [1]. Developed by Robert Guthrie in the 1960s, the first

NBS test used a blood sample collected from a heel prick onto filter paper (now known as the Guthrie card) to test for phenylketonuria [2]. While some conditions (such as congenital hypothyroidism and cystic fibrosis) were added in the 1970s and 80s [3], the 1990s saw an expansion of the number of conditions included in NBS panels with the introduction of tandem mass spectrometry technology [4]. Today, NBS programs around the world are highly successful, operating in many countries at relatively low cost with near-universal uptake [5]. The level and detail of informed consent required for traditional NBS varies by jurisdiction; in many countries, consent for traditional NBS is implied [6], yet overall, population trust and uptake remain high [7].

Standard NBS (stdNBS) acts as a screening test, meaning subsequent diagnostic testing is usually required to confirm a diagnosis [7]. In some cases, the diagnostic testing is genetic in nature; such NBS programs typically follow a protocol of first-tier biochemical testing (commonly tandem mass spectrometry), followed by genetic or genomic sequencing as a second-tier confirmatory/diagnostic test as appropriate, such as for cystic fibrosis [5,8,9]. However, some countries are either considering or beginning to include genetic testing as part of the first-line testing in NBS for conditions, such as spinal muscular atrophy [10,11].

Recent dramatic reductions in the timeframes in which genomic sequencing can deliver results, as well as the price, mean its application in time-sensitive screening programs such as NBS is becoming a reality [7]. Genomic newborn screening (gNBS) provides a single assay for the testing of many genetic conditions that would benefit from detection in infancy, but which do not have biochemical markers measurable by traditional NBS methodologies [12].

gNBS has sparked considerable discussion in the literature. Expert ethicists and clinicians in the field have suggested that we may not yet be ready for the implementation of gNBS [7,13] and position statements from leading bodies worldwide also urge caution at this time [14–18]. Yet, inclusion of genomic sequencing in NBS programs is not only inevitable [19,20], but already occurring [21]. Jurisdictions including the US (through the Guardian study, BabySeq, BeginNGS, and Early Check), England (Generation Study), Belgium (Baby Detect), France (PERIGENOMED), the EU (Screen4Care), and Australia (BabyScreen+) are all piloting gNBS programs as part of research studies [22,23].

To date, the inclusion of conditions in NBS programs has been based on the goal of identifying newborns with serious conditions who are likely to benefit from treatment early in life [22,24]. Yet with gNBS, the potential to screen for more conditions means that these parameters are being questioned [25–27].

Some work has been conducted using a variety of methodologies exploring parents' and the public's preferences and perspectives on gNBS in the US [20,28–41], Canada [42–44], the UK [45,46] and New Zealand [47]. Surveys have been conducted with Australian parents exploring their views [48,49]; however, to date, no in-depth qualitative work has been conducted with members of the Australian public.

As gNBS programs are developed around the world, there is an increasing need to address the ethical and social issues that such initiatives raise [22]. This study therefore aimed to explore the Australian public's perspectives and values regarding key gNBS characteristics and preferences for gNBS service delivery.

2. Materials and Methods

We recruited English-speaking members of the Australian public over 18 years of age. Advertisements were distributed via social media posts on Facebook. Individuals who were interested in participating were directed to a website where they could register their interest and provide contact details. FL then telephoned potential participants to ask a series of screening questions to confirm eligibility and maximise diversity in focus group participation (e.g., diversity of age, gender, parental status, and geographical distribution). Screened individuals were sent further information about the study via email, invited to sign an online consent form, and provide their availabilities if they wished to participate.

Participants were provided with a AUD 75 voucher as remuneration for their time at focus group completion.

Sampling aimed for heterogeneity in participant characteristics, including age; gender; location (by state and metropolitan/rural location); parental status; and country of birth and language spoken at home (as measures of cultural and linguistic diversity). Recruitment continued until sufficient heterogeneity was achieved and until minimal new data were generated addressing the study aims.

Prior to the focus groups, participants were asked to watch a 3 min video [50] to provide them with background information about the topics that would be discussed. The video included information about what DNA and genomic sequencing are, and how genomic sequencing can lead to disease detection. It also outlined what stdNBS in Australia involves and briefly introduced the idea of using genomics in NBS. Focus groups explored participants' preferences and values regarding key gNBS characteristics and preferences for gNBS service delivery. The degree to which concepts such as the uncertainty and sensitivity of gNBS, targeted versus broader testing approaches, and the potential test outcomes were covered varied between focus groups depending on the discussion. The focus group guide is included as Supplementary Material.

Focus groups were facilitated by DV with support from FL and conducted via Zoom. Both DV and FL are skilled qualitative researchers with experience in focus group methodology and training in genetic counselling. None of the participants were known to the researchers.

Focus groups were recorded using the Zoom recording function and transcribed by FL. Interview transcripts were analysed by using inductive context analysis, whereby content categories are generated from the data, rather than predetermined [51]. Coding continued iteratively until all data relevant to the research question had been coded into categories and subcategories. Findings were discussed by DV and FL to ensure rigour. Data analysis was managed using NVivo (released March 2023) [52].

This study was reviewed and approved by The Royal Children's Hospital Human Research Ethics Committee (HREC ID: 91392). Participants provided voluntary, informed consent.

3. Results

3.1. Participant Demographics

We had 643 people express interest in the study and managed to contact and confirm eligibility in 155 of them. No potential participants were excluded.

Seventy-five members of the Australian public aged 23–72 participated in 1 of 15 focus groups (range 2–8 per group). The participant characteristics are summarised in Table 1. We had representation from 7/8 states/territories across Australia. Thirteen participants self-reported they were medical or allied health professionals. Seventeen participants disclosed they had a child with a genetic condition. Eleven participants were on parental leave at the time of the focus group.

Table 1. Participant characteristics.

	n (%)
Age	
Mean	42
Range	23–72
Metro/rural	
Metro	61 (81%)
Regional/rural	14 (19%)

Table 1. *Cont.*

	n (%)
Children	
Y	62 (83%)
N	13 (17%)
Country of birth	
Australia	61 (81%)
Other	14 (19%)
Language spoken at home	
English only	60 (80%)
Language other than English	15 (20%)
Gender	
Female	66 (88%)
Male	9 (12%)
TOTAL	75

3.2. General Support for gNBS

Below, we present quantitative and qualitative data. Participants were polled at the beginning and end of each focus group to both facilitate discussion, and gauge if perspectives on gNBS changed over the course of the discussion. Quotes are used to illustrate our qualitative findings. An ellipsis (…) reflects where a significant portion of speech has been removed, and square brackets represent where a word has been replaced for clarity or to protect participant anonymity. Quotes are deidentified to protect participant anonymity; codes are used to identify participants based on their focus group number (e.g., FG1 P1 refers to focus group 1, participant 1).

All focus groups were asked whether they thought genomics should be used in newborn screening programs. Prior to the discussion, the majority (77%) of participants thought that genomics should be used, with 23% stating they were unsure. Following the focus group, the same number of participants thought that genomics should be used, however, in contrast to the beginning of the session, a proportion (7%) thought it should not be used.

Half of the focus groups were asked whether a NBS program that includes genomics should be run any differently to stNBS programs. Just under half (46%) of the participants expressed the view that a gNBS program should be run differently to a stdNBS program prior to the discussion. After the discussion, most (74%) thought it should be run differently.

The results of the polls are shown in Table 2.

Table 2. Results of the poll.

		Pre-Discussion *n* (%)	**Post-Discussion** *n* (%)
Do you think genomics should be used in newborn screening programs?	Yes	58 (77%)	57 (77%)
	No	0	5 (7%)
	Not sure	17 (23%)	12 (16%)
	TOTAL	75	74
Should a newborn screening program that includes genomics be run any differently to standard newborn screening programs?	Yes	18 (46%)	29 (74%)
	No	9 (23%)	8 (21%)
	Not sure	12 (31%)	2 (5%)
	TOTAL	39	39

Qualitative data showed that participants were generally supportive of introducing genomic sequencing into newborn screening, with several stating that the adoption of such revolutionary and beneficial technology was a moral obligation.

> *"Personally, I think if the technology is there for us to screen and find anomalies of whatever sort early, I think we should use it." [FG3 P1]*

3.3. Perceived Benefits of gNBS

Participants consistently highlighted receiving an early diagnosis as the leading benefit of implementing gNBS (Table 3, Quote 1). This was frequently linked to the potential for early treatment and intervention, or to access other forms of assistance, such as peer support (Table 3, Quote 2).

Table 3. Benefits of gNBS.

Perceived Benefit	Illustrative Quote(s)
Benefits of early diagnosis	*Quote 1: "I think the other thing I'm really conscious of is that there will be medical and pharmaceutical interventions and therapeutic interventions in relation to some genetic conditions which, if undertaken at the earliest opportunity, will have more positive implications for children and their families in the long term." [FG1 P8]* *Quote 2: "And also, getting support from other families. . .A lot of groups are on Facebook and things like that these days. . .you can hear how other people have gone through it and how they've survived it and all those sorts of things, or how they're coping with it and what they're using to cope with it and those sorts of things." [FG9 P3]* *Quote 3: ". . .you can go through years of testing and hospitalisation trying to find an answer to a question about what's going on with your child, and that would certainly make it easier if that could be available early on." [FG3 P1]* *Quote 4: "I also imagine that for families that have to care for a loved one in this space, if they know ahead of time that there's going to be a financial burden on them, it allows them to plan a little bit better if they know earlier." [FG4 P6]* *Quote 5: "I kind of think knowledge is power regardless of what it is. Like you might not be able to alter things medically or like get the right treatment, whether or not it's like the right kind of changes to make for your family, whether you're a working mum and you decide to stop working or you've got other children that you need to care for and you might need some extra care. Might not necessarily be able to like make a decision medically about how to help your child, but how to help your own lifestyle and your own family. I think there's other kinds of decisions that you can make around like news." [FG15 P3]*
Research and knowledge benefits	*Quote 6:"I think it's important because it gives an indication of actually how prevalent it is and that can help drive the funding and the research into it. If it's not necessarily monitored then we don't know just how rare it is. . ." [FG8 P5]* *Quote 7: "I'd like to think that the data could be used for more research but also for governments to plan and services to plan and if there's going to show that there's going to be more of particular disorders or illnesses, then that can be planned for future sort of care or services. . .For that individual child but for a population as well." [FG12 P3]*
Benefits for reproductive planning and the broader family	*Quote 8: ". . .it would be good if they were aware of it for future children. Because some people have children very close together. . .And I've seen many cases where people end up with three children with the same genetic condition, because they had three children in four years or five years, before any symptoms were recognised." [FG5 P4]* *Quote 9: "I think there are other implications for families in terms of your broader family, if you find things out that are inherited. . ." [FG1 P1]*

Participants also reflected on either their own or friends/families' experiences of the diagnostic odyssey, suggesting that receiving an earlier diagnosis would reduce the stress associated with lengthy diagnoses (Table 3, Quote 3).

Furthermore, participants foresaw that receiving an early diagnosis would allow parents more time to prepare, both emotionally and practically (Table 3, Quotes 4 and 5).

Participants highlighted the potential benefits of gNBS to research and the ability to increase knowledge about rare genetic conditions (Table 3, Quote 6). They mentioned that an improved understanding of genetic conditions would lead to better resource allocation, such as government funding, to support patients and families with these conditions (Table 3, Quote 7).

Benefits of gNBS for other family members were also raised by participants. This included the ability to inform parents, siblings, and extended family members that there was a genetic condition within the family and explain how this knowledge could be used in pregnancy planning (Table 3, Quotes 8 and 9).

3.4. Potential Challenges with gNBS

Participants were concerned about the potential psychological impact that a diagnosis from gNBS could have on parents of newborns. They reflected that having a newborn was already a stressful time for new parents and were concerned about the added stress that an early genetic diagnosis might have on the family (Table 4, Quote 1). This was particularly the case for uncertain gNBS results and untreatable conditions (Table 4, Quote 2).

Table 4. Potential challenges with gNBS.

Potential Challenges	Illustrative Quote(s)
Possible impact of gNBS on parents	*Quote 1: "When you're handed a baby it's so overwhelming, there's so many new things already. I think adding another one then could just be overwhelming." [FG4 P5]* *Quote 2: "...unless it's completely accurate and we know what's really likely to happen, it's that, the alarm factor and who wants to be unnecessarily alarmed or feel unnecessarily alarmed if the accuracy of the initial testing is not as great as it should be?" [FG9 P1]* *Quote 3: "...but if the parent has a condition that can be pretty asymptomatic, what effect is that going to have on the parent if they find out they do have this condition even if they have had no complications of this condition prior and then they have a child with this condition and are very severely affected?...Would there be some like guilt there?" [FG2 P1]* *Quote 4: "...I'm just concerned that people who are presented with these situations very early on, is that going to affect their emotional attachment and bonding with their child?" [FG7 P2]*
Data security, privacy, discrimination and insurance concerns	*Quote 5: "...how's the information going to be stored, like particularly in this digital world around cyber and security and all that stuff. How long will it be stored? Who's got access to it and who could have access to it down the track?" [FG8 P3]* *Quote 6: "...if a child comes back saying that they have a higher chance of getting something, is that then going to affect their private health insurance? It'll now either cost them more or they won't be able to get covered for that?" [FG12 P5]*

In addition to psychological impact, participants recognised that a diagnosis in a child might also have clinical implications for the parents as asymptomatic or mildly affected carriers of the condition (Table 4, Quote 3).

Relatedly, some participants discussed the potential negative impact of a diagnosis from gNBS on parent–child bonding (Table 4, Quote 4).

Participants expressed concern for the security of their and their child's genomic data following gNBS (Table 4, Quote 5). They were particularly concerned about how the data might be used to discriminate against individuals in terms of insurance and employment later in life (Table 4, Quote 6). Because of this, they expressed that there should be strict regulations and processes for how genomic data are stored, shared, and accessed.

3.5. When to Discuss and Obtain Consent for gNBS

Most participants agreed that the availability of gNBS should be raised and discussed during pregnancy, rather than at, or soon after, the birth of the child (Table 5, Quote 1). Participants noted that birth and the immediate newborn period was a busy and stressful time for parents, and that this was therefore not an ideal time to be discussing something as complex at gNBS.

Table 5. When, who and what: Discussing and consent for gNBS.

	Illustrative Quote(s)
gNBS should be discussed during pregnancy	*Quote 1: "I feel when it comes time for the heel prick test, it's just like, "Do you want to get the heel prick test done?" and you go, "Yeah, sure," and your baby's 48 h old, and you've just given birth and you're a bit sleep deprived, and there's not that considered decision making. So I think the earlier the information can be given, and time for consideration and research, the better." [FG11 P3]* *Quote 2: "...maybe a public campaign about screening for particular conditions...not just people having babies, but educating the community about why this would be really important." [FG13 P6]* *Quote 3: "...perhaps education packages for people who are trying to become pregnant as well, so they've got more of a chance to learn more about it..." [FG1 P4]* *Quote 4: "I kind of wonder whether that first appointment where women have just found out they're pregnant or they're planning to become pregnant, I wonder whether that would that be a good point where you are not necessarily, have any brochures yet. I mean obviously you get to the point in pregnancy where you are just getting so much information..." [FG1 P2]* *Quote 5: "I would prefer this sort of information to be disseminated and discussed probably in the third trimester of pregnancy...because it stays relevant. If it was maybe discussed any earlier it might sort of get lost in amongst other things that are happening during pregnancy..." [FG6 P3]* *Quote 6: "...the education just can't depend on one person. It needs to be multiple people that you trust." [FG13 P3]*
Consent for gNBS should be obtained during pregnancy	*Quote 7: "I don't think it would be fair to put it onto someone who's just given birth, whether we go ahead and test. So you need time. You need time to think and make a choice, an informed choice." [FG14 P5]* *Quote 8: "I think you can maybe do an early consent and then re-confirm at collection because they may change their mind and decide they would want to do it when they said they didn't want to do it or something." [FG7 P1]*
Who should discuss gNBS	*Quote 9: "...in terms of who this information I suppose is given, or who gives this information, I would say it would be best coming from an obstetrician or maybe a midwife if that's...who's looking after the pregnancy. Maybe GPs..." [FG6 P3]* *Quote 10: "Maybe GPs, again depending on their knowledge and that sort of thing, they're probably not the most appropriate person to be making this sort of I suppose recommendations. Maybe they can make the parents or the parent aware that this is available, but in terms of going into it further, they're general practitioners, they're not specialised." [FG6 P3]* *Quote 11: "Midwife is a good option, but again, it would all depend on how much knowledge she has and how much she can share, and also the workload that she has. So that could be one of the drawbacks." [FG13 P3]* *Quote 12: "...in an ideal world, it would be someone that had, like a genetic counsellor or someone with that type of background. But obviously that is probably more costly..." [FG1 P1]* *Quote 13: "I don't think it really matters who does it, as long as it's somebody that's well educated and experienced in providing education to parents." [FG7 P2]*
What parents need to know about gNBS	*Quote 14: "I think as much information as possible should be given to parents. It might be overwhelming but you would rather tell them than not tell them..." [FG6 P3]* *Quote 15: "...many people learn in many different ways, and that it won't be a one size fits all...You have language barriers, cultural barriers, so it needs to be inclusive, you need to consult with community groups and present information in different ways if it's going to be effective." [FG3 P1]* *Quote 16: "...talking about what conditions are covered but what are the ones that possibly aren't covered. There's obviously thousands and thousands...you obviously can't financially and logistically maybe test for all of those conditions. But there are, obviously, still letting people know there are conditions out there that we're not able to test for at this point of time too... I think just letting them know it's not a be-all, end-all, we're not testing everything." [FG4 P1]* *Quote 17: "...just some idea of the process that the testing will take place...if everything's okay you won't hear, or you will hear that everything's okay. If anything comes up, you'll be put in touch with a genetic counsellor, just some idea of what to expect in the next weeks after the testing." [FG3 P1]* *Quote 18: "...how's the information going to be stored...How long will it be stored? Who's got access to it and who could have access to it down the track?" [FG8 P3]* *Quote 19: "I think written information is only as good as how capable the person that's reading it is able to read, so yeah, a couple of different mediums would be good, and the ability to ask questions rather than just being, you know, just online, having a face-to-face conversation with someone and being able to ask questions that are pertinent to the parent." [FG7 P2]*

The exact timepoint at which gNBS should be discussed with soon-to-be parents raised many differing opinions. Some participants thought that gNBS should be discussed as early as possible, with some even suggesting implementing public education campaigns or raising it with couples trying to conceive (Table 5, Quotes 2 and 3).

However, others commented that various stages of pregnancy—from the first confirmation of pregnancy appointment to sometime in the third trimester—were appropriate times to have the conversation (Table 5, Quotes 4 and 5).

Some suggested that gNBS should be raised and discussed multiple times and potentially by multiple specialists to allow parents to fully understand the screening process (Table 5, Quote 6).

For similar reasons, many participants articulated that formal consent should also be obtained prior to birth (Table 5, Quote 7).

Some participants raised the concept of implementing two stages of consent, whereby parents provided formal, written consent prior to the birth, but that there was a process of 'rechecking' consent at the time of sample collection (Table 5, Quote 8).

3.6. Who Should Discuss gNBS

Participants were asked who they thought gNBS should be discussed by. Many suggested members of the existing prenatal care team, including the general practitioner (GP), obstetrician, midwife, hospital staff, or maternal and child health nurse (Table 5, Quotes 9, 10 and 11).

It was expressed that familiarity and rapport were important to have with the person discussing gNBS, and so someone that parents already have an existing relationship with would be best placed to discuss gNBS.

Some participants raised concerns that GPs were not adequately trained to discuss genomics or rare diseases with their patients.

Despite commonly proposing obstetricians or midwives as the most appropriate health professional to discuss gNBS, some participants were concerned that midwives might not have the training required to discuss gNBS in detail.

Other participants commented that discussions about gNBS required specialist expertise from someone like a genetic counsellor (Table 5, Quote 12).

Irrespective of who was responsible for discussing gNBS with parents, participants recognised that they needed to have the skills and training to provide accurate and comprehensive information, and to answer any questions that might arise (Table 5, Quote 13).

3.7. What Parents Need to Know about gNBS

Participants generally expressed that as much information as possible should be given to parents, and that discussions about gNBS should be detailed (Table 5, Quote 14).

However, others recognised that parents might be overwhelmed by receiving too much information, and instead, the detail of informed consent discussions should be tailored to the needs of each individual parent and family (Table 5, Quote 15).

There were also specific aspects of the screening test that participants thought parents should be made aware of. These included things such as which conditions were being tested for and which were not (Table 5, Quote 16).

With regard to processes, participants explained that parents needed to be made aware of what happens after gNBS, either in the case of a negative or positive result. This included an explanation of the timeframe, including when to expect to hear from a health professional regarding the child's result (Table 5, Quote 17).

Participants agreed that parents should know what would happen to their child's data, including where it would be stored, for how long, and who would have access to it (Table 5, Quote 18).

Participants wanted other resources to support parents in understanding and making a decision about gNBS for their child. As well as sufficient opportunities to ask questions of their health professional, participants suggested pamphlets, websites, a hotline, or even a genetic counsellor as alternative sources of information about gNBS (Table 5, Quote 19).

3.8. Type of Consent

When asked what type of consent gNBS should require, participants compared this with their experiences of consent for other tests and investigations (Table 6, Quote 1).

Table 6. Type of consent.

	Illustrative Quote(s)
Comparison with consent for other relevant healthcare interventions	*Quote 1: "...like vaccinations. They're not really mandated, but they're, I suppose people make it difficult not to have them. And then there's the argument which is it can be negligent not to vaccinate your children. But the choice is still there." [FG14 P2]* *Quote 2: "...in regards to consent I think it needs to be different because there is also, in and above the child or the baby themselves, there may be ramifications for the immediate and extended family of any results that are found and how they may be communicated to other members of the family." [FG1 P4]* *Quote 3: "I don't think the consent process should be any different because at the time you're providing consent or not you would have gone through all the information about genomic testing and what it involves. So your, if you do have any questions, absolutely, feel free to ask but I think the consent process in itself shouldn't really differ from the newborn screening test as it currently is." [FG6 P3]*
Perceptions that gNBS should be mandated	*Quote 4: "...if it's going to make such massive differences to children's, baby's lives, and potentially provide life-saving treatment, then do the parents really need to consent, or is it just something that should be done? But I guess superficially, yes, I think it should be a matter of consent." [FG7 P2]* *Quote 5: "I believe an opt-out system is probably the best the best option I guess. There will be parents who have certain cultural or religious beliefs where they don't want blood taken from their child. I've worked with people who will refuse certain medical procedures for their very young children because it's their perception that it goes against their religion. And I think there is a risk if you don't respect that, you start to get the fringe people out there that start making a big fuss on social media and in the news...you need to be seen to be doing the right thing..." [FG8 P5]* *Quote 6: "I think it would go without saying that you could always revoke consent at any stage even if the test has been sent off you can revoke it while it's being processed so you don't find out the results if that was what you desire." [FG6 P2]*
Views about informed consent	*Quote 7: "I think the choice, it's a good choice, both having the choice to do or not to do. I don't think it should be mandated, if it's introduced...because it's a personal decision...I just think choice is probably a good thing." [FG14 P2]*
Perspectives on whether both parents need to consent for gNBS	*Quote 8: "I'd say explicit consent and from both parents because of the implication that a genetic condition might have for either parent and also for siblings of that child...I actually believe that both parents should give consent in all areas. And so if you can't obtain both parents' consent at that time it should be either that the sample can be taken but not tested is maybe a possibility until consent can be obtained from the other parent." [FG6 P4]* *Quote 9: "I would say if either parent gives consent maybe the testing could be done and it's, and if the results could maybe be conveyed to the parent that did give consent...So if mum wants to know about it and dad doesn't, for example, then maybe the testing could go ahead rather than not go ahead at all and only whoever gave consent in the first place is informed of those results." [FG6 P3]*

Several suggested that the choice about whether to have gNBS should be like the choice about whether to vaccinate against COVID-19. Others recognised that many things happen in hospital without explicit parental consent, and questioned whether gNBS should be any different. Yet some suggested that because most things for children did in fact require explicit consent, so should gNBS.

Reflecting specifically on their experience of stdNBS, most parents believed that consent for gNBS should be different (Table 6, Quote 2). Those that believed it should be the same assumed that existing consent processes for stdNBS were robust and in-depth (Table 6, Quote 3).

Some groups discussed whether gNBS should be mandated, whereby parents would have no choice but for their child to receive screening (Table 6, Quote 4). However, most thought that this was not appropriate, and that parents should instead be given the opportunity to opt-out (Table 6, Quote 5).

Irrespective of a parent's decision, participants thought that they should be able to withdraw their consent at any time in the process (Table 6, Quote 6).

Participants generally agreed that gNBS should require explicit and informed consent from parents prior to being administered (Table 6, Quote 7). They explained that choice was important in both protecting parents' autonomy, but also in facilitating trust in a population-based screening program.

Whether both parents needed to consent for gNBS for it to occur was a contentious issue in the focus group discussions. Some participants demonstrated strong views that both parents should be involved (Table 6, Quote 8). However, others ecognized that this was not always practical or possible, and that therefore only one parent's consent should be required (Table 6, Quote 9).

Illustrative quotes are shown in Table 6.

4. Discussion

Our findings show that, after education and discussion, the members of the Australian public we engaged with were generally supportive of including genomic sequencing in NBS. This is in line with other studies reporting positive public and parental attitudes towards, and high interest in, gNBS, such as in the US, Canada and New Zealand [22,53]. Likewise, Genomics England demonstrated wide support for implementing genomic sequencing into NBS programs in their large-scale public deliberative approach [45,54]. Surveys with parents of healthy children enrolled in a randomised clinical trial of gNBS in the US also showed general support for population-wide implementation of gNBS for every newborn [39], and several studies report that parents express hypothetical interest in receiving genomic information about their newborn [29,30]. Of note, our participants thought a gNBS program should be run differently to stdNBS, which mainly related to the consent process as we discuss further below.

4.1. There Is Support for gNBS Provided Potential Risks Can Be Addressed

Participants in our study saw many benefits of gNBS, including early diagnosis, progression of medical research, and wider family benefits. However, participants were also cognisant of several potential risks associated with gNBS, such as data security, privacy, and the potential for discrimination. Research with parents and clinicians in the US demonstrate that both groups perceive both benefits and risks associated with gNBS; one of the major risks identified is the potential for psychological distress as a result of screening [20,37]. Our participants were also worried about the potential negative psychological impact of an early genetic diagnosis on parents and on parent–child bonding. Reassuringly, recent research from the BabySeq Project shows that families experience no sustained negative psychosocial effects from gNBS [55,56]. Interestingly, previous work suggests that parents perceive greater benefits and fewer risks associated with gNBS than clinicians [20,37], implying that our concerns may not be reflected by the wider public.

The concerns for genomic data security and privacy, and potential avenues for discrimination in employment and insurance raised by our participants are similar to those identified in a survey with parents conducted in the US [20]. Because of the very nature of gNBS programs, it is difficult to predict what changes in regulation may occur throughout the lifetime of today's newborns, raising challenges for ensuring informed consent and maintaining trust in such programs. Relatedly, others have raised concerns about the potential infringement of the child's autonomy by removing the child's ability to make their own decisions about knowing their genomic information later in life [37].

4.2. Explicit Consent Should Be Required for gNBS

Although others in the literature have raised the timing of information provision and consent for gNBS as a concern [22], to our knowledge, this is the first study to gauge public opinion on the issue. Focus group participants agreed overwhelmingly that gNBS should be raised and discussed during pregnancy, probably more than once by multiple practitioners, and that at least a first stage of consent should also be implemented before birth.

Participants explained that a familiar face, that is, a member of the existing care team, would be best placed to have these discussions about gNBS with prospective parents. However, they raised concerns for the level of knowledge and skill required to have these conversations, suggesting that some professional education or training is required prior to the implementation of gNBS. Other population screening programs—such as expanded reproductive carrier screening—raise similar issues with health professional preparedness and a need for training [57]. In fact, the widespread adoption of genomic technologies across many specialty areas of medicine is generating considerable discussion about the need to upskill non-genetics health professionals to support patients [58]. Other authors have suggested that midwives in particular will play a significant role in the delivery of gNBS, and that any changes to NBS practice should therefore include multifaceted education programs aimed at such key stakeholders [59].

Participants in our study desired tailored informed consent discussions, covering as much or as little detail about gNBS as each parent required, which corresponds with a tiered and layered approach suggested by others in relation to diagnostic genomics [60]. There were, however, some key aspects that participants expressed should be communicated to all parents, including which conditions were being screened; the process following gNBS (particularly if a result suggesting a high chance for a genetic condition was identified); and what would happen to the child's data. Participants also expressed that additional resources in varied formats could be useful to communicate complex information to families.

In Australia, NBS is voluntary and free for all infants, with uptake being close to 100% [49]. For gNBS, parents are likely to require more information to ensure that consent is informed and to maintain such high trust and coverage [7]. One concern is that implementing a more detailed and potentially burdensome informed consent process into NBS would reduce participation, thereby reducing the intended benefits of the program overall [36]. Although our participants appreciated this, they maintained that explicit, informed consent should be required for gNBS (rather than, for example, implicit consent or mandated screening) to facilitate trust in the program. Surveys with parents enrolled in a randomised clinical trial of gNBS in the US also suggest that parents see informed consent as more important for gNBS than for stdNBS [39]. Reassuringly, early studies obtaining explicit informed consent do not report a reduction in the uptake of gNBS compared to stdNBS [36,48,53]. However, some have suggested that introducing gNBS initially as a separate screening test to stdNBS may mitigate some of this risk [22].

4.3. Members of the Public Hold Less Conservative Views than Health Professionals

Our data support the general trend that views of the public about gNBS are less conservative than those of health professionals, who frequently report that gNBS is not currently ready for population-wide implementation [13,49,61–63]. Previous qualitative work also shows that while Australian healthcare professionals do not feel it is currently appropriate to incorporate genomic sequencing into NBS, they believe it will be implemented in the next decade [13].

One possible reason for this discrepancy is that parents and the public do not fully appreciate the complexities and potential challenges relating to gNBS. Certainly, one potential limitation of this study is that we deliberately provided limited information about how gNBS might be implemented prior to the focus groups so as not to bias their views. Topics such as the possibility of identifying variants of uncertain significance or late onset forms of disease using gNBS could be challenging for members of the public to understand. However, our participants raised many of the issues that concern HPs, indicating they do appreciate the nuances to some degree. This may suggest that perhaps HPs are overly concerned about these issues, or indicate higher levels of genetic exceptionalism within healthcare workers than the public. However, implementation of any gNBS program should consider the desires of the general population alongside those of experts.

5. Conclusions

Genomic sequencing has the potential to drastically increase the scope of existing NBS programs. Including genomic sequencing in NBS programs could help to identify conditions that traditional biochemical screening cannot [7] and overcome some of the current limitations of biochemical screening in premature and unwell infants [22]. Furthermore, the population-wide genomic data that would be generated from gNBS would also allow for research into the diagnosis, treatment and management of genetic diseases, as well as allow early access to clinical trials for those diagnosed through gNBS [22].

Implementation of such an ambitious population-wide screening program as gNBS is being considered in several contexts around the world. However, doing so without addressing parental concerns is likely to reduce trust and subsequently uptake of the program [39]. Engaging stakeholders in potential changes to NBS programs is therefore vital in maintaining a high participation rate [49] as well as in informing the design of programs so that they are tailored to local contexts.

Supplementary Materials: The following supporting information can be downloaded at: https://www.mdpi.com/article/10.3390/ijns10010006/s1.

Author Contributions: Conceptualization: F.L., S.B., C.G. (Clara Gaff), L.D., A.D.A., C.G. (Christopher Gyngell), I.G., R.P., S.L., Z.S. and D.F.V.; Data collection: F.L. and D.F.V.; Formal analysis: F.L. and D.F.V.; Funding acquisition: S.B., C.G. (Clara Gaff), L.D., A.D.A., C.G. (Christopher Gyngell), I.G., J.S., S.L., Z.S. and D.F.V.; Methodology: F.L. and D.F.V.; Project administration: F.L., Z.S. and D.F.V.; Writing—original draft: F.L. and D.F.V.; Writing—review and editing: F.L., S.B., C.G. (Clara Gaff), L.D., A.D.A., C.G. (Christopher Gyngell), I.G., R.P., J.S., S.L., Z.S. and D.F.V. All authors have read and agreed to the published version of the manuscript.

Funding: The authors acknowledge the infrastructure funding received from the Victorian State Government through the Operational Infrastructure Support (OIS) Program. This work was funded by the Australian Government through the Medical Research Future Fund, as part of the Genomics Health Futures Mission (Grant number GHFM2015937). This research was funded in whole, or in part, by the Wellcome Trust [Grant number WT203132/Z/16/Z]. For the purpose of open access, the author has applied a CC BY public copyright license to any Author Accepted Manuscript version arising from this submission.

Institutional Review Board Statement: The study was conducted in accordance with the Declaration of Helsinki, and approved by The Royal Children's Hospital Human Research Ethics Committee (HREC ID: 91392).

Informed Consent Statement: Informed consent was obtained from all subjects involved in the study.

Data Availability Statement: The datasets generated during the current study are available from the corresponding author upon reasonable request.

Acknowledgments: The authors thank the participants for their involvement.

Conflicts of Interest: The authors declare no conflicts of interest.

References

1. Berg, J.S.; Agrawal, P.B.; Bailey, D.B.; Beggs, A.H.; Brenner, S.E.; Brower, A.M.; Cakici, J.A.; Ceyhan-Birsoy, O.; Chan, K.; Chen, F. Newborn sequencing in genomic medicine and public health. *Pediatrics* **2017**, *139*, e20162252. [CrossRef]
2. Guthrie, R.; Susi, A. A simple phenylalanine method for detecting phenylketonuria in large populations of newborn infants. *Pediatrics* **1963**, *32*, 338–343. [CrossRef] [PubMed]
3. Department of Health and Aged Care. About Newborn Bloodspot Screening. Available online: https://www.health.gov.au/our-work/newborn-bloodspot-screening/about (accessed on 4 September 2023).
4. Sweetman, L. Newborn screening by tandem mass spectrometry (MS-MS). *Clin. Chem.* **1996**, *42*, 345–346. [CrossRef]
5. Therrell, B.L.; Padilla, C.D.; Loeber, J.G.; Kneisser, I.; Saadallah, A.; Borrajo, G.J.; Adams, J. Current status of newborn screening worldwide: 2015. *Semin. Perinatol.* **2015**, *39*, 171–187. [CrossRef]
6. Hanley, W.B. Newborn screening in Canada–Are we out of step? *Paediatr. Child Health* **2005**, *10*, 203–207. [CrossRef]
7. Vears, D.F.; Savulescu, J.; Christodoulou, J.; Wall, M.; Newson, A.J. Are We Ready for Whole Population Genomic Sequencing of Asymptomatic Newborns? *Pharmacogenomics Pers. Med.* **2023**, *16*, 681–691. [CrossRef] [PubMed]

8. Smon, A.; Repic Lampret, B.; Groselj, U.; Zerjav Tansek, M.; Kovac, J.; Perko, D.; Bertok, S.; Battelino, T.; Trebusak Podkrajsek, K. Next generation sequencing as a follow-up test in an expanded newborn screening programme. *Clin. Biochem.* **2018**, *52*, 48–55. [CrossRef]
9. Wang, H.; Yang, Y.; Zhou, L.; Wang, Y.; Long, W.; Yu, B. NeoSeq: A new method of genomic sequencing for newborn screening. *Orphanet J. Rare Dis.* **2021**, *16*, 481. [CrossRef] [PubMed]
10. Kariyawasam, D.S.; D'Silva, A.M.; Sampaio, H.; Briggs, N.; Herbert, K.; Wiley, V.; Farrar, M.A. Newborn screening for spinal muscular atrophy in Australia: A non-randomised cohort study. *Lancet Child Adolesc. Health* **2023**, *7*, 159–170. [CrossRef]
11. Müller-Felber, W.; Blaschek, A.; Schwartz, O.; Gläser, D.; Nennstiel, U.; Brockow, I.; Wirth, B.; Burggraf, S.; Röschinger, W.; Becker, M. Newbornscreening SMA–From Pilot Project to Nationwide Screening in Germany. *J. Neuromuscul. Dis.* **2023**, *10*, 55–65. [CrossRef] [PubMed]
12. Kingsmore, S.F.; BeginNGS Consortium. Dispatches from Biotech beginning BeginNGS: Rapid newborn genome sequencing to end the diagnostic and therapeutic odyssey. *Am. J. Med. Genet. Part C Semin. Med. Genet.* **2022**, *190*, 243–256. [CrossRef] [PubMed]
13. Cao, M.; Notini, L.; Ayres, S.; Vears, D.F. Australian healthcare professionals' perspectives on the ethical and practical issues associated with genomic newborn screening. *J. Genet. Couns.* **2023**, *32*, 376–386. [CrossRef]
14. Friedman, J.M.; Cornel, M.C.; Goldenberg, A.J.; Lister, K.J.; Sénécal, K.; Vears, D.F.; Friedman, J.M.; Cornel, M.C.; Al-Thihli, K.; Borry, P.; et al. Genomic newborn screening: Public health policy considerations and recommendations. *BMC Med. Genom.* **2017**, *10*, 9. [CrossRef]
15. Howard, H.C.; Knoppers, B.M.; Cornel, M.C.; Clayton, E.W.; Sénécal, K.; Borry, P. Whole-genome sequencing in newborn screening? A statement on the continued importance of targeted approaches in newborn screening programmes. *Eur. J. Hum. Genet.* **2015**, *23*, 1593–1600. [CrossRef] [PubMed]
16. Cornel, M.C. New recommendations for the Dutch neonatal screening programme. A report from the Health Council of the Netherlands. *Ned. Tijdschr. Voor Geneeskd.* **2015**, *159*, A9115.
17. ACMG Board of Directors. Points to consider in the clinical application of genomic sequencing. *Genet. Med. Off. J. Am. Coll. Med. Genet.* **2012**, *14*, 759–761.
18. Borghesi, A.; Mencarelli, M.A.; Memo, L.; Ferrero, G.B.; Bartuli, A.; Genuardi, M.; Stronati, M.; Villani, A.; Renieri, A.; Corsello, G.; et al. Intersociety policy statement on the use of whole-exome sequencing in the critically ill newborn infant. *Ital. J. Pediatr.* **2017**, *43*, 100. [CrossRef]
19. Tarini, B.A.; Goldenberg, A.J. Ethical issues with newborn screening in the genomics era. *Annu. Rev. Genom. Hum. Genet.* **2012**, *13*, 381–393. [CrossRef] [PubMed]
20. Pereira, S.; Robinson, J.O.; Gutierrez, A.M.; Petersen, D.K.; Hsu, R.L.; Lee, C.H.; Schwartz, T.S.; Holm, I.A.; Beggs, A.H.; Green, R.C. Perceived benefits, risks, and utility of newborn genomic sequencing in the BabySeq Project. *Pediatrics* **2019**, *143*, S6–S13. [CrossRef] [PubMed]
21. Hussain, Z. Over£ 175m investment in genomic research aims to detect more genetic disorders at birth. *BMJ* **2022**, *379*, o2996. [CrossRef] [PubMed]
22. Stark, Z.; Scott, R.H. Genomic newborn screening for rare diseases. *Nat. Rev. Genet.* **2023**, *24*, 755–766. [CrossRef]
23. Pichini, A.; Ahmed, A.; Patch, C.; Bick, D.; Leblond, M.; Kasperaviciute, D.; Deen, D.; Wilde, S.; Garcia Noriega, S.; Matoko, C.; et al. Developing a National Newborn Genomes Program: An Approach Driven by Ethics, Engagement and Co-design. *Front. Genet.* **2022**, *13*, 866168. [CrossRef]
24. Bick, D.; Ahmed, A.; Deen, D.; Ferlini, A.; Garnier, N.; Kasperaviciute, D.; Leblond, M.; Pichini, A.; Rendon, A.; Satija, A.; et al. Newborn Screening by Genomic Sequencing: Opportunities and Challenges. *Int. J. Neonatal Screen.* **2022**, *8*, 40. [CrossRef] [PubMed]
25. Parisi, M.A.; Caggana, M.; Cohen, J.L.; Gold, N.B.; Morris, J.A.; Orsini, J.J.; Urv, T.K.; Wasserstein, M.P. When is the best time to screen and evaluate for treatable genetic disorders?: A lifespan perspective. *Am J Med Genet C Semin Med Genet.* **2023**, *193*, 44–55. [CrossRef]
26. Holm, I.A.; McGuire, A.; Pereira, S.; Rehm, H.; Green, R.C.; Beggs, A.H.; BabySeq Project Team. Returning a Genomic Result for an Adult-Onset Condition to the Parents of a Newborn: Insights from the BabySeq Project. *Pediatrics.* **2019**, *143*, S37–S43. [CrossRef] [PubMed]
27. Chung, W.K.; Berg, J.S.; Botkin, J.R.; Brenner, S.E.; Brosco, J.P.; Brothers, K.B.; Currier, R.J.; Gaviglio, A.; Kowtoniuk, W.E.; Olson, C.; et al. Newborn screening for neurodevelopmental diseases: Are we there yet? *Am. J. Med. Genet. C Semin. Med. Genet.* **2022**, *190*, 222–230. [CrossRef]
28. Tarini, B.A.; Singer, D.; Clark, S.J.; Davis, M.M. Parents' interest in predictive genetic testing for their children when a disease has no treatment. *Pediatrics* **2009**, *124*, e432–e438. [CrossRef] [PubMed]
29. Goldenberg, A.J.; Dodson, D.S.; Davis, M.M.; Tarini, B.A. Parents' interest in whole-genome sequencing of newborns. *Genet. Med.* **2014**, *16*, 78–84. [CrossRef]
30. Waisbren, S.E.; Bäck, D.K.; Liu, C.; Kalia, S.S.; Ringer, S.A.; Holm, I.A.; Green, R.C. Parents are interested in newborn genomic testing during the early postpartum period. *Genet. Med. Off. J. Am. Coll. Med. Genet.* **2015**, *17*, 501. [CrossRef]
31. Joseph, G.; Chen, F.; Harris-Wai, J.; Puck, J.M.; Young, C.; Koenig, B.A. Parental views on expanded newborn screening using whole-genome sequencing. *Pediatrics* **2016**, *137*, S36–S46. [CrossRef]

32. Lewis, M.A.; Paquin, R.S.; Roche, M.I.; Furberg, R.D.; Rini, C.; Berg, J.S.; Powell, C.M.; Bailey, D.B., Jr. Supporting parental decisions about genomic sequencing for newborn screening: The NC NEXUS decision aid. *Pediatrics* **2016**, *137*, S16–S23. [CrossRef] [PubMed]
33. Waisbren, S.E.; Weipert, C.M.; Walsh, R.C.; Petty, C.R.; Green, R.C. Psychosocial factors influencing parental interest in genomic sequencing of newborns. *Pediatrics* **2016**, *137*, S30–S35. [CrossRef]
34. DeLuca, J.M. Public Attitudes Toward Expanded Newborn Screening. *J. Pediatr. Nurs. Nurs. Care Child. Fam.* **2018**, *38*, e19–e23. [CrossRef] [PubMed]
35. Lewis, M.A.; Stine, A.; Paquin, R.S.; Mansfield, C.; Wood, D.; Rini, C.; Roche, M.I.; Powell, C.M.; Berg, J.S.; Bailey, D.B. Parental preferences toward genomic sequencing for non-medically actionable conditions in children: A discrete-choice experiment. *Genet. Med.* **2018**, *20*, 181–189. [CrossRef]
36. Genetti, C.A.; Schwartz, T.S.; Robinson, J.O.; VanNoy, G.E.; Petersen, D.; Pereira, S.; Fayer, S.; Peoples, H.A.; Agrawal, P.B.; Betting, W.N. Parental interest in genomic sequencing of newborns: Enrollment experience from the BabySeq Project. *Genet. Med.* **2019**, *21*, 622–630. [CrossRef] [PubMed]
37. Moultrie, R.R.; Paquin, R.; Rini, C.; Roche, M.I.; Berg, J.S.; Powell, C.M.; Lewis, M.A. Parental views on newborn next generation sequencing: Implications for decision support. *Matern. Child Health J.* **2020**, *24*, 856–864. [CrossRef]
38. Paquin, R.S.; Peinado, S.; Lewis, M.A.; Biesecker, B.B.; Rini, C.; Roche, M.; Butterfield, R.M.; Powell, C.M.; Berg, J.S.; Bailey, D.B., Jr. A behavior-theoretic evaluation of values clarification on parental beliefs and intentions toward genomic sequencing for newborns. *Soc. Sci. Med.* **2021**, *271*, 112037. [CrossRef]
39. Armstrong, B.; Christensen, K.D.; Genetti, C.A.; Parad, R.B.; Robinson, J.O.; Blout Zawatsky, C.L.; Zettler, B.; Beggs, A.H.; Holm, I.A.; Green, R.C. Parental attitudes toward standard newborn screening and newborn genomic sequencing: Findings from the BabySeq study. *Front. Genet.* **2022**, *13*, 867371. [CrossRef]
40. Pereira, S.; Gutierrez, A.M.; Robinson, J.O.; Christensen, K.D.; Genetti, C.A.; Zawatsky, C.L.B.; Hsu, R.L.; Zettler, B.; Uveges, M.K.; Parad, R.B. Parents' decision-making regarding whether to receive adult-onset only genetic findings for their children: Findings from the BabySeq Project. *Genet. Med.* **2023**, *25*, 100002. [CrossRef]
41. Roman, T.S.; Crowley, S.B.; Roche, M.I.; Foreman, A.K.M.; O–Daniel, J.M.; Seifert, B.A.; Lee, K.; Brandt, A.; Gustafson, C.; DeCristo, D.M.; et al. Genomic Sequencing for Newborn Screening: Results of the NC NEXUS Project. *Am. J. Hum. Genet.* **2020**, *107*, 596–611. [CrossRef]
42. Etchegary, H.; Dicks, E.; Green, J.; Hodgkinson, K.; Pullman, D.; Parfrey, P. Interest in newborn genetic testing: A survey of prospective parents and the general public. *Genet. Test. Mol. Biomark.* **2012**, *16*, 353–358. [CrossRef] [PubMed]
43. Etchegary, H.; Dicks, E.; Hodgkinson, K.; Pullman, D.; Green, J.; Parfey, P. Public attitudes about genetic testing in the newborn period. *J. Obstet. Gynecol. Neonatal Nurs.* **2012**, *41*, 191–200. [CrossRef] [PubMed]
44. Bombard, Y.; Miller, F.A.; Hayeems, R.Z.; Barg, C.; Cressman, C.; Carroll, J.C.; Wilson, B.J.; Little, J.; Avard, D.; Painter-Main, M.; et al. Public views on participating in newborn screening using genome sequencing. *Eur. J. Hum. Genet.* **2014**, *22*, 1248–1254. [CrossRef]
45. Van Mil, H. Implications of Whole Genome Sequencing for Newborn Screening: A Public Dialogue. 2021. Available online: https://assets.publishing.service.gov.uk/media/60e584418fa8f50c79779207/WGS_for_newborn_screening_FINAL_ACCESSIBLE.pdf (accessed on 4 September 2023).
46. Kinsella, S.; Hopkins, H.; Cooper, L.; Bonham, J.R. A public dialogue to inform the use of wider genomic testing when used as part of newborn screening to identify cystic fibrosis. *Int. J. Neonatal Screen.* **2022**, *8*, 32. [CrossRef] [PubMed]
47. Kerruish, N. Parents' experiences 12 years after newborn screening for genetic susceptibility to type 1 diabetes and their attitudes to whole-genome sequencing in newborns. *Genet. Med.* **2016**, *18*, 249–258. [CrossRef] [PubMed]
48. Downie, L.; Halliday, J.; Lewis, S.; Lunke, S.; Lynch, E.; Martyn, M.; Gaff, C.; Jarmolowicz, A.; Amor, D.J. Exome sequencing in newborns with congenital deafness as a model for genomic newborn screening: The Baby Beyond Hearing project. *Genet. Med.* **2020**, *22*, 937–944. [CrossRef] [PubMed]
49. White, S.; Mossfield, T.; Fleming, J.; Barlow-Stewart, K.; Ghedia, S.; Dickson, R.; Richards, F.; Bombard, Y.; Wiley, V. Expanding the Australian Newborn Blood Spot Screening Program using genomic sequencing: Do we want it and are we ready? *Eur. J. Hum. Genet.* **2023**, *31*, 703–711. [CrossRef]
50. Biomedical Ethics Research Group. Implementing Genomics into Newborn Screening Programs. January 2023. Available online: https://www.youtube.com/watch?v=Lht9OIf2560 (accessed on 4 September 2023).
51. Vears, D.F.; Gillam, L. Inductive content analysis: A guide for beginning qualitative researchers. *Focus Health Prof. Educ. A Multi-Discip. J.* **2022**, *23*, 111–127. [CrossRef]
52. QSR International Pty Ltd. *NVivo Qualitative Data Analysis Software, Version 14*; QSR International Pty Ltd.: Doncaster, VIC, Australia, 2023.
53. Downie, L.; Halliday, J.; Lewis, S.; Amor, D.J. Principles of Genomic Newborn Screening Programs: A Systematic Review. *JAMA Netw. Open* **2021**, *4*, e2114336. [CrossRef]
54. Genomics England. New Public Dialogue Finds Support for the Use of Whole Genome Sequencing in Newborn Screening—Providing That the Right Safeguards and Resources Are in Place. 2021. Available online: https://www.genomicsengland.co.uk/news/public-dialogue-genomics-newborn-screening (accessed on 4 September 2023).

55. Pereira, S.; Smith, H.S.; Frankel, L.A.; Christensen, K.D.; Islam, R.; Robinson, J.O.; Genetti, C.A.; Zawatsky, C.L.B.; Zettler, B.; Parad, R.B. Psychosocial Effect of Newborn Genomic Sequencing on Families in the BabySeq Project: A Randomized Clinical Trial. *JAMA Pediatr.* **2021**, *175*, 1132–1141. [CrossRef]
56. Wojcik, M.H.; Zhang, T.; Ceyhan-Birsoy, O.; Genetti, C.A.; Lebo, M.S.; Yu, T.W.; Parad, R.B.; Holm, I.A.; Rehm, H.L.; Beggs, A.H. Discordant results between conventional newborn screening and genomic sequencing in the BabySeq Project. *Genet. Med.* **2021**, *23*, 1372–1375. [CrossRef] [PubMed]
57. Best, S.; Long, J.; Theodorou, T.; Hatem, S.; Lake, R.; Archibald, A.; Freeman, L.; Braithwaite, J. Health practitioners' perceptions of the barriers and enablers to the implementation of reproductive genetic carrier screening: A systematic review. *Prenat. Diagn.* **2021**, *41*, 708–719. [CrossRef] [PubMed]
58. Nisselle, A.; King, E.A.; McClaren, B.; Janinski, M.; Metcalfe, S.; Gaff, C.; Australian Genomics Workforce & Education Working Group. Measuring physician practice, preparedness and preferences for genomic medicine: A national survey. *BMJ Open* **2021**, *11*, e044408. [CrossRef] [PubMed]
59. Nisselle, A.; Bishop, M.; Charles, T.; Morrissy, S.; King, E.; Metcalfe, S.; Gaff, C. Lessons learnt from implementing change in newborn bloodspot screening processes over more than a decade: Midwives, genetics and education. *Midwifery* **2019**, *79*, 102542. [CrossRef] [PubMed]
60. Bunnik, E.M.; Janssens, A.C.J.W.; Schermer, M.H.N. A tiered-layered-staged model for informed consent in personal genome testing. *Eur. J. Hum. Genet.* **2013**, *21*, 596–601. [CrossRef] [PubMed]
61. Iskrov, G.; Ivanov, S.; Wrenn, S.; Stefanov, R. Whole-genome sequencing in newborn screening—Attitudes and opinions of Bulgarian pediatricians and geneticists. *Front. Public Health* **2017**, *5*, 308. [CrossRef]
62. Ulm, E.; Feero, W.G.; Dineen, R.; Charrow, J.; Wicklund, C. Genetics professionals' opinions of whole-genome sequencing in the newborn period. *J. Genet. Couns.* **2015**, *24*, 452–463. [CrossRef]
63. Wu, X.; Yang, Y.; Zhou, L.; Long, W.; Yu, B. Are We Ready for Newborn Genetic Screening? A Cross-Sectional Survey of Healthcare Professionals in Southeast China. *Front. Pediatr.* **2022**, *10*, 875229. [CrossRef]

International Journal of
Neonatal Screening

MDPI

Article

Charting the Ethical Frontier in Newborn Screening Research: Insights from the NBSTRN ELSI Researcher Needs Survey

Yekaterina Unnikumaran [1,†], Mei Lietsch [1,2] and Amy Brower [1,3,4,*]

1 American College of Medical Genetics and Genomics (ACMG), Bethesda, MD 20814, USA; yunnikumaran@gmail.com (Y.U.); mei-lietsch@uiowa.edu (M.L.)
2 Carver College of Medicine, University of Iowa, Iowa City, IA 52242, USA
3 Genetic Medicine, Munore-Meyer Institute, University of Nebraska Medical Center, Omaha, NE 68106, USA
4 Department of Health Professions., Creighton University School of Medicine, Omaha, NE 68178, USA
* Correspondence: amybrower@creighton.edu
† Current address: TechStream Analytics LLC, Silver Spring, MD 20904, USA.

Abstract: From 2008 to 2024, the Newborn Screening Translational Research Network (NBSTRN), part of the National Institute of Child Health and Human Development (NICHD) Hunter Kelly Newborn Screening Program, served as a robust infrastructure to facilitate groundbreaking research in newborn screening (NBS), public health, rare disease, and genomics. Over its sixteen years, NBSTRN developed into a significant international network, supporting innovative research on novel technologies to screen, diagnose, treat, manage, and understand the natural history of more than 280 rare diseases. The NBSTRN tools and resources were used by a variety of stakeholders including researchers, clinicians, state NBS programs, parents, families, and policy makers. Resources and expertise for the newborn screening community in ethical, legal, and social issues (ELSI) has been an important area of focus for the NBSTRN and this includes efforts across the NBS system from pilot studies of candidate conditions to public health implementation of screening for new conditions, and the longitudinal follow-up of NBS-identified individuals to inform health outcomes and disease understanding. In 2023, the NBSTRN conducted a survey to explore ELSI issues in NBS research, specifically those encountered by the NBS community. Since NBS research involves collaboration among researchers, state NBS programs, clinicians, and families, the survey was broadly designed and disseminated to engage all key stakeholders. With responses from 88 members of the NBS community, including researchers and state NBS programs, the survey found that individuals rely most on institutional and collegial resources when they encounter ELSI questions. Most survey responses ranked privacy as extremely or very important in NBS research and identified the need for policies that address informed consent in NBS research. The survey results highlight the need for improved collaborative resources and educational programs focused on ELSI for the NBS community. The survey results inform future efforts in ELSI and NBS research in the United States (U.S.) and the rest of the world, including the development of policies and expanded ELSI initiatives and tools that address the needs of all NBS stakeholders.

Keywords: newborn screening; ethical; legal; social issues; ELSI; research; rare disease; NBSTRN; privacy; informed consent; public health

1. Introduction

The landscape of medical research is underscored by ever-present ethical, legal, and social issues (ELSI). As a fundamental aspect of all scientific inquiries, ELSI considerations play an indispensable role in guiding the ethical conduct, legal framework, and social implications of research endeavors. Although consideration of ELSI is firmly established across the medical research spectrum [1], their integration into the realm of newborn screening (NBS) research, which inherently requires collaboration between academic, clinical, public health, patient, and family communities, remains an area in which more cohesive and comprehensive implementation is needed [2–4].

For 16 years, the Newborn Screening Translational Research Network (NBSTRN) was a robust infrastructure dedicated to facilitating and expanding groundbreaking NBS research [5,6]. Founded in 2008 as a key component of the Hunter Kelly Newborn Screening Program at the Eunice Kennedy Shriver National Institutes of Child Health and Human Development (NICHD) through a contract with the American College of Medical Genetics and Genomics (ACMG), NBSTRN grew into an international network involved in supporting cutting-edge research, population-based pilots, and longitudinal studies to discover novel technologies to screen, diagnose, treat, and manage rare disease across the lifespan [7–13]. NBSTRN tools and resources have been used by a variety of stakeholders, including researchers, clinicians, state NBS programs, parents, families, and policy makers working across the NBS system of basic, translational, and clinical research, prenatal education, neonatal screening, clinical diagnosis, treatment, and lifelong care [14–21].

Resources and expertise for the NBS community in ethical, legal, and social issues (ELSI) has been an important area of focus for the NBSTRN, and this includes efforts across the NBS system from pilot studies of candidate conditions to public health implementation of screening for new conditions, and the longitudinal follow-up of NBS-identified individuals to inform health outcomes and disease understanding [4,22,23]. In 2023, to better understand ELSI issues in NBS research encountered by the NBS community, the NBSTRN conducted a survey of the NBS community. Because NBS research involves collaboration between researchers, state NBS programs, clinicians, and families, the survey was designed for all stakeholders and widely disseminated to reach all these groups. We describe the survey design, execution, results, and key takeaways to inform future efforts in ELSI and NBS research in the United States (U.S.) and the rest of the world.

1.1. ELSI across the NBS System

In the U.S., NBS is led by the state public health departments and is recognized as one of the most triumphant public health initiatives. Since the inception of the first successful screen for phenylketonuria (PKU) in the 1960s, state NBS programs have expanded their list of conditions to include screenings for up to 81 conditions [24], with the goal of facilitating early intervention for affected newborns. The decision-making power regarding condition inclusion within NBS programs lies with state NBS programs, and the makeup of screening panels are informed by the Recommended Uniform Screening Panel (RUSP). The RUSP is a list of disorders that the Secretary of the Department of Health and Human Services (HHS) recommends for states to screen. A federal advisory committee coordinates a process of nomination, evidence review, and recommendation which evaluates information provided by nominators and assesses the net benefit of screening all newborns, the certainty of the evidence regarding the net benefit, the feasibility of implementing a comprehensive program of screening for the condition, and the readiness of public health programs to implement such a program of expanded screening, including an assessment of costs to the newborn screening programs to expand screening for a condition under review [25–27].

The past two decades have witnessed a rapid expansion in NBS capabilities fueled by technological advancements in tools to screen and diagnose, including sequencing, and novel approaches to treatment, including precision medicine [15,19,28–30]. This technological expansion and complexity of NBS research underscore the urgent requirement to address ELSI considerations across each component of NBS from parental education, sample collection and screening, communication of results, confirmatory testing, treatment, and long-term follow-up [31,32]. This is particularly critical given the multi-dimensional scope of NBS research, which includes pilot studies to evaluate candidate conditions for the RUSP nomination, review, and public health implementation [33–38]. The RUSP process reveals the intricate relationship between ELSI elements and NBS, as well as the interplay between researchers, state NBS programs, clinicians, and families. As a whole, this prioritizes ELSI as a crucial component of the NBS system. This includes the differences in disease expression, symptoms, severity, and outcomes resulting from population-based screening; the preparedness of state programs for screening expansion; the increasing complexity of care coordination for conditions with varying clinical onsets and treatment urgency; the integration of trauma-informed care to support families impacted by the screening process, and equitable access to timely diagnosis, treatment, and life-long care and management regardless of the location of birth [39–42].

1.2. NBSTRN Efforts to Facilitate ELSI in NBS

In the U.S., the RUSP is an established a system of nomination, review, and endorsement to establish a list of conditions recommended for NBS [24]. The evidence review includes an assessment of the potential benefits and harms of NBS informed by NBS research that includes pilot and natural history studies led by academia, public health, and advocacy groups. NBSTRN served as a coordinating center for several pilot and natural history studies and found that most pilot studies involved collaboration between researchers, clinicians, and state NBS programs. We observed that the approaches to informed consent, institutional board review (IRB), and consumer input varied across pilot sites [9,10]. In 2019, the NBSTRN Bioethics and Legal Workgroup (WG) conducted a series of professional and public discussions to begin to address the observed differences in pilot studies with the goal of identifying important ELSI challenges and facilitating the integration of ELSI into NBS pilot studies [4]. This effort identified nine key ELSI questions that could be integrated into pilot studies to ultimately help the NBS program to better understand the potential impact of screening for a new condition on newborns and families. To facilitate the continued exploration of ELSI in NBS, we designed a survey in 2023 to gather input on ELSI needs in NBS research for all stakeholders in the NBS community.

2. Materials and Methods

We developed an online survey to assess the ELSI challenges in NBS research and identify the resources that are used or of interest to the NBS community, including researchers, state NBS programs, clinicians, advocacy groups, and individuals living with and parents of an individual with a disease identified through NBS. The survey was designed using a series of online meetings and communications with the NBSTRN Bioethics and Legal Workgroup and consisted of one open-ended question and thirteen multiple choice questions written in English. Identifying information was not included in the survey. The survey was developed, validated, and disseminated using Research Electronic Data Capture (REDCap) ([43], Appendix). An electronic link to the survey was disseminated to a convenience sample consisting of the NBSTRN network that included individuals who had registered for the NBSTRN website, participated in events, and received the NBSTRN newsletter. The survey was deployed during the NBSTRN Network Meeting on 18 May 2023, and this was followed by a comprehensive outreach campaign that included social media engagement, directed emails to the NBSTRN network members, and listserv announcements. To ensure a wide reach within the NBSTRN community, broader dissemination efforts continued, and the survey remained open until 25 August 2023. The Accumulated data were exported from REDCap® (https://projectredcap.org/software/, accessed on 15 August 2024), and the percentage of participants who selected each response was computed for the thirteen binary and/or categorical response options. Three staff members independently reviewed the text responses for the open-ended question and identified themes.

The privacy and confidentiality of the survey respondents were prioritized throughout the study. Personal identifiers were removed from the dataset to protect the anonymity of the participants. Data were stored securely and only accessible to authorized personnel directly involved in the study.

3. Results

Eighty-eight (N = 88) individuals accessed the 13-question survey, and a data quality check found that 98% (86/88) answered all questions. Incomplete surveys were included in the analysis for the questions that were completely answered. Figure 1 presents the results of twelve multi-choice questions (Q1–11, Q13) using GraphPad Prism 6 [44]. The themes identified from the open-ended question (Q12) are listed in Table 1.

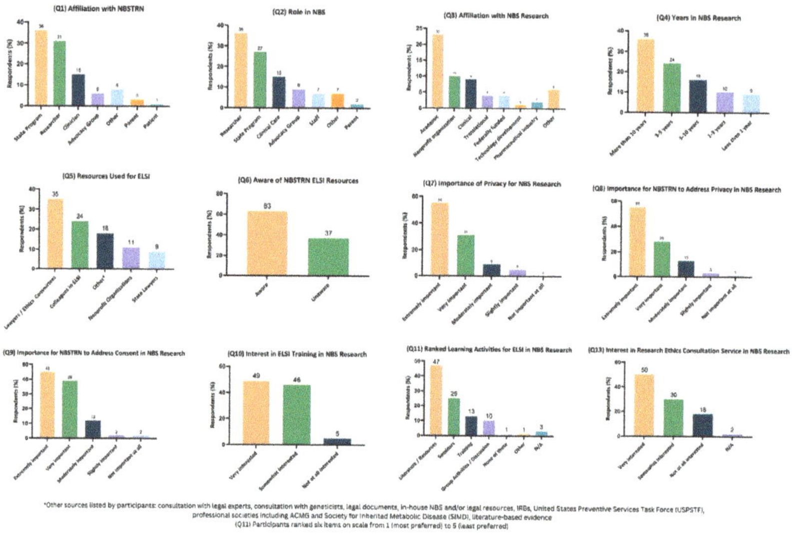

Figure 1. Results from multiple choice questions Q1 to Q11 and Q13 (the results are reported in descending order, from left to right). Not Applicable (N/A).

Table 1. Areas for ELSI Considerations identified in the open-ended question.

Theme	Number of Mentions (n = 41)	Percentage of All Responses
Informed consent	14	34%
Usage and standardization of data	9	22%
Usage and storage of dried blood spots (DBS)	6	15%
Policy	6	15%
The NBS process	6	15%
Privacy	4	10%
Population diversity of data and samples	4	10%

Of those who accessed the survey, 36% (32/88) identified their role in NBS research as researcher, 27% as state program (24/88%), 15% (13/88) as clinical care, and 9% (8/88) as advocacy (Figure 1, Q2). A total of 81% (71/88) has been involved in NBS research for three or more years, and 86% (75/88) identified privacy as either an extremely or very important ethical issue in NBS research (Figure 1, Q4, Q7). When encountering legal or ethical issues related to NBS research, 35% (31/88) typically seek information or guidance from institutional lawyers or ethics committees within their organization, 24% (21/88) utilized colleagues, 18% (16/88) other resources including the literature, 11% (10/88) nonprofit organizations, and 9% (8/88) utilized state lawyers with expertise in healthcare law (Figure 1, Q5). A total of 63% (55/88) were aware of the NBSTRN ELSI resources, and 80% (60/88) were somewhat or very interested in a research ethics consultation service that helps to answer ethical issues around the ethical issues surrounding NBS research (Figure 1, Q6, Q13).

To examine differences between the individual stakeholder groups related to ELSI information or guidance, we compared the responses to Q5, "When encountering legal or ethical issues related to newborn screening research, where do you typically seek information or guidance", by self-identified stakeholder groups: 55% (16/29) of self-identified researchers sought information or guidance from colleagues conducting ethical research. A total of 58% (14/24) of self-identified state NBS program members sought information or guidance from institutional lawyers or ethics committees within their organization and 25% (6/24) consulted with state lawyers specialized in healthcare law. A total of 46% (6/13) self-identified clinicians sought guidance from institutional lawyers.

Forty-seven percent (41/88) of participants answered the open-ended question (Question 12; Supplementary Survey S1): "What are the ethical, legal, or social issues that you face in your own work? Explain." Seven common themes were identified by three staff members who reviewed the text responses. Table 1 details the seven themes and the frequency with which they were mentioned by the participants. Informed consent was a theme identified by 34% (14/41) participants.

4. Discussion and Future Efforts

NBS research is a crucial area that aims to presymptomatically identify and treat rare, often life-threatening conditions early in a child's life. This research is essential because early intervention can significantly improve health outcomes and quality of life through the discovery of novel technologies to screen, diagnose treat, and manage disease. Given the complexity and rarity of these diseases, coupled with population-based screening that is coordinated by state NBS programs, collaboration among various stakeholders to plan, carry out, disseminate, and implement research findings is critical. Including the consideration of ELSI in the NBS research is also important and our survey of a convenience sample of the NBS community found overwhelming interest in training or educational activities related to ethical issues in NBS research and identified a need for improved collaborative frameworks, tools and educational programs focused on ELSI for the NBS community. Sixty-three percent (56/88) of respondents self-identified as either researchers or state NBS programs. This reinforces the experience of many that research in NBS involves both collaboration between researchers and state NBS programs. Therefore, to address ELSI in NBS research, we should consider the concerns and needs that these groups have in common as well as those that are unique to researchers based in academia or foundations, public health team members working in state departments of health, and clinical care providers in hospitals and community based centers.

Across all stakeholder groups, the participants identified privacy and informed consent as key issues to address in NBS research. Almost all (95%, 83/88) respondents were somewhat or very interested in a research ethics consultation service focused on the ethical issues surrounding NBS research. The preference for educational formats that facilitate direct engagement and real-time discussion reveals a potential gap in the current educational offerings that are focused on static content. In summary, the survey results inform future efforts in ELSI and NBS research in the U.S. and have relevance to the rest of the world, including the development of policies and expanded ELSI frameworks and tools that address the needs of all NBS stakeholders.

These future efforts to support ELSI in NBS research will be important as the number of diseases, treatments, and technologies increase and the complexities surrounding ELSI issues continue to grow. In addition, groups around the world are researching ways to integrate genomics to screen, diagnose, and design interventions in newborns and children, and this heightens the need for robust, coordinated, and widely disseminated ELSI efforts and policies [45]. Informed by the sixteen years of discussions, collaborations, and workgroups of the NBSTRN, Table 2 lists nine suggested key areas for future efforts and provides examples to illustrate how targeted projects can address ELSI considerations in NBS research by leveraging patient-centric resources, participatory research models, public education and engagement, and collaborative education programs. The NBSTRN of diverse stakeholders across the NBS community from public health partners to clinicians, patients, parents, families, researchers, and advocacy groups continually highlighted the importance of a focus on privacy, informed consent, interdisciplinary collaboration, social acceptance, and ongoing education. This broad approach to ELSI in NBS research coupled with innovative initiatives that consider local, regional, and county-wide policies and practices will help to ensure that ELSI aspects are comprehensively integrated into NBS research around the world. In the U.S., the continued collaboration between the National Institutes of Health (NIH), the Centers for Disease Control and Prevention (CDC), and the Health Resources and Services Administration (HRSA) will be vital in supporting these efforts to advance ELSI in NBS research and ensure the successful implementation of evolving best practices. Each of these agencies brings unique strengths and expertise to the table, creating a comprehensive approach that addresses scientific discovery, translational research, public health implementation and surveillance, and clinical and community-based care across the lifespan delivery aspects [46]. In conclusion, the NBSTRN ELSI survey results demonstrate that the NBS community recognizes the important of ELSI in NBS research infrastructure and calls upon all stakeholders and federal partners to invest in a future where rare disease research is prioritized and supported across research, clinical care, and state NBS programs.

Table 2. Nine suggested areas for future efforts to advance ELSI in NBS research for the worldwide NBS community.

Key Area	Description	Example(s)
ELSIs in NBS Research	Funded efforts to develop, validate, pilot, and implement accessible, patient-centric resources that address the burgeoning ELSI challenges identified by the NBS research community. Emphasis would be placed on privacy and informed consent tools, catering to the nuanced requirements of rare disease research.	Establish a global consortium dedicated to addressing ELSIs specific to genomic newborn screening. The consortium would develop guidelines, share best practices, and support collaborative research projects. This could be used to develop an online platform called the "Patient-Centric ELSI Resource Hub" to create, validate, pilot, and implement resources addressing ELSI challenges in NBS. Key features are privacy and informed consent tools, personalized education materials for parents, interactive FAQs, and case studies tailored to rare diseases. Users include researchers, clinicians, parents, and patient advocacy groups. This hub would ensure that parents are well-informed about privacy and consent issues, and it would help researchers address ELSI challenges effectively, promoting ethical and transparent research practices.
Innovative NBS Research Approaches	Design NBS research using a participatory research model that involves parents and communities in the design and implementation of research studies ensuring that their perspectives and needs are considered, an incorporating trauma-informed care to address emotional impacts. Forming interdisciplinary research teams that include ethicists, legal scholars, sociologists, and community representatives to address ELSI issues comprehensively. Developing tools and methodologies to assess the impact of ELSI considerations in NBS programs, ensuring continuous improvement and responsiveness to emerging challenges.	Create councils consisting of patients and family members affected by conditions identified through NBS and NBS research. These councils would provide insights into real-world impacts of screening programs and help to guide ELSI policies and practices. Establish a consortium called the "Participatory NBS Research Consortium" that uses a participatory research model involving parents and communities in the design and implementation of NBS research. Activities focus on engaging parents and community representatives in research design, forming interdisciplinary teams with ethicists, legal scholars, sociologists, and community representatives and developing assessment tools for ELSI impact. Researchers, community representatives, ethicists, legal scholars, and sociologists would be members. This consortium would ensure that research studies are designed with input from those directly affected, leading to more ethically sound and socially acceptable research outcomes.

Table 2. *Cont.*

Key Area	Description	Example(s)
Enhancing Social Acceptance and Engagement	Developing comprehensive education and outreach programs to inform the public about the benefits, risks, and ethical considerations of newborn screening, fostering a greater acceptance and informed participation. Providing cultural competence training for healthcare providers to ensure sensitive and respectful communication with families from diverse backgrounds. Creating platforms for public engagement where stakeholders, including parents, patient advocacy groups, and the public, can discuss and influence newborn screening policies and practices.	Launch nationwide and worldwide campaigns to educate the public about NBS research, focusing on ELSI implications. Use multimedia platforms, community events, and partnerships with advocacy groups to research diverse audiences and create the "Newborn Screening Education and Outreach Initiative". Activities include creating educational materials and campaigns, cultural competence training for healthcare providers, and establishing public engagement platforms for discussion and policy influence. Collaborators include healthcare providers, educators, patient advocacy groups, and public health officials. This initiative would foster a greater public understanding and acceptance of NBS, ensure respectful and sensitive communication with diverse families, and provide a forum for public input on NBS policies.
Collaborative Education Programs	With an expressed preference for interactive and structured learning found in our survey, supporting the establishment of seminars and workshops. These would serve to disseminate current ELSI practices and foster a collaborative learning environment, integrating patient advocacy groups in the educational design to ensure patient-relevant outcomes.	Establish dedicated research centers focused on studying the ELSI aspects of NBS research. These centers would conduct interdisciplinary research, provide training for healthcare professionals, and offer policy recommendations. Develop a series of seminars and workshops called the "ELSI in NBS Seminar Series" to disseminate current ELSI practices and foster a collaborative learning environment. The format consists of interactive sessions with case studies, panel discussions, and breakout groups, co-designed with patient advocacy groups to ensure relevance and impact. Participants include researchers, clinicians, patient advocates, legal experts, and ethicists. This seminar series would promote ongoing education on ELSI issues, facilitate collaboration across disciplines, and ensure that patient perspectives are integrated into educational efforts.
Digital Engagement Platforms	Investments could be allocated towards developing digital platforms for ELSI education and discussion. These platforms would encourage cross-disciplinary collaboration and facilitate real-time dialogue among researchers, clinicians, and patient groups.	A dedicated online platform called the "Newborn Screening ELSI Hub" could be developed to provide a space for education and discussion around the ethical, legal, and social implications of newborn screening. The platform would include forums for real-time dialogue, webinars hosted by experts in the field, interactive case studies, and a repository of educational materials, such as articles, videos, and guidelines. Researchers, clinicians, ethicists, patient advocacy groups, and parents could be the targeted users. This platform would facilitate cross-disciplinary collaboration, ensuring that diverse perspectives are considered in ELSI discussions and decision-making processes.

Table 2. *Cont.*

Key Area	Description	Example(s)
Ethics Consultation Services	Recognizing the need for ongoing support in navigating ethical complexities, programs such as the Rare Diseases Clinical Research Network (RDCRN) could establish a consultative service within its consortia. This service would be tasked with providing expert advice on ethical considerations in clinical trial design and implementation, especially for rare diseases where the ethical landscape can be particularly complex.	The Rare Diseases Clinical Research Network (RDCRN) could establish an Ethical Consultation Unit within its consortia to provide expert advice on ethical issues in clinical trials, particularly those involving rare diseases. The unit would offer consultations on trial design, informed consent processes, data management, and the handling of incidental findings. It would also provide training sessions for researchers and support for navigating ethical review boards. The unit would comprise bioethicists, legal experts, patient advocates, and experienced clinicians. This service would ensure that ethical considerations are thoroughly addressed in the planning and execution of clinical trials, enhancing the integrity and acceptability of research projects.
Legal and Regulatory Navigation Tools	Considering the diverse regulatory environments encountered across research sites, funding could be targeted to the development of tools that aid rare disease researchers in understanding and complying with local and international regulations, thereby ensuring the ethical conduct of rare disease research.	The RDRN could be a comprehensive digital tool designed to help researchers to understand and comply with varying legal and regulatory requirements across different regions. Interactive maps showing regulatory landscapes, step-by-step guides for compliance, templates for necessary documentation, and a database of region-specific legal requirements and ethical guidelines. Researchers, regulatory affairs specialists, and clinical trial coordinators could be the targeted users. By simplifying the navigation of complex legal environments, the RDRN would facilitate smoother and more ethically compliant research processes, reducing delays and legal risks.
Data Sharing and Privacy Initiatives	With big data playing an increasingly critical role in research, funding could support the creation of protocols and best practices that ensure the ethical use and sharing of data, while respecting patient privacy and the specific confidentiality concerns associated with rare diseases in the newborn screening space.	Develop a "SecureDataShare Protocol" to ensure the ethical use and sharing of data in newborn screening research, with a strong emphasis on protecting patient privacy. Key features include encryption standards for data storage and transfer, protocols for anonymizing sensitive information, consent management systems that allow patients to control their data usage, and guidelines for ethical data sharing practices. Collaborators could be IT specialists, bioethicists, data protection officers, and patient advocacy groups. This initiative would enhance trust in research by ensuring that patient data are handled with the highest ethical standards, while still enabling valuable scientific collaborations.
Policy Development and Advocacy	Developing comprehensive policy frameworks that integrate ethical, legal, and social considerations into all aspects of newborn screening programs. Advocating for sustained funding and resources to support ELSI research and the implementation of best practices in newborn screening. Facilitating collaboration between policymakers, researchers, healthcare providers, and patient advocacy groups to ensure that policies are well-rounded and effectively implemented.	A task force dedicated to developing and advocating for policies that integrate ethical, legal, and social considerations into all aspects of newborn screening programs. Activities include conducting policy analysis, drafting policy recommendations, organizing advocacy campaigns, and facilitating stakeholder meetings. Members could be policymakers, researchers, healthcare providers, patient advocates, and legal experts. This task force would ensure that newborn screening programs are guided by comprehensive, well-rounded policies that reflect the needs and concerns of all stakeholders, leading to more effective and ethically sound screening practices.

Supplementary Materials: The following supporting information can be downloaded at: https://www.mdpi.com/article/10.3390/ijns10030064/s1, Supplementary Survey S1.

Author Contributions: Conceptualization, Y.U., M.L. and A.B.; formal analysis, Y.U., M.L. and A.B.; data curation, Y.U., M.L. and A.B.; writing—original draft preparation, Y.U., M.L. and A.B.; writing—review and editing, Y.U., M.L. and A.B.; visualization, Y.U. and M.L.; supervision, A.B.; project administration, A.B.; funding acquisition, A.B. All authors have read and agreed to the published version of the manuscript.

Funding: This project was wholly funded with Federal funds from the NICHD, National Institutes of Health, Department of Health and Human Services, under Contract No. HHSN275201800005C.

Institutional Review Board Statement: The research presented in this article was conducted in accordance with the highest ethical standards and best practices in the field of newborn screening (NBS) research. The Newborn Screening Translational Research Network (NBSTRN) and the National Institute of Child Health and Human Development (NICHD) Hunter Kelly Newborn Screening Program are committed to the responsible and ethical conduct of research, particularly when it involves vulnerable populations, such as newborns and their families.

Informed Consent Statement: Informed consent and Institutional Review Board (IRB) approval was not required for this survey study as it did not involve the collection of identifiable personal information or pose any risk to participants.

Data Availability Statement: All data are available within this article.

Acknowledgments: This paper and the research it presents could not have been accomplished without the exceptional support of the NBSTRN Bioethics and Legal Workgroup. Special thanks are due to Flavia Chen; Ed Goldman; Aaron J. Goldenberg; Ingrid Holm; and Stacey Pereira. Their contributions were vital to the development of the ELSI Researcher Needs Survey, and their invaluable comments and feedback greatly enriched the reporting, results, and analysis of the survey data.

Conflicts of Interest: The authors declare no conflicts of interest.

References

1. ELSIhub. Available online: https://elsihub.org/ (accessed on 2 December 2023).
2. Nicholls, S.G.; Wilson, B.J.; Etchegary, H.; Brehaut, J.C.; Potter, B.K.; Hayeems, R.; Chakraborty, P.; Milburn, J.; Pullman, D.; Turner, L.; et al. Benefits and burdens of newborn screening: Public understanding and decision-making. *Pers. Med.* **2014**, *11*, 593–607. [CrossRef] [PubMed]
3. Taylor-Phillips, S.; Stinton, C.; Di Ferrante Ruffano, L.; Seedat, F.; Clarke, A.; Deeks, J.J. Association between use of systematic reviews and national policy recommendations on screening newborn babies for rare diseases: Systematic review and meta-analysis. *BMJ* **2018**, *361*, k1612. [CrossRef] [PubMed]
4. Goldenberg, A.J.; Lloyd-Puryear, M.; Brosco, J.P.; Therrell, B.; Bush, L.; Berry, S.; Brower, A.; Bonhomme, N.; Bowdish, B.; Chrysler, D.; et al. Including ELSI research questions in newborn screening pilot studies. *Genet. Med.* **2019**, *21*, 525–533. [CrossRef] [PubMed]
5. Brower, A.; Chan, K. Special issue: Newborn screening research. *Am. J. Med. Genet. Part C Semin. Med. Genet.* **2022**, *190*, 135–137. [CrossRef] [PubMed] [PubMed Central]
6. Brower, A.; Chan, K.; Taylor, J.; Wiebenga, R.; Tona, G.; Unnikumaran, Y.; Barnes, L. Accelerating the Pace of Newborn Screening Research to Advance Disease Understanding and Improve Health Outcomes: Key Efforts of the Newborn Screening Translational Research Network (NBSTRN). *Del. J. Public Health* **2021**, *7*, 36–37. [CrossRef] [PubMed] [PubMed Central]
7. Lekstrom-Himes, J.; Augustine, E.F.; Brower, A.; Defay, T.; Finkel, R.S.; McGuire, A.L.; Skinner, M.W.; Yu, T.W. Data sharing to advance gene-targeted therapies in rare diseases. *Am. J. Med. Genet. Part C Semin. Med. Genet.* **2023**, *193*, 87–98. [CrossRef] [PubMed]
8. Lekstrom-Himes, J.; Brooks, P.J.; Koeberl, D.D.; Brower, A.; Goldenberg, A.; Green, R.C.; Morris, J.A.; Orsini, J.J.; Yu, T.W.; Augustine, E.F. Moving away from one disease at a time: Screening, trial design, and regulatory implications of novel platform technologies. *Am. J. Med. Genet. Part C Semin. Med. Genet.* **2023**, *193*, 30–43. [CrossRef]
9. Brower, A.; Chan, K.; Williams, M.; Berry, S.; Currier, R.; Rinaldo, P.; Caggana, M.; Gaviglio, A.; Wilcox, W.; Steiner, R.; et al. Population-Based Screening of Newborns: Findings From the NBS Expansion Study (Part One). *Front. Genet.* **2022**, *13*, 867337. [CrossRef] [PubMed] [PubMed Central]
10. Chan, K.; Brower, A.; Williams, M.S. Population-based screening of newborns: Findings from the newborn screening expansion study (part two). *Front. Genet.* **2022**, *13*, 867354. [CrossRef] [PubMed] [PubMed Central]
11. Brower, A.; Chan, K.; Hartnett, M.; Taylor, J. The Longitudinal Pediatric Data Resource: Facilitating Longitudinal Collection of Health Information to Inform Clinical Care and Guide Newborn Screening Efforts. *Int. J. Neonatal Screen.* **2021**, *7*, 37. [CrossRef] [PubMed] [PubMed Central]

12. Chan, K.; Hu, Z.; Bush, L.W.; Cope, H.; Holm, I.A.; Kingsmore, S.F.; Wilhelm, K.; Scharfe, C.; Brower, A. NBSTRN Tools to Advance Newborn Screening Research and Support Newborn Screening Stakeholders. *Int. J. Neonatal Screen.* **2023**, *9*, 63. [CrossRef] [PubMed] [PubMed Central]
13. Talebizadeh, Z.; Hu, V.; Shababi, M.; Brower, A. Landscape Analysis of Neurodevelopmental Comorbidities in Newborn Screening Conditions: Challenges and Opportunities. *Int. J. Neonatal Screen.* **2024**, *10*, 4. [CrossRef] [PubMed]
14. Köhler, S.; Gargano, M.; Matentzoglu, N.; Carmody, L.C.; Lewis-Smith, D.; Vasilevsky, N.A.; Danis, D.; Balagura, G.; Baynam, G.; Brower, A.M.; et al. The Human Phenotype Ontology in 2021. *Nucleic Acids Res.* **2021**, *49*, D1207–D1217. [CrossRef] [PubMed] [PubMed Central]
15. Berg, J.S.; Agrawal, P.B.; Bailey, D.B., Jr.; Beggs, A.H.; Brenner, S.E.; Brower, A.M.; Cakici, J.A.; Ceyhan-Birsoy, O.; Chan, K.; Chen, F.; et al. Newborn Sequencing in Genomic Medicine and Public Health. *Pediatrics* **2017**, *139*, e20162252. [CrossRef] [PubMed]
16. Hartnett, M.J.; Lloyd-Puryear, M.A.; Tavakoli, N.P.; Wynn, J.; Koval-Burt, C.L.; Gruber, D.; Trotter, T.; Caggana, M.; Chung, W.K.; Armstrong, N.; et al. Newborn Screening for Duchenne Muscular Dystrophy: First Year Results of a Population-Based Pilot. *Int. J. Neonatal Screen.* **2022**, *8*, 50. [CrossRef] [PubMed] [PubMed Central]
17. Tavakoli, N.P.; Gruber, D.; Armstrong, N.; Chung, W.K.; Maloney, B.; Park, S.; Wynn, J.; Koval-Burt, C.; Verdade, L.; Tegay, D.H.; et al. Newborn screening for Duchenne muscular dystrophy: A two-year pilot study. *Ann. Clin. Transl. Neurol.* **2023**, *10*, 1383–1396. [CrossRef] [PubMed] [PubMed Central]
18. Wilhelm, K.; Edick, M.J.; Berry, S.A.; Hartnett, M.; Brower, A. Using Long-Term Follow-Up Data to Classify Genetic Variants in Newborn Screened Conditions. *Front. Genet.* **2022**, *13*, 859837. [CrossRef] [PubMed] [PubMed Central]
19. Lietsch, M.; Chan, K.; Taylor, J.; Lee, B.H.; Ciafaloni, E.; Kwon, J.M.; Waldrop, M.A.; Butterfield, R.J.; Rathore, G.; Veerapandiyan, A.; et al. Long-Term Follow-Up Cares and Check Initiative: A Program to Advance Long-Term Follow-Up in Newborns Identified with a Disease through Newborn Screening. *Int. J. Neonatal Screen.* **2024**, *10*, 34. [CrossRef]
20. Gruber, D.; Lloyd-Puryear, M.; Armstrong, N.; Scavina, M.; Tavakoli, N.P.; Brower, A.M.; Caggana, M.; Chung, W.K. Newborn screening for Duchenne muscular dystrophy-early detection and diagnostic algorithm for female carriers of Duchenne muscular dystrophy. *Am. J. Med. Genet. Part C Semin. Med. Genet.* **2022**, *190*, 197–205. [CrossRef]
21. Milko, L.V.; Chen, F.; Chan, K.; Brower, A.M.; Agrawal, P.B.; Beggs, A.H.; Berg, J.S.; Brenner, S.E.; Holm, I.A.; Koenig, B.A.; et al. FDA oversight of NSIGHT genomic research: The need for an integrated systems approach to regulation. *NPJ Genom. Med.* **2019**, *4*, 32. [CrossRef]
22. Lloyd-Puryear, M.A.; Crawford, T.O.; Brower, A.; Stephenson, K.; Trotter, T.; Goldman, E.; Goldenberg, A.; Howell, R.R.; Kennedy, A.; Watson, M. Duchenne Muscular Dystrophy Newborn Screening, a Case Study for Examining Ethical and Legal Issues for Pilots for Emerging Disorders: Considerations and Recommendations. *Int. J. Neonatal Screen.* **2018**, *4*, 6. [CrossRef] [PubMed]
23. Botkin, J.R.; Lewis, M.H.; Watson, M.S.; Swoboda, K.J.; Anderson, R.; Berry, S.A.; Bonhomme, N.; Brosco, J.P.; Comeau, A.M.; Goldenberg, A.; et al. Parental permission for pilot newborn screening research: Guidelines from the NBSTRN. *Pediatrics* **2014**, *133*, e410–e417. [CrossRef] [PubMed]
24. Recommended Uniform Screening Panel (RUSP). Available online: https://www.hrsa.gov/advisory-committees/heritable-disorders/rusp (accessed on 27 November 2023).
25. Calonge, N.; Green, N.S.; Rinaldo, P.; Lloyd-Puryear, M.; Dougherty, D.; Boyle, C.; Watson, M.; Trotter, T.; Terry, S.F.; Howell, R.R. Advisory Committee on Heritable Disorders in Newborns and Children Committee report: Method for evaluating conditions nominated for population-based screening of newborns and children. *Genet. Med. Off. J. Am. Coll. Med. Genet.* **2010**, *12*, 153–159. [CrossRef]
26. Kemper, A.R.; Green, N.S.; Calonge, N.; Lam, W.K.; Comeau, A.M.; Goldenberg, A.J.; Ojodu, J.; Prosser, L.A.; Tanksley, S.; Bocchini, J.A., Jr. Decision-making process for conditions nominated to the recommended uniform screening panel: Statement of the US Department of Health and Human Services Secretary's Advisory Committee on Heritable Disorders in Newborns and Children. *Genet. Med. Off. J. Am. Coll. Med. Genet.* **2014**, *16*, 183–187. [CrossRef] [PubMed]
27. Chan, K.; Brower, A.; Ganiats, T.G. The "Other E" in ELSI: The Use of Economic Evaluation to Inform the Expansion of Newborn Screening. *Arch. Pediatr.* **2024**, *9*, 307. [CrossRef]
28. Hale, J.E.; Darras, B.T.; Swoboda, K.J.; Estrella, E.; Chen, J.Y.H.; Abbott, M.A.; Hay, B.N.; Kumar, B.; Counihan, A.M.; Gerstel-Thompson, J.; et al. Massachusetts' Findings from Statewide Newborn Screening for Spinal Muscular Atrophy. *Int. J. Neonatal Screen.* **2021**, *7*, 26. [CrossRef]
29. Milko, L.V.; O'Daniel, J.M.; DeCristo, D.M.; Crowley, S.B.; Foreman, A.K.M.; Wallace, K.E.; Mollison, L.F.; Strande, N.T.; Girnary, Z.S.; Boshe, L.J.; et al. An Age-Based Framework for Evaluating Genome-Scale Sequencing Results in Newborn Screening. *J. Pediatr.* **2019**, *209*, 68–76. [CrossRef]
30. Ceyhan-Birsoy, O.; Murry, J.B.; Machini, K.; Lebo, M.S.; Yu, T.W.; Fayer, S.; Genetti, C.A.; Schwartz, T.S.; Agrawal, P.B.; Parad, R.B.; et al. Interpretation of Genomic Sequencing Results in Healthy and Ill Newborns: Results from the BabySeq Project. *Am. J. Hum. Genet.* **2019**, *104*, 76–93. [CrossRef]
31. Tarini, B.A.; Goldenberg, A.J. Ethical issues with newborn screening in the genomics era. *Annu. Rev. Genom. Hum. Genet.* **2012**, *13*, 381–393. [CrossRef] [PubMed] [PubMed Central]
32. Esquerda, M.; Palau, F.; Lorenzo, D.; Cambra, F.J.; Bofarull, M.; Cusi, V.; Grup Interdisciplinar En Bioetica. Ethical questions concerning newborn genetic screening. *Clin. Genet.* **2021**, *99*, 93–98. [CrossRef]

33. Hasegawa, L.; Fergus, K.; Ojeda, N.; Au, S. Parental Attitudes Toward Ethical and Social Issues Surrounding the Expansion of Newborn Screening Using New Technologies. *Public Health Genom.* **2011**, *14*, 298–306. [CrossRef]
34. Dhondt, J.L. Expanded newborn screening: Social and ethical issues. *J. Inherit. Metab. Dis.* **2010**, *33*, 211–217. [CrossRef]
35. Bailey, D.B.; Skinner, D.; Davis, A.M.; Whitmarsh, I.; Powell, C. Ethical, legal, and social concerns about expanded newborn screening: Fragile X syndrome as a prototype for emerging issues. *Pediatrics* **2008**, *121*, e693–e704. [CrossRef] [PubMed]
36. Goldenberg, A.; Dodson, D.; Davis, M.; Tarini, B.A. Parents' interest in whole-genome sequencing of newborns. *Genet. Med.* **2014**, *16*, 78–84. [CrossRef] [PubMed]
37. King, J.S.; Smith, M.E. Whole-Genome Screening of Newborns? The Constitutional Boundaries of State Newborn Screening Programs. *Pediatrics* **2016**, *137* (Suppl. S1), S8–S15. [CrossRef]
38. Goldenberg, A.J.; Sharp, R.R. The Ethical Hazards and Programmatic Challenges of Genomic Newborn Screening. *JAMA* **2012**, *307*, 461–462. Available online: https://www.ncbi.nlm.nih.gov/pmc/articles/PMC3868436/ (accessed on 17 August 2024).
39. Brunelli, L.; Sohn, H.; Brower, A. Newborn sequencing is only part of the solution for better child health. *Lancet Reg. Health Am.* **2023**, *25*, 100581. [CrossRef] [PubMed]
40. Chapman, A.R.; Brunelli, L.; Forman, L.; Kaempf, J. Promoting children's rights to health and well-being in the United States. *Lancet Reg. Health. Am.* **2023**, *25*, 100577. [CrossRef]
41. Brunelli, L.; Chan, K.; Tabery, J.; Brower, A.; Binford, W. A children's rights framework for personalized medicine: Solutions to healthcare equity by pivoting to newborn screening and sequencing. *Genet. Med. Open* **2024**, *2*, 101804. [CrossRef]
42. Brunelli, L.; Chan, K.; Tabery, J.; Binford, W.; Brower, A. A Children's Rights Framework for Genomic Medicine: Newborn Screening as a Use Case. *Med. Res. Arch.* **2024**, *12*, 5167. [CrossRef] [PubMed]
43. Research Electronic Data Capture (RedCap) Repository. Available online: https://www.project-redcap.org/ (accessed on 17 August 2024).
44. GraphPad. Available online: https://www.graphpad.com/search/?&searchquery=cite&doc0=1 (accessed on 17 August 2024).
45. Bick, D.; Ahmed, A.; Deen, D.; Ferlini, A.; Garnier, N.; Kasperaviciute, D.; Leblond, M.; Pichini, A.; Rendon, A.; Satija, A.; et al. Newborn Screening by Genomic Sequencing: Opportunities and Challenges. *Int. J. Neonatal Screen.* **2022**, *8*, 40. [CrossRef] [PubMed]
46. Minear, M.A.; Phillips, M.N.; Kau, A.; Parisi, M.A. Newborn screening research sponsored by the NIH: From diagnostic paradigms to precision therapeutics. *Am. J. Med. Genet. Part C Semin. Med. Genet.* **2022**, *190*, 138–152. [CrossRef] [PubMed] [PubMed Central]

MDPI AG
Grosspeteranlage 5
4052 Basel
Switzerland
Tel.: +41 61 683 77 34

International Journal of Neonatal Screening Editorial Office
E-mail: ijns@mdpi.com
www.mdpi.com/journal/ijns

www.ingramcontent.com/pod-product-compliance
Lightning Source LLC
Chambersburg PA
CBHW061607210926
51850CB00009B/2237
9783725876938